D1544450

TEXTBOOK OF
CLINICAL NEUROPHARMACOLOGY

Textbook of
Clinical Neuropharmacology

Harold L. Klawans, M.D.
Associate Chairman
Department of Neurological Sciences
Rush-Presbyterian-St. Lukes Medical Center; and
Professor
Departments of Neurological
Sciences and Pharmacology

William J. Weiner, M.D.
Associate Professor
Departments of Neurological
Sciences and Pharmacology

in conjunction with

Paul A. Nausieda, M.D.
Assistant Professor
Departments of Neurological
Sciences and Pharmacology

Christopher G. Goetz, M.D.
Assistant Professor
Department of Neurological Sciences

Rush University, Chicago, Illinois

Raven Press ■ New York

Raven Press, 1140 Avenue of the Americas, New York, New York 10036

Great care has been taken to maintain the accuracy of the information contained in this volume. However, Raven Press cannot be held responsible for errors or for any consequences arising from the use of the information contained herein.

Library of Congress Cataloging in Publication Data

Klawans, Harold L.
  Textbook of clinical neuropharmacology.

  Includes bibliographical references and index.
  1. Neuropharmacology.   I. Weiner, William J.
II. Title.   [DNLM: 1. Psychopharmacology.
QV   77   K63t]
RM315.K56   615'.78   81–12156
ISBN 0–89004–430–9   AACR2

Preface

In writing this textbook, we have attempted to present a single, coherent overview of the basics of neuropharmacology and the clinical applications of such knowledge. The book is intended for all physicians, both neurologists and non-neurologists, who participate in the care of patients with neurologic disorders. At the same time, we hope it will be useful in the teaching of neuropharmacology to medical students and residents alike.

Since clinicians and students interested in the evaluation and treatment of patients with dysfunction of the nervous system are the primary audience for this book, many classes of agents that affect neurologic function but are not used for specific therapy of neurologic and/or psychiatric disorders, such as: 1) general anesthetics, 2) local anesthetics, 3) analgesics, and 4) drugs that primarily affect the peripheral nervous system have not been included.

In order to best carry out our purposes we have organized the text as far as possible along clinical lines (i.e. by disease or disorder being treated, not by class of agent). Each chapter discusses the pathophysiology of a disorder and the mechanism of action of the drugs used in treating the disorder. These two basic approaches are then integrated into a discussion of clinical pharmacologic (e.g. pharmacokinetics, blood levels, etc.) and practical therapeutic issues. Obviously, this cannot be done for all disorders or all drugs, for basic knowledge is often lacking.

A review of the table of contents and the chapters themselves reveals a number of disorders that have been excluded from discussion in this volume for lack of appropriateness:

1) Infectious diseases. These agents are not neuropharmacologic agents per se. 2) Deficiency diseases. These disorders, varying from vitamin deficiencies to hypothyroidism (in which there is a deficiency of thyroid hormone due to disease of the thyroid gland), are often included in textbooks of therapeutics of neurologic disorders. This however is not a textbook of therapeutics, and replacement of deficiency is not of sufficient neuropharmacologic interest to warrant inclusion. 3) Systemic diseases. Also excluded are systemic diseases of the nervous system in which involvement of the nervous system is part of the primary illness and treatment of the neurologic disorder consists of treatment of the primary disease. For example, we have chosen not to discuss the use of steroids and other agents in the treatment of collagen diseases involving the nervous system. This is consistent with our view that this is a textbook of neuropharmacology, not of general pharmacology with special reference to the nervous system.

Drugs used in the treatment of such nonneurologic and nonpsychiatric disorders are discussed only if they cause specific neurotoxicity, e.g. vincristine-induced peripheral neuropathy is included, but coma due to aspirin overdose is not.

The references cited in this volume are intentionally nonencyclopedic. In general, references that are accessible and potentially useful to the clinician have been chosen on the following principles:

1) When possible, non-English language sources have been avoided.

2) When possible, widely disseminated sources have been chosen for citation over less widely available ones.

3) Clinical papers have been given preference over preclinical ones.

4) Selected reviews including both clinical and preclinical data have been listed where possible and marked with an asterisk (*). (These are often a good starting point for readers desiring more preclinical data.)

H. L. K.

Acknowledgments

This textbook has had a three year gestation period. Much of it was finally compiled or edited during a three month sabbatical I spent at Neve Ilan in the Judean Hills outside of Jerusalem. To all those in Neve Ilan who assisted in the work there, TODAH RABBAH. Special thanks are also due to Paula Klawans, Pat Gerdes, and Madelyn Glanton, who together did that typing which was not completed in Israel.

Dr. Alan Edelson of Raven Press is thanked for his continued support and encouragement from the stages of preliminary planning to the production of the final product. The continued support of our Chairman, Dr. Maynard M. Cohen, in this as in all our previous work has been indispensable.

I personally want to thank Donald Calne for reviewing many of the chapters. His suggestions helped us greatly in preparing our final texts.

As always, special thanks are due to Ms. Genevieve Logan without whose organizational genius we would never have completed this project.

Contents

Chapter 1

Parkinsonism

Parkinsonism is a symptom complex composed of four separate clinical manifestations: (a) resting tremor; (b) rigidity, or increased resistance to passive movement; (c) akinesia or bradykinesia; (d) loss of normal postural reflexes.

CHOLINERGIC MECHANISMS

The medical treatment of parkinsonism began over 100 years ago when Ordenstein, a student of Charcot, suggested the use of belladonna alkaloids in the treatment of Parkinson's disease. These drugs were known to cause dryness of the mouth and were given to parkinsonian patients to alleviate their excessive salivation. Unexpectedly, these belladonna alkaloids had a beneficial effect on the rigidity and tremor of parkinsonism.

The second class of drugs that was found to be of value in the treatment of parkinsonism was the antihistamines. Diphenylhydramine is the most widely used such agent, but other related agents such as orphenadrine and chlorphenoxamine are also employed.

The long-established value of the belladonna alkaloids, combined with the discovery that certain antihistamines were beneficial, led to a vigorous search for other drugs. This search focused on a variety of synthetic spasmolytic agents and resulted in the introduction of several new drugs. It is believed by many that these newer preparations have a somewhat better ratio of therapeutic to side effects. Trihexyphenidyl can be considered the prototype of this class of synthetic alkaloids, which includes cycrimine, biperiden, and procyclidine.

Benztropine was synthesized in anticipation that the antiparkinsonian activity of both the belladonna alkaloids and the antihistamines could be combined into a single molecule which would then prove to be a valuable therapeutic agent. The molecule that was synthesized does combine chemical features of both of these classes, possesses both atropine-like and antihistaminic properties, and is clinically useful.

Later, it was discovered that an antihistamine of the phenothiazine series, promethazine, was of some value and that a phenothiazine without any known antihistaminic properties, ethopropazine, also appeared to benefit patients with parkinsonism. The structures of typical examples of each class of these agents are shown in Table 1.

After the observation of their efficacy, belladonna alkaloids were used in the treatment of parkinsonism for 75 years without a great deal of speculation as to

TABLE 1.

Class of Drugs	Example	Structure
Belladonna alkaloids	Scopolamine	HOH_2C, $CH-C-O-CH$ ... $CH_2-CH-CH$ ... $N-CH_3$ ... $CH_2-CH-CH$ ... O
Antihistamines	Diphenylhydramine	$HC-O-CH_2CH_2-N$ ... CH_3 / CH_3
Synthetic alkaloids	Trihexyphenidyl	$HO-C-CH_2CH_2-N$
Combined anticholinergic-antihistamine	Benztropine	$CH_2-CH-CH_2$ ... $CH-O-CH$ ... $N-CH_3$ ... $CH_2-CH-CH_2$
Phenothiazines with antihistamine properties	Promethazine	S ... $N-CH_2CH-N$ ... CH_3 ... CH_3 / CH_3
Phenothiazines without antihistamine properties	Ethopropazine	S ... $N-CH_2CH-N$ ... CH_3 ... C_2H_5 / C_2H_5

why they seemed to work. In 1945, Feldberg theorized that a central acetylcholine–atropine antagonism could be invoked to explain the usefulness of the anticholinergic agent atropine in parkinsonism (16). The concept that antagonism of acetylcholine within the brain improves parkinsonism presupposes that some altered or increased effect of acetylcholine is involved in producing the symptoms of parkinsonism. Over the next two decades the combined efforts of a number of investigators demonstrated that the effectiveness of a wide variety of antiparkinsonian agents is related to their ability to antagonize acetylcholine within the CNS.

In the mid 1950s, tremorine, a cholinomimetic agent, was found to produce tremors in mice (14). Antiparkinsonian drugs were able to antagonize this tremor, and it was suggested that tremorine-induced tremor would be a convenient model for experimental evaluation of antiparkinsonian agents.

If human parkinsonian tremor is related to central hypersensitivity to acetylcholine, then effective antiparkinsonian drugs should be specific antagonists of acetylcholine both centrally and peripherally. Ahmed and Marshall tested this hypothesis with belladonna alkaloids and synthetic antispasmodics as well as a number of antihistamines and phenothiazines (1). They found a definite relationship between antiparkinsonian activity and both peripheral acetylcholine inhibition and antitremorine potency. They concluded that this supported the view that the pathophysiology of parkinsonism is associated in some way with acetylcholine, possibly in its role as a transmitter within the CNS. Tremorine-induced tremor should not be taken as a perfect analog of the parkinsonian tremor. The validity of this model is much more pharmacologic than anatomic. It allows one to test for central acetylcholine antagonism but does not define the exact central site of that antagonism.

The hypothesis that the standard antiparkinsonian drugs owe their effectiveness to central acetylcholine antagonism was not well tested in patients with parkinsonism until 1967. Duvoisin reasoned that if the hypothesis of central antagonism were correct, then centrally acting cholinergic agents should exacerbate the signs and symptoms of parkinsonism and antagonize the therapeutic effects of anticholinergics (12). He studied the response to physostigmine and quaternary anticholinesterases as well as benztropine and scopolamine in parkinsonian patients. In most cases, physostigmine given intravenously produced a definite worsening of all the parkinsonian manifestations already present without giving rise to any signs or symptoms not previously present. This effect of physostigmine could be reversed by either benztropine or scopolamine. None of these effects could be demonstrated with quaternary anticholinesterases, which do not cross into the CNS. This elegant study demonstrated that there is a direct and mutual antagonism of physostigmine and anticholinergic agents on the manifestation of parkinsonism and that this antagonism takes place centrally. Duvoisin did much more than just reconfirm a 25-year-old notion. He extended the theory by suggesting that this antagonism takes place in a specific site, the striatum, that is, the caudate nucleus and the putamen. The striatum contains the highest concentration of acetylcholine in the entire nervous system. It also possesses the highest concentrations in the brain of the enzymes necessary for acetylcholine synthesis (choline acetylase) and degradation (acetylcholinesterase). These facts suggest that the striatum is a reasonable site for involvement of the cholinergic system. Duvoisin also suggested that the involvement of the cholinergic mechanism is not primary but is secondary to the involvement of another possible CNS transmitter, dopamine.

Whereas muscarinic blockade is clearly the major factor contributing to the therapeutic action of anticholinergic agents, it has been suggested that inhibition of active reuptake of dopamine may contribute to the efficacy of these agents. Under normal circumstances the activity of dopamine and striatal dopamine receptors is terminated by reuptake into the presynaptic dopaminergic nerve terminal. This active reuptake mechanism is inhibited by many but not all of the anticholinergic agents that are employed to treat parkinsonism (9). Blockade of this reuptake system would allow the transmitter to remain in the synaptic cleft where it could continue to act on postsynaptic receptors.

Anticholinergic agents have significant therapeutic effect on tremor and rigidity, but akinesia and loss of postural reflexes (the most disabling clinical features of parkinsonism) usually respond poorly if at all. There is no real evidence that any one anticholinergic drug is specifically effective for any one particular parkinsonian symptom. Sometimes a combination of two anticholinergic agents seems better than one, but it is rarely of any value to give more than two anticholinergics at the same time. The initial therapeutic response to anticholinergic drugs is sometimes poorly sustained, suggesting the development of tolerance. It is usual to start patients with a low dose, which is gradually increased until a satisfactory response is obtained or unwanted effects are encountered. Minor side effects such as dryness of the mouth, constipation, and slight blurring of vision are so common as to be ubiquitous and usually must be tolerated in order to have an antiparkinsonian effect. Older patients appear to be much more sensitive to the central side effects of these agents, and great care must be exercised in using these agents in elderly individuals. These central side effects include alterations in mentation, especially memory loss and confusion. This often presents as interruption in thinking or talking (speech arrests). Hallucinations, which are usually visual, are quite common, and agitation, dysphoria, or lethargy can also occur, as can a frank toxic psychosis. Patients with dementia, which frequently accompanies parkinsonism, are usually very sensitive to such central side effects.

A number of common anticholinergic side effects are produced by blockade of muscarinic synapses of the parasympathetic system. These include dryness of the mouth; defective ocular accommodation; mydriasis, which can precipitate glaucoma; constipation; and retention of urine. The last can of course lead to acute retention of urine in patients with prostatic hypertrophy.

DOPAMINERGIC MECHANISMS

Dopamine (3,4-dihydroxyphenylethylamine) is one of the three catecholamines found in man. Dopamine is chemically the simplest of the three catecholamines, although the other two, epinephrine (adrenaline) and norepinephrine (noradrenalin), came into clinical prominence much earlier. The first step in the synthesis of catecholamines is the conversion of tyrosine to levodopa (L-3,4-dihydroxyphenyl-alanine) by tyrosine hydroxylase (see Fig. 1).

This enzyme reaction is the rate-limiting step in the production of catecholamines from tyrosine. End-product inhibition (feedback) of this step has been shown *in vitro* and *in vivo*. Levodopa is then decarboxylated to form dopamine. The enzyme that carries out this process is either a relatively nonspecific enzyme that can decarboxylate a variety of substrates, or one of a group of closely related enzymes that have yet to be clearly separated from one another. Because of the lack of specificity, this enzyme is referred to as aromatic amino acid decarboxylase, or dopa decarboxylase. When synthesized, dopamine is taken up into storage granules. In neurons that synthesize dopamine, no further biochemical process occurs until dopamine is released. In norepinephrine-synthesizing neurons, dopamine is then converted to norepinephrine by dopamine β-hydroxylase. Neurons that synthesize dopamine but not norepinephrine do not contain this enzyme. In the adrenal medulla epinephrine is formed from norepinephrine by phenylethanolamine-*N*-methyltrans-ferase.

Two major enzyme systems are involved in the degradation of catecholamines: monoamine oxidase and catecholamine-*O*-methyltransferase. These may act singly or in sequence, with either acting initially (Fig. 2). Monoamine oxidase catalyzes

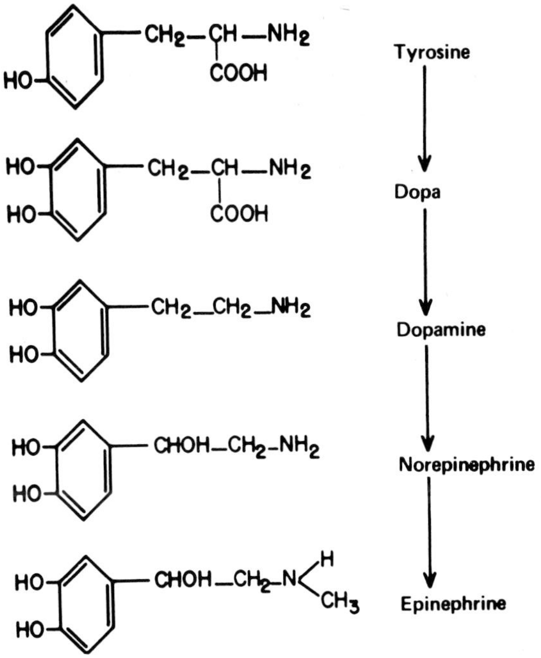

FIG. 1.   Main pathway of biosynthesis of catecholamines.

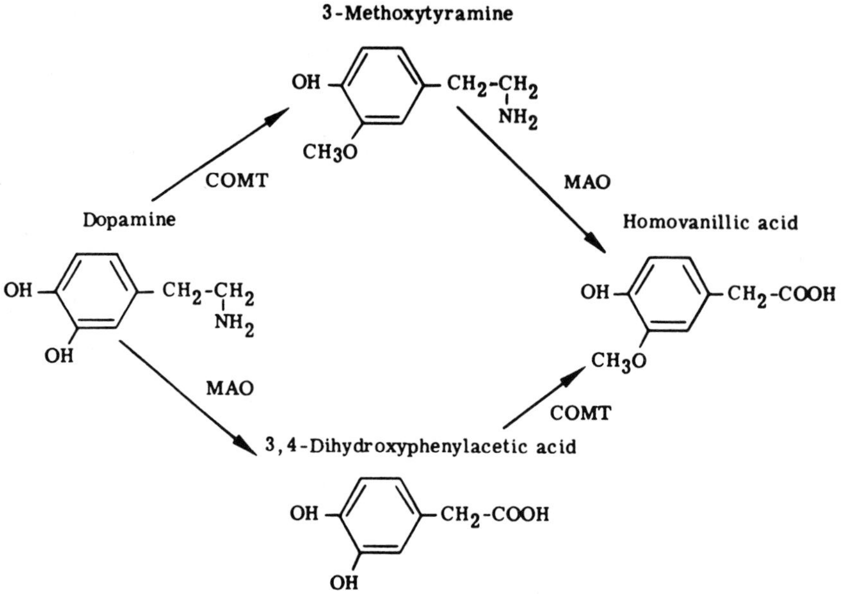

FIG. 2. Major pathway for catabolism of dopamine. MAO, monoamine oxidase; COMT, catecholamine-*O*-methyltransferase.

the oxidative deamination of catecholamines and various other aromatic monoamines to their aldehyde derivatives, which are then rather rapidly oxidized to the corresponding acid. The product in the case of dopamine is DOPAC (3,4-dihydroxyphenylacetic acid). DOPAC is then acted on by catecholamine-*O*-methyltransferase to produce homovanillic acid (HVA). The reverse sequence can also occur, with catecholamine-*O*-methyltransferase acting before monoamine oxidase to form 3-methoxytyramine. HVA is the major breakdown product of dopamine in the CNS.

Monoamine oxidase is localized primarily within the neuron, where it acts on intracellularly released catecholamines. Catecholamine-*O*-methyltransferase acts initially on extracellularly released catecholamines. Since inhibition of these enzymes does not produce marked potentiation of the effect of released catecholamines, some other mechanism must be responsible for the physiologic inactivation of released catecholamines. It appears that catecholamines are inactivated by being removed from the site of action on the postsynaptic cell by a specific active transport mechanism located in the presynaptic neuron itself. In the catecholamine system, then, physiologic inactivation by reuptake plays the same role that enzymatic inactivation by degradation plays in the cholinergic system.

The notion that dopamine has a specific function in the CNS dates from 1959, when it was noted that dopamine accounted for approximately half of the total catecholamine content of the brain and that the regional distributions of dopamine and norepinephrine were markedly different. The dopamine-rich areas like the striatum can have almost 100 times as much dopamine as norepinephrine, whereas the norepinephrine-rich hypothalamus contains approximately 10-fold as much norepinephrine as dopamine. This marked variation in the ratio of these two amines from area to area is not consistent with the idea that the role of dopamine in all areas is to serve only as a precursor of norepinephrine.

After the development of fluorescent microscopic techniques, two distinct types of fluorescence were discovered within the neurons of a number of brainstem nuclei. These techniques delineate the exact cellular location of monoamines including dopamine, norepinephrine, and serotonin and have demonstrated that the substantia nigra is one of the most impressive nuclear areas containing neurons with a marked green (catecholamine) fluorescence owing to its high concentration of dopamine. In contrast, no fluorescent nerve cell bodies have been found in the striatum, which contains the highest concentration of dopamine in the brain. The dopamine in the striatum is located within a dense meshwork of very fine, closely packed nerve terminals. Anatomic experiments in several species have demonstrated a nigrostriatal dopamine-containing tract with cell bodies in the substantia nigra and axon terminations in the striatum.

The existence of this previously unsuspected nigrostriatal neuronal system in which dopamine may act as the neurotransmitter is of interest in relation to Parkinson's disease and postencephalitic parkinsonism. In both of these conditions it is generally accepted that the most conspicuous sites of pathology are the pigmented nuclei of the brainstem, notably the substantia nigra. If the nerve cell bodies of the dopamine-containing neurons located in the substantia nigra are affected in these diseases, then the distal ends of these neurons should be decreased. By 1966, Hornykiewicz and his associates had examined the brains of 40 patients who had died from either idiopathic or postencephalitic parkinsonism (17). In all instances the dopamine content of the striatum was greatly reduced, as was the dopamine content of the substantia nigra and globus pallidus. The levels of norepinephrine and serotonin in the caudate were slightly decreased.

Knowledge of the nigrostriatal dopaminergic pathway makes it possible to understand the influence of several drugs on the extrapyramidal system. Reserpine frequently causes parkinson-like syndromes in man. In many animals reserpine produces a state of rigidity and akinesia called "reserpine-induced catalepsy." By analogy to various clinical conditions, it is assumed that this syndrome results from action on extrapyramidal centers. Reserpine depletes dopamine from the striatum and other dopamine-rich regions by blocking the uptake of intracellular dopamine into its storage granules. This has led to the suggestion that reserpine-induced parkinsonism is due to dopamine deficiency.

Certain neuroleptic phenothiazines and butyrophenones also cause parkinsonism. Phenothiazines block some peripheral actions of catecholamines, and they appear to have a similar action centrally. Van Rossum has proposed that chlorpromazine and other neuroleptic agents act by blocking dopamine receptors in the CNS (18). Competitive inhibition of dopamine at the dopamine receptors blocks the action of this transmitter at these receptors. Neuroleptic-induced parkinsonism is thought to be related to this dopaminergic blocking action of these agents.

If decreasing the amount of dopamine acting at dopamine receptors produces parkinsonism, increasing the amount of dopamine acting at these same receptors may well be beneficial to parkinsonian patients. It is generally accepted that the therapeutic efficacy of levodopa is due to the production of increased amounts of dopamine within the blood–brain barrier. This presupposes that the levodopa is decarboxylated to dopamine in the relatively dopaminergically denervated striatum. There is some reason to think that this may occur, since sufficient levels of the enzyme that carries out this decarboxylation are still present in the striatum of such patients.

It has been shown that levodopa therapy increases the CSF level of HVA. Since HVA content in the CSF is thought to reflect dopamine metabolism within the CNS, this increase is thought to be a reflection of increased dopamine utilization in patients receiving levodopa and supports the theory that the effectiveness of levodopa is related to dopamine formed and acting within the blood–brain barrier. Interpretation of spinal fluid HVA data is complicated by the fact that some HVA may be formed at the blood–brain barrier and may reflect dopamine formation at the barrier and not within the brain.

Detailed biochemical studies of patients who have died while receiving levodopa for Parkinson's disease have demonstrated increased concentrations of both dopamine and HVA in the striatum as well as in other areas of the brain that normally have a low concentration of dopamine. This supports the idea that dopamine is formed from levodopa in parkinsonian patients, although its formation is not limited to the nigrostriatal neuronal system.

DOPAMINE–ACETYLCHOLINE BALANCE

Some degree of dopaminergic denervation of striatal neurons is a constant feature of parkinsonism. If the striatal neurons receive antagonistic dopaminergic and cholinergic innervations, then alterations of a single system would result in an imbalance in the overall system. This supposed imbalance between the input of the cholinergic and dopaminergic systems to the neurons of the striatum explains a variety of observations. The first of these is drug-induced parkinsonism. Reserpine depletes the striatum of dopamine and therefore swings the balance in favor of the unaffected cholinergic input analogous to the imbalance suggested for Parkinson's disease itself. Levodopa reverses this reserpine effect. The compound α-methyl-*p*-tyrosine also depletes the brain of dopamine and aggravates parkinsonism. Chlorpromazine and haloperidol are thought to act as blocking agents at the dopamine receptor site. A block of these receptors shifts the balance in the same direction. Levodopa would not as easily overcome this blockade and therefore is not as effective in this form of drug-induced parkinsonism.

The standard therapy of parkinsonism can also be explained by the theory of neurotransmitter imbalance. The central antagonism of acetylcholine by atropine would tend to bring the two systems back toward balance by inhibiting the intact system. The same mechanism can explain the action of a variety of agents with known central anticholinergic effects. This includes such diverse agents as anti-histamines, synthetic alkaloids, and certain phenothiazines. These agents are all useful in both neuroleptic- and reserpine-induced parkinsonism as well as in naturally occurring parkinsonism.

The usefulness of levodopa depends on its conversion to dopamine, which then acts on dopaminergic receptors. This tends to restore the normal dopaminergic–cholinergic balance, which was shifted in the cholinergic direction by the loss of dopamine.

Agents that increase the activity of the acetylcholine within the CNS do not result in parkinsonism when given to normal individuals or to patients with other extra-pyramidal diseases without antiparkinsonian manifestations. The same agents, how-ever, do result in marked exacerbation of symptoms when given to patients with parkinsonism. Only symptoms already present in parkinsonian patients are aggra-vated by the administration of physostigmine. If the dopamine loss in a patient does not produce rigidity, increased acetylcholine activity will not produce rigidity. These observations suggest that dopamine loss must be present in order to make it possible for increasing central cholinergic activity to produce any of the signs or symptoms of parkinsonism.

DOPAMINERGIC AGENTS

A variety of pharmacologic approaches has been used in an attempt to increase the activity of dopamine or dopamine-like substances at striatal dopamine receptors. Three separate classes of agents have been tried and are now in use. These are:

1. *Precursors of dopamine.* Dopamine is formed by the decarboxylation of le-vodopa, which is a naturally occurring amino acid and is itself pharmacologically inert. Any efficacy levodopa has depends entirely on its conversion to active cate-cholamines, specifically dopamine. Levodopa is now the most widely used and effective agent in the treatment of parkinsonism.

The early evidence for the effectiveness of levodopa came from two studies carried out in the early 1960s. Birkmayer and Hornykiewicz gave 50 to 150 mg of levodopa i.v. to 20 patients (5a). All subjects showed decreased akinesia. This effect reached a peak in 2 to 3 hr and persisted up to 24 hr. Monoamine oxidase inhibition enhanced these results whereas dopamine, D-DOPA, and 5-hydroxytryp-tophan, the analogous serotonin precursor, were without effect. The following year Barbeau reported decreased rigidity following oral levodopa and some reduction of akinesia if monoamine oxidase inhibitors were also given (1a). In the late 1960s, Cotzias et al. (11) demonstrated that larger doses of levodopa given over prolonged periods of time had a remarkable and sustained beneficial effect. They originally treated 16 severely debilitated parkinsonian patients with large doses of oral DL-DOPA ranging from 3 to 16 g/day and reported complete or marked improvement in several of the individual manifestations of parkinsonism and felt that rigidity responded to lower doses than tremor. This therapy resulted in several instances of granulocytopenia, leading these investigators to switch to levodopa, which had equally striking beneficial results without adverse blood reactions.

The long-term efficacy of levodopa is limited by numerous side effects, but it remains the most powerful single antiparkinsonian agent.

2. *Indirect dopamine agonists.* Only one agent, amantadine, is felt to work in this manner. An indirect agonist is a drug that itself does not act at a receptor but increases the degree of naturally occurring agonist (neurotransmitters) receptor site interaction.

3. *Direct-acting agonists.* These agents have the ability to act directly on the striatal dopamine receptor. Bromocriptine is the primary example of such agents.

Since levodopa causes numerous side effects that are felt to be due to the activity of dopamine formed and acting outside the blood–brain barrier, two other types of agents have been used to modify the side effects of levodopa. These are: (a) peripheral DOPA decarboxylase inhibitors and (b) peripheral dopamine receptor site antagonists. Since these drugs do not cross the blood–brain barrier, their entire effect is peripherally mediated.

LEVODOPA

Levodopa is readily absorbed from the gastrointestinal tract, annd most of it is metabolized outside the CNS and excreted in the urine as HVA and DOPAC. Its half-life varies from 45 to 90 min or more between individuals and may also depend on duration of previous exposure. Levodopa has significant efficacy against all of the major signs and symptoms of parkinsonism. The usually therapeutic regime consists of anywhere from 1.6 to 6 g/day in divided doses with a mean daily dose of between 3 and 3.5 g/day. Most patients are begun on 250 mg t.i.d. p.c. and can have their dosage slowly increased by 250 mg weekly.

The initial enthusiasm that levodopa administration aroused following its intro-duction into clinical use has been somewhat tempered by clinical experience. Several recent studies concerned with large populations of parkinsonian patients who have been followed for 6 or more years while receiving levodopa have indicated that, although there is a definite tendency for disability to increase over the years, many patients remain improved after many years of chronic administration. In addition, some of these studies indicate that the mortality associated with idiopathic Par-kinson's disease has been lessened by the use of levodopa. At present, this agent remains the mainstay of therapy in Parkinson's disease despite the many problems associated with its chronic administration. Levodopa is now often used with a peripheral dopadecarboxylase inhibitor. Such agents inhibit the formation of do-pamine from levodopa outside the blood–brain barrier. As a result of this, less levodopa is metabolized so the patient actually takes less levodopa. At the same time those side effects owing to the formation of catecholamines outside the blood–brain barrier are decreased. Two such agents are in wide use: Sinemet (le-vodopa/carbidopa) and Madopar (levodopa/benseramide). Only Sinemet is available in the U.S.

Dyskinesias

Levodopa-induced dyskinesias are characterized clinically by choreiform movements of the limbs, hands, trunk, and lingual–facial–buccal musculature. Occasionally abnormal contractions of the abdominal and thoracic musculature may occur. These abnormal involuntary movements may occasionally be of slower or of longer duration and may appear to be more choreoathetoid or dystonic in nature. The incidence of levodopa-induced dyskinesias ranges from 40 to 90% of treated patients. The prevalence of levodopa-induced dyskinesias seems clearly related to the duration of high-dosage levodopa therapy (20). Sinemet, the levodopa–carbidopa combination that has been helpful in delineating central from peripheral dopamine effects because of its inhibition of peripheral dopa decarboxylase activity, induces dyskinesias with at least the same regularity as levodopa itself. There is, in fact, some suggestion that Sinemet may induce dyskinetic movements at an earlier time than levodopa alone. There is also a direct relationship between duration of parkinsonism and the development of the dyskinesias. The longer the patient has had parkinsonism, the greater the likelihood of developing levodopa-induced hyperkinetic movements. In individual patients the dyskinesias often begin and are more pronounced on the side first affected by parkinsonism. Although levodopa-induced movements may be clearly dose-related in an individual patient, there is absolutely no correlation between a given dose of levodopa and the induction of dyskinesias in the parkinsonian population as a whole.

The precise mechanisms that result in levodopa-induced dyskinesias are unknown. Several investigators believe that these movements are an example of denervation hypersensitivity of dopamine receptor sites. Since the initial successful high-dose levodopa trials in 1967, it has been proposed that the induction of these abnormal movements is more related to a pathologically altered CNS substrate than to levodopa itself (11). The apparently low incidence of levodopa-induced dyskinesias in normal individuals has suggested that the occurrence of levodopa-induced dyskinesias in parkinsonian patients is a result of the action of dopamine on neurons which are altered in a manner that increases their susceptibility to levodopa-induced abnormal movements. It has been proposed that one of the mechanisms underlying such an alteration of neuronal response could be a denervation hypersensitivity of striatal dopamine receptors. In parkinsonian patients the degeneration of the substantia nigra would produce dopaminergic denervation of the striatal dopamine receptors.

Evidence to support the hypothesis that dopamine denervation and subsequent dopamine receptor-site hypersensitivity are related to the development of levodopa-induced dyskinesias in parkinsonism comes from clinical studies relating the duration of Parkinson's disease to the incidence of drug-induced dyskinesia. Presumably, a longer duration of parkinsonism would entail more chronic denervation and therefore a greater degree of dopamine hypersensitivity.

It would be unreasonable to maintain that levodopa could never produce abnormal movements in normal individuals. "Normal" in this instance means individuals who have no signs, symptoms, or history of extrapyramidal dysfunction and who have never received major neuroleptics. Neuronal degenerative changes in the striatum do occur during the aging process, and movements similar to those induced by levodopa can and do occur spontaneously in some older people. If it is assumed that dopamine is involved in the production of these movements, levodopa may bring them out in some percentage of elderly patients. Larger doses may occasionally elicit these movements in younger patients, but this is quite rare. In fact, experimental evidence shows that extremely high doses of levodopa can produce dyskinetic facial movements in normal monkeys. The dosage employed to produce these abnormal movements, however, when translated into milligram/kilogram terms, is almost always far in excess of any therapeutic levodopa regime employed in patients.

These theories of denervation hypersensitivity, although attractive, are incomplete. Several clinical observations suggest that denervation hypersensitivity cannot be the sole mechanism underlying the development of levodopa-induced dyskinesia. The first of these is the fact that the prevalence of dyskinesias is directly related to the duration of therapy. Since denervation would not be expected to increase steadily during levodopa therapy, this is difficult to explain on the basis of denervation hypersensitivity. There is a direct relationship between the duration of dyskinesias and their severity in many patients. The dyskinesias are often quite mild at first but increase in severity with time. This increase often includes a wider distribution (e.g., from solely lingual–facial–buccal movements to involvement of the trunk and/or limbs), as well as an increase in the degree of the original movements.

There is often an inverse relationship between the duration of dyskinesias and the dosage of levodopa that elicits the abnormal movements; that is, the longer the levodopa dyskinesias have been present, the lower the dose of levodopa needed to produce them. The levodopa-induced excessive dopamine stimulation in these patients appears to alter striatal dopaminergic sensitivity and thereby decreases the threshold dosage of levodopa necessary to elicit dyskinesias. None of these observations is consistent with the denervation hypersensitivity hypothesis. It is most likely that the chronic dopamine agonist may alter subsequent response to dopamine, a form of dopamine-agonist-induced hypersensitivity (21).

If levodopa-induced abnormal movements are related to the action of dopamine at striatal dopamine receptor sites, then the therapeutic approach to the management of these dyskinesias involves either decreasing the dopaminergic input to the striatum or increasing the cholinergic input. A reduction in levodopa dosage invariably alleviates these dyskinetic movements. There have been no reported cases of levodopa inducing a permanent dyskinesia in Parkinson's disease.

When levodopa is reduced, however, there is often an increase in parkinsonism. This loss of levodopa efficacy makes many if not most patients reluctant to accept a lowered levodopa dosage. A certain degree of dyskinesia should be tolerated in patients who are achieving important functional improvements in mobility; however, since the chronic agonism of prolonged high-dosage levodopa therapy may play a role in the pathogenesis of these movements, an early reduction in the amount of levodopa administered may in the long run be beneficial if the resultant loss of efficacy is mild and tolerable.

A second approach that has been advocated is the use of dopaminergic blocking agents. Although the administration of phenothiazines or butyrophenones can effectively stop levodopa-induced dyskinesias, the use of these neuroleptics in large doses will also effectively block all dopaminergic activity and result in loss of the therapeutic effects of the levodopa (12). The observation that levodopa-induced improvement in parkinsonism can occur independently of levodopa-induced dyskinesias and vice versa, as well as the fact that levodopa-induced improvement and dyskinesias can occur concomitantly in the same patient, suggests that there may be two separate dopamine receptor-site populations involved in improvement and dyskinesia. There are distinct populations of striatal neurons that respond in a different manner to iontophoretic dopamine application. If dopamine-facilitated receptors are blocked more easily then dopamine-inhibited receptors, it might be possible, with low doses of neuroleptics, to block differentially the dopamine-facilitated receptor and thus decrease dyskinesia while not blocking the dopamine-inhibited receptor and thus not interfering with the efficacy of levodopa in the treatment of Parkinson's disease. Unfortunately, as a practical therapeutic maneuver, the use of haloperidol or other neuroleptics is not a successful approach to levodopa-induced dyskinesia.

A third way to alter the function of striatal cells that contain the abnormally responsive dopaminergic receptors is to alter the cholinergic input to these cells. This might have some influence on levodopa-induced dyskinesia. Duvoisin demonstrated that in most parkinsonian patients physostigmine increased parkinsonism secondary to an increased central activity of acetylcholine. This abnormal responsiveness to physostigmine is often lost during long-term levodopa therapy. Physostigmine can improve chorea presumably because of the effect of acetylcholine in the striatum. If levodopa-induced dyskinesias are attributable to an abnormal response to dopamine by striatal dopamine receptors, it seemed reasonable to ask if physostigmine might improve these movements without any associated increase in parkinsonism. We have given intravenous physostigmine to 6 patients with levodopa-induced dyskinesias (20). This improved the movements in 4 patients. In 2 of the 4 patients in whom movements were improved there was no increase in parkinsonism, whereas in the other 2 the signs and symptoms of parkinsonism became more prominent. Tarsy and co-workers also administered physostigmine to patients with levodopa-induced dyskinesias with similar results (38).

At present, the concept of dopamine–acetylcholine balance has only one definite practical application: in relationship to levodopa-induced dyskinesias. Decreasing central anticholinergic medications may improve levodopa-induced dyskinesia. Although some observers have not found this to be true (40), our observations suggest that decreasing the level of anticholinergic medication does decrease levodopa-induced dyskinesias in approximately one-third of the patients, often without any overall loss of therapeutic benefit.

Since almost all patients with parkinsonism prefer to be mildly to moderately choreatic than to be significantly parkinsonian, the practical therapeutic question remains if there is any danger in maintaining a mild-to-moderate dyskinetic state. Often with milder forms, patients will not be at all disturbed by lingual–facial–buccal dyskinesias or occasional limb movements, and it will be the family or the physician who first draws attention to these movements. There are, of course, more clinical implications for the patient with levodopa-induced dyskinesias than the cosmetics of how he or she appears. Clinical observers have pointed out that if no alteration in therapy is undertaken when mild dyskinetic movements appear, there will usually be an increase in the severity of these movements in the area already involved. In addition, there will be spread of the dyskinesias to involve more areas. For example, lingual–facial–buccal dyskinesias, which are usually the first sign of levodopa-induced dyskinesias, will spread to a more generalized choreiform disorder. The more flagrant generalized choreiform movements can be as disabling as the bradykinesia of parkinsonism. It appears most judicious to alter the pathogenesis of levodopa-induced dyskinesias by use of the methods discussed previously in order to prevent not only increased severity of the initial abnormal involuntary movements but their spread into a more generalized disorder as well.

Possible additional evidence to support the concept that increased cholinergic influences can decrease levodopa-induced dyskinesia comes from a report that the administration of dimethylaminoethanol (deanol), an agent reported to increase central cholinergic activity by conversion to acetylcholine, resulted in excellent improvement in levodopa-induced dyskinesia without increased parkinsonism in 9 of 11 patients (31). It appears, however, that the efficacy of deanol in the treatment of levodopa-induced dyskinesias is much more limited than originally reported. In a later study of 17 parkinsonian patients, deanol showed very limited if any efficacy in regard to long-term suppression of the dyskinesias (26). Even more significantly, there was very little evidence that deanol increased parkinsonian symptoms, casting doubt on the central effect of this agent.

More recently attempts have been made to use choline and lecithin to increase striatal acetylcholine synthesis but the long-term efficacy of these approaches remains unproven.

On–Off Phenomena

Although some degree of fluctuation in motor performance in parkinsonian patients was described prior to the levodopa era, including the more astounding episodes of "kinesia paradoxica," the widespread use of levodopa has resulted in numerous descriptions of a unique problem of oscillation in motor performance in patients on chronic levodopa therapy. In a matter of minutes a patient enjoying normal or near-normal mobility may suddenly revert to a severe degree of parkinsonism. The reappearance of tremor, loss of postural reflexes, and akinesia usually without rigidity may persist from 30 min to 3 or 4 hr. Levodopa-induced dyskinesias may herald the onset or termination of the off period in some patients. The on and off cycles may occur from once a day to three to four times during waking hours with more and more time spent in the off period. This phenomenon is primarily associated with long-term levodopa therapy. Most patients experiencing this problem usually do so after 2 years of treatment. The combined use of levodopa and a peripheral decarboxylase inhibitor does not prevent this problem and may in fact induce it sooner than treatment with levodopa alone. Although it may be that only a minority of patients receiving chronic therapy develop on–off phenomena, there is also some indication that the longer the duration of high-dosage levodopa therapy, the higher the frequency of the phenomena. There are at least two separate types of on–off phenomena: (a) end-of-dose akinesia in which the duration of efficacy of each dose becomes shorter and akinesia appears between doses, and (b) "classic" on–off phenomena, not temporally related to time of previous dose.

Various postulates have been advanced to explain the occurrence of on–off phenomena, ranging from altered neural substrate secondary to progression of the parkinsonism to numerous pharmacologic abnormalities. Among those proposed have been progressive loss of nigral neurons with secondary axonal collateral sprouting of remaining intact neurons so that the physiologic field of influence of each nigral neuron is greatly enlarged, with subsequent loss of synchronizing of function; the formation of "false" neurotransmitters produced via interaction of dopamine and carbonyl reagents; and chronic excess of transmitter leading to alterations in receptor-site responsiveness. Although there is no direct evidence for any of these theories, the abrupt nature of the oscillation in performance is suggestive of some type of physiologic imbalance. The alteration in function could be related to fluctuating levels of dopamine available to act in the striatum. If this were so, the question would still remain as to why the on–off phenomenon appears only after chronic therapy. The demonstration that apomorphine, a dopamine receptor agonist, can reverse the motor symptomatology in parkinsonian patients during the off period lends credence to the idea that off periods are related to fluctuations in dopamine availability. It is extremely difficult to investigate central fluctuations in dopamine metabolism in patients. Peripheral metabolic studies are easier to perform, and there are some clinical observations to suggest that it is in fact peripheral fluctuations of dopamine that relate to off periods. Specific measurements of plasma levodopa and the correlation of these values with the clinical state of the patient have been undertaken on several occasions. In a study of a single patient, Calne et al. correlated high levels of plasma levodopa with increasing dyskinesias and facial hypokinesia (7). These symptoms improved as plasma levodopa levels returned toward a more therapeutic range. There have been several additional reports, involving larger numbers of patients, which tend to correlate off periods with low plasma levodopa levels and on periods with higher plasma levodopa levels (7,15,37). Additional impetus to the concept that fluctuating plasma levodopa is related to on–off is provided by a report which demonstrated that while the plasma levodopa level was held constant the oscillations were not seen. At present, this has no practical clinical implications since there are no effective sustained-release levodopa modalities.

If on–off responses were related entirely to peripheral metabolism of levodopa, then use of peripheral dopa decarboxylase inhibitors would be expected to eliminate some of the myriad factors that influence plasma levodopa levels and thereby eliminate some such episodes. If plasma levodopa levels can still be generally correlated with on–off effects when levodopa is administered with a peripheral dopa decarboxylase inhibitor remains to be seen. Although there have been reports that the use of peripheral inhibitors attenuates but does not eliminate on–off effects, most observers do not believe that the peripheral inhibitors make any long-term contribution to the management of on–off problems. The observations cast a great deal of doubt on the role of peripheral levodopa metabolism in these phenomena.

Because basic understanding of the mechanisms involved in the on–off effect is lacking, it is difficult to formulate a truly rational approach to the management of the problem. The most common suggestions involve either spreading out the chronic dosage of levodopa being administered by the use of more frequent smaller doses each day or slowing reduction of the total daily maintenance dose. Some investigators believe that altering dose delivery schedules has little or no effect on on–off, whereas others believe that this maneuver with slight dose reduction is worthwhile. Part of this difference of opinion is probably related to the use of different criteria for the diagnosis of on–off. At least three types of fluctuations in performance are seen in parkinsonian patients:

(a) Patients who appear virtually to run out of gas just before each dose. In such patients there is often a good correlation between levodopa level and clinical performance. Giving more frequent doses is often efficacious in such end-of-dose akinesias.

(b) Patients with classic on–off in which a temporal relationship between doses and akinesias cannot be defined. In such patients we have not noted any benefit from increasing the number of doses.

(c) Patients with episodic freezing as part of their parkinsonism. This is more likely to respond to an increase in the total dosage of levodopa.

The ability of apomorphine to reverse off periods, thereby seemingly demonstrating that it is not dopamine receptors that are unresponsive during these times, may prove to be significant in the future management of these patients. Apomorphine itself is not a practical therapeutic tool because of its mode of administration and its side effects; however, other newly developed direct-acting dopamine receptor agonists may provide a more successful answer. The use of bromocriptine in such patients may prove to be a significant advance in therapy (see below).

The effectiveness of amantadine in parkinsonism is apparently related to its effect on dopaminergic transmission. Its efficacy in the therapy of parkinsonian patients has been established when it is administered both by itself and in combination with levodopa. One interesting effect that has been repeatedly observed is that a single 100-mg amantadine dose will at times almost completely eliminate the cyclic on–off symptoms. Unfortunately, this effect has been short-lived, persisting for only 1 to 3 months.

Loss of Efficacy

The dramatic improvement in functional capacity seen in patients during the first year of therapy is often not maintained in subsequent years. Several recent review articles reporting 5- and 6-year follow-up experience with chronic levodopa therapy have documented that the percentage of patients achieving remarkable improvement in their functional abilities decreases with the chronicity of treatment. However, these same studies also point out that, although excellent improvement compared to pretreatment capacities is less common the longer the duration of therapy, even after many years most patients are better than they were prior to treatment. The reason for this gradual loss of efficacy during chronic levodopa therapy is not known. Progression of the basic degenerative process in parkinsonian brain involving both pre- and postsynaptic structures is most likely the major factor.

Observations of individual patients provide clear instances in which loss of efficacy to levodopa seems to be related not to progression of disease but to unspecified pharmacologic alterations. A given patient may experience gradual loss of efficacy over a period of 1 to 3 months, returning very nearly to base-line pretreatment performance despite adequate therapy with levodopa and other agents. When such patients are hospitalized and withdrawn from levodopa for 3 to 4 days and then reintroduced to levodopa, there can be a reachievement of therapeutic benefit often at lower dosages than were required before the "drug holiday." There must be a pharmacologic reason in those patients who respond favorably to this maneuver; however, this phenomenon has been poorly studied to date. Possible explanations advanced for the occurrence of this phenomenon include the build-up of "minor" metabolites of dopamine that interfere with transmitter function, chronic agonism of receptor sites leading to altered responsiveness, and chronic agonist receptor interaction resulting in "tying up" of active receptor sites so that no active sites are available for response.

Loss of efficacy, which is a major problem in levodopa therapy, should be divided into that associated with probable progression of disease and that associated with pharmacologic phenomena. In a given patient experiencing these difficulties, a drug holiday, while the patient is hospitalized, can be an important clinical maneuver in the management of this problem.

Psychiatric Side Effects

The mental status of patients with Parkinson's disease who receive chronic levodopa therapy has become increasingly important. A distinction must be drawn between mental changes related to progression of disease and/or aging and those mental changes that are clearly pharmacologically induced. Although dementia was not originally described as part of the clinical spectrum of Parkinson's disease, the association of dementia with this disorder was well known before the advent of the levodopa era. The incidence of dementia in Parkinson's disease prior to levodopa therapy, the observation that most patients who became severely demented on chronic levodopa were already experiencing mild dementia prior to treatment, the failure of levodopa or anticholinergic withdrawal to reverse dementia, and the pathologic evidence of a more widespread degenerative process involving far more CNS areas than the substantia nigra alone all suggest that the mental changes characterized as dementia are not related to the pharmacologic treatment of the disorder but are probably associated with advancement and progression of the basic disorder. This is not true of the psychotic behavior seen during levodopa therapy.

Levodopa-induced psychosis occurs in two separate clinical situations: early in the course of treatment, when it is seen in patients with a previous history of mental disease, and after several years of treatment, when it occurs in patients with no history of psychiatric disorders.

When levodopa-induced psychosis occurs early in the course of levodopa therapy it usually happens within a few weeks after the levodopa regimen has started. Almost invariably the patient has had a past history of severe psychiatric disorders, and most often the diagnosis has been schizophrenia (20). The manifestations of levodopa-induced psychoses in such patients can be quite variable. They often resemble the previous psychotic manifestations the patient had, although in our experience most of these patients exhibit some element of paranoid thinking after taking levodopa, even if such thinking has not been present previously. These patients frequently have a formal thought disorder as well as all other manifestations of schizophrenia.

This levodopa-induced exacerbation of preexisting schizophrenia has been ob- served in two patient populations. The first group includes those patients who were receiving neuroleptic treatment for their psychoses and, on developing drug-induced parkinsonism, were given levodopa. The phenomenon is probably analogous to the exacerbation of schizophrenic symptoms by amphetamine and methylphenidate, both of which act by increasing the activity of dopamine within the striatum. Psychiatric symptoms exacerbated by the levodopa are invariably reversible when the levodopa is discontinued. The high incidence of levodopa-induced exacerbation of preexisting schizophrenia in this group of patients, however, serves as an absolute contraindication to prescribing levodopa for drug-induced parkinsonism. The second group consists of patients who had past histories of psychoses but were not being treated for those disorders at the time they were given levodopa for idiopathic parkinsonism. After treatment with levodopa for idiopathic parkinsonism, the psy- choses reappeared. This, again, is almost always self-limited and usually quickly reverses when levodopa is withdrawn. A past history of schizophrenia should be considered a contraindication to the use of levodopa in a parkinsonian patient, since there will be an occasional patient in this group in whom the psychosis will last for several months after the levodopa is discontinued.

Levodopa is also able to induce a psychosis in parkinsonian patients without any history of psychiatric disorders. Although cerebral cortical atrophy accompanied by dementia is common in parkinsonian patients and may predispose to this com- plication, levodopa-induced psychosis also occurs in parkinsonian patients without any evidence of dementia. This usually occurs after several years of levodopa therapy and is definitely related to two other types of levodopa-induced mental alterations: dreams and hallucinations.

Three types of dream alterations occur in chronic parkinsonian patients receiving levodopa over a long period. These occur in at least one-third of all patients taking levodopa for at least 2 years. We have classified them as vivid dreams, night terrors, and nightmares (32).

Vivid dreams. Levodopa-related dreams are qualitatively quite vivid, seemingly real, temporally condensed, internally organized and coherent, often affectively neutral, with a frequent theme of persons and events from the dreamer's remote past. These dreams are qualitatively different from the patient's previous dream experiences and are by far the most common type of levodopa-induced dreams.

Night terrors. Since patients are always amnesic during these experiences, night terrors are reported by other members of the family. Typically the patient screams, calls out, and thrashes around during sleep. He may awaken screaming but remain amnesic in regard to why he screamed or why he woke up. Approximately 5% of chronic levodopa patients have such experiences.

Nightmares. These are classic, frightening, often paranoid nightmares, and—like the vivid dreams described above—are considered by the patients to be distinctly different from other dreams. Approximately 5% of chronic levodopa patients report nightmares.

Approximately one-half of the patients on levodopa for 2 or more years develop hallucinations. The hallucinatory phenomena usually are stereotyped in each patient; they are often nocturnal, nonthreatening, and recurrent. The hallucinations are predominantly visual (at times with a secondary auditory component) and are superimposed on a clear sensorium. They usually conform to boundaries imposed by actual concurrent sensory input and often concern individuals and experiences that were significant in the patient's past. At times, the hallucinations blend indistinguishably with the dream phenomena possessing similar themes. At least two-thirds of these hallucinations are associated with levodopa-induced dreams.

Levodopa-induced psychosis almost invariably develops later in the course of therapy in patients who already have levodopa hallucinations and dreams. The psychotic phenomena that we have observed have all been paranoid in nature. They are characterizable as a pure paranoid delusional system, superimposed on a clear sensorium, with no other qualities of thought disorder present. A rare patient will develop a full-blown schizophreniform psychosis and an occasional patient will progress from paranoid psychosis to a confusional toxic psychosis. Approximately 3% of the patients who have been treated with levodopa for 2 or more years experience psychoses each year.

All levodopa-induced psychotic states are associated with vivid dreams and/or hallucinations. Almost invariably these have been present for weeks or months prior to any psychotic behavior. Levodopa-induced confusional psychosis has been found to be usually associated with preexisting paranoid nonconfusional psychosis.

Overall, then, this suggests a progression of medication-induced psychiatric symptomatology from striking dreams, to dreams plus hallucinatory experiences, to a pure paranoid delusional system, and, finally, to a confusional state super-imposed on the rest. The actual onset of psychiatric symptoms varies in these patients from insidious to acute. Although the onset is occasionally triggered by an increase in levodopa dosage, usually it is not associated with any alteration in maintenance therapy (32).

The first step to take in managing these side effects is to attempt to prevent their occurrence. This can best be done by keeping the daily dose of levodopa or levodopa–carbidopa as low as possible while obtaining therapeutic efficacy. This will, one hopes, decrease the incidence or at least delay the onset. By themselves neither the dreams nor the hallucinations are bothersome to the patient. There is the possibility, however, that their progressive course will become a problem.

Many patients with such problems are on anticholinergic medications, and these can cause similar hallucinations as well as make the levodopa-related hallucinations worse. When confusion occurs in conjunction with hallucinations, one should sus-pect that the hallucinations are related to anticholinergic therapy, and the anti-cholinergic drugs should be withdrawn. If possible, this should be done slowly, over a week to 10 days, in order to avoid the rebound worsening of parkinsonism that may be caused by sudden withdrawal of the anticholinergics. If a patient is hallucinating, the anticholinergic agents should be reduced even if there is no confusional state. Amantadine hydrochloride, like the anticholinergics, can both cause and exacerbate hallucinations and should be reduced or withdrawn when hallucination occurs. Amantadine-induced hallucinations are usually associated with confusion or obtundation.

If adjustment of anticholinergics or amantadine fails to reduce psychotic symp-toms adequately, consideration must, of course, be given to reducing the levodopa dosage. Because this will usually result in decreased therapeutic efficacy, in many patients it may be necessary to maintain the levodopa dosage level despite the existence and possibility of progression of dreams and hallucinations. Fortunately in most patients psychiatric symptoms do not progress beyond the dream–hallucination stage.

When psychosis occurs, therapeutic intervention is, of course, required. If the psychosis is confusional, one should be suspicious that anticholinergic agents or amantadine may be playing a role, and these drugs should be withdrawn first. This is especially true if there is no paranoid component and the patient has not gone through the usual progression of levodopa-induced psychosis. If the patient does not improve by these manipulations, levodopa administration should be stopped.

The psychosis tends to clear within days after levodopa withdrawal. Usually by this time the patient's parkinsonism is much worse and requires antiparkinsonian therapy. Our usual practice is to restart the patient on half the previous dosage. If this is tolerated well, the dosage can be slowly increased as necessary, to two-thirds or three-quarters of the previous dose. Because of the drug holiday effect, such patients often do well on a lower dose.

The occurrence of a paranoid psychosis often tempts the physician to use neu-roleptics. This should be avoided if at all possible, since these drugs worsen the patient's parkinsonian manifestations. If a neuroleptic is necessary to control behavior, low doses are usually sufficient, and the drug can usually be stopped after a few days. Because of the lower incidence of drug-induced parkinsonism, we use thioridazine in such patients.

Levodopa-Induced Myoclonus

We have described a levodopa-induced movement disorder that is distinct from the previously discussed levodopa-induced choreiform disorder (23). The movements characteristic of the former consist of myoclonic jerking of the entire body and extremities sometimes associated with the more common levodopa-induced choreiform movements and sometimes occurring independently of the more typical choreoathethoid movements. All patients experiencing this levodopa-induced myoclonus had been receiving levodopa for at least 1 year when the movements developed. Pharmacologic investigation of these myoclonic jerks revealed that increasing levodopa increased the myoclonus in all patients. Neither the withdrawal or addition of anticholinergics nor a trial of propranolol altered the myoclonus. Methysergide, a serotonin antagonist, reduced the myoclonic jerking in all of the patients and completely stopped it in 58%. It is noteworthy that the antagonism of serotonergic activity, which alleviated the myoclonus, did not alter the degree of the more lingual–facial–buccal dyskinesias produced by levodopa. There is both clinical and laboratory evidence that some types of myoclonus are related to a levodopa-induced alteration in serotonin activity.

Nausea, Vomiting, Anorexia

One of the most common problems in levodopa therapy is the occurrence of nausea and vomiting. This side effect of therapy can occur with the initial dose of levodopa and is most troublesome during initiation and build-up of adequate maintenance of dosages. Nausea and vomiting may also appear for the first time when high dose levels of levodopa are reached. It has been common clinical experience for 30 to 80% of patients to report nausea and vomiting during early therapy. Fortunately, if levodopa therapy is introduced gradually, tolerance to these side effects develops in the majority of the patients, although 10 to 17% on chronic levodopa treatment may continue to experience occasional gastrointestinal disturbance.

The pharmacologic activity of dopamine that is related to the production of nausea and vomiting is the effect of dopamine on chemoreceptors in the area postrema. The area postrema, the "vomiting center," is physiologically outside of the blood–brain barrier and is sensitive to noxious influences circulating within the vascular system. The neuronal receptors in the area postrema are sensitive to dopamine. The systemically formed dopamine stimulates the postrema and produces emesis. Support for this mechanism of action of levodopa-induced vomiting comes from the remarkable success of peripheral dopa decarboxylase inhibition in limiting the degree of emesis connected with levodopa therapy (4). By preventing the formation of dopamine outside the blood–brain barrier, these agents markedly reduce access of dopamine to the area postrema and thereby prevent nausea and vomiting.

The management of levodopa-related gastrointestinal distress should first be handled by gradual dose induction when beginning therapy; levodopa should always be administered with meals or snacks. If nausea and vomiting remain a therapeutic problem, then the combined administration of carbidopa (dopa decarboxylase inhibitor) and levodopa results in an approximate 75% reduction in the amount of levodopa that must be administered to a parkinsonian patient to achieve the same antiparkinsonian effect as levodopa alone. Although this treatment is effective in preventing nausea, vomiting, and anorexia in a vast majority of patients, there are still some patients who continue to have these gastrointestinal problems. The treatment of this persistent levodopa-related nausea and emesis must not include phenothiazine antiemetics. Although these agents are effective in reducing the vomiting as a result of their dopamine receptor blocking activity, they also block central dopamine receptors and interfere with therapy in Parkinson's disease. The successful treatment of levodopa-induced nausea and vomiting with diphenidol, a trihexyphenidyl analog with little anticholinergic and no antiparkinsonian effect has been reported (13). Diphenidol strongly antagonizes the effect of apomorphine on the emesis center. Similar clinical experience with hydroxyzine has been reported.

Cardiac Arrhythmias

Levodopa has been demonstrated to have an effect on the myocardium in experimental animals that includes alterations in contractile force, tachycardia, and arrhythmias. These have all been related to dopamine and not to levodopa itself. The use of peripheral dopa decarboxylase inhibitors has been shown to reduce markedly such arrhythmias. Cardiac arrhythmias have been reported to occur in patients receiving levodopa, and the use of peripheral dopa decarboxylase inhibition has also been demonstrated to prevent these dysrhythmias (39). In a specific patient in whom it can be demonstrated that a levodopa-related arrhythmia exists, or in a patient with preexistent cardiac arrhythmias, the possibly deleterious effect of peripherally formed dopamine can be eliminated by the use of peripheral decarboxylase inhibitors (34). In general, the potential for cardiac arrhythmias in a patient receiving levodopa should be borne in mind; in practice, however, this potential problem occurs quite infrequently.

Blood Pressure Alterations

Chronic levodopa therapy frequently causes hypotension. In particular, orthostatic hypotension has been repeatedly observed. Calne and his colleagues have divided the hypotensive effect of levodopa into what they believe is a peripherally mediated impairment of baroreceptor responses, which contributes to the orthostatic component, and a centrally mediated effect on resting blood pressure. This division of the effect of levodopa was accomplished by the study of patients on and off peripheral decarboxylase inhibitors (8). In this study the use of carbidopa tended to decrease levodopa-induced orthostatic hypotension without eliminating the levo-dopa-induced reduction in basal blood pressure. If the orthostatic hypotension related to levodopa therapy is clearly a peripheral effect of dopamine, then the use of peripheral decarboxylase inhibitors should have clinical advantages in patients with this problem. Most studies do indicate a mild decrease in orthostatic blood pressure problems with such combination therapy. Fortunately, patients with the problem of orthostatic hypotension tend to develop tolerance to this effect of levodopa both in terms of the unpleasant clinical sensations associated with transient hypotension and in terms of actual measured hypotension.

Although the incidence of postural hypotension tends to decline with length of levodopa treatment and the severity of the hypotensive symptoms in patients with this problem tends to improve, there are still some patients in whom the postural hypotensive effect is dose-limiting. Improvement of motor performance in these people may be greatly hindered by the inability to administer appropriate dosages of levodopa alone or in combination because of this problem. First, patients must be instructed to rise from supine positions slowly and with awareness of their problem. Elastic stockings and mild increases in sodium intake may be enough to circumvent the hypotensive problem. If these simpler solutions are ineffective, 9-α-fluorocortisol acetate (fludrocortisone) can be used. This agent causes an increase in intravascular volume and tends to decrease postural hypotension.

As initially mentioned, levodopa remains the mainstay of pharmacologic man-agement of Parkinson's disease. Combination therapy (decarboxylase inhibitor–levodopa) is useful in the management of nausea and vomiting associated with levodopa and in levodopa-related cardiac arrhythmias, and it is of possible benefit in the management of postural hypotension. It is of little or no value in the management of patients with centrally mediated side effects and rarely adds to functional ability of a patient who is well managed on levodopa alone. There are some indications that combined therapy, although able to induce a quicker thera-peutic response than levodopa alone, may induce the dose-limiting central side effects earlier than levodopa alone. At this time, the practice of initiating therapy with levodopa alone in parkinsonian patients requiring dopaminergic therapy re-mains sound. If an indication for decarboxylase inhibition arises, the patient can be quickly and safely switched to combined therapy, thereby avoiding the possibility of introducing some of the long-term therapeutic problems of levodopa adminis-tration at an even earlier time.

Because most of the severe dose- and eventually efficacy-limiting side effects of levodopa therapy are clearly related to the duration of levodopa therapy with regard to both their incidence and severity, it is obvious that levodopa is not the initial treatment of choice for parkinsonism but should be used only in patients with significant disability despite other therapy.

Drug Holiday

As discussed, patients who are experiencing prominent central dopaminergic side effects should be instructed to lower their antiparkinsonian medication dosage.

Often, a simple reduction in one or several drugs will abate the side effects without precipitating significant decline in motor function. In a large number of patients, however, even small decreases in a drug will cause prominent exacerbation of the parkinsonian features, so that the lower dose is unacceptable because of parkinsonism and the higher dose is equally unacceptable because of side effects. In such patients, Klawans et al. have introduced the concept of a drug holiday in which patients are admitted to the hospital and stop their antiparkinsonian medication for 4 to 7 days. Then, the medications are slowly reintroduced. Follow-up studies indicate that, after the holiday, patients can be maintained on lower doses of medication and tend to show enhanced antiparkinsonian efficacy and reduced side effects for up to 1 year. During the hospitalization, patients show a usual precipitous decline when receiving no medication so that expert physical therapy, respiratory therapy, and nursing care are paramount. The physiologic or pharmacologic basis underlying the effectiveness of a period of transient drug withdrawal is unknown. Alteration of dopaminergic receptor site sensitivity has been postulated as being responsible for drug-related side effects observed after chronic dopaminergic therapy. It has been suggested that long-term dopaminergic stimulation results in postsynaptic supersensitivity, postsynaptic desensitization, or presynaptic desensitization, and hence that the drug holiday may abort the development of one or more of these.

PERIPHERAL DECARBOXYLASE INHIBITORS

Levodopa is pharmacologically inert. Both its efficacy and its side effects depend on its metabolic products. As early as 1967, it was suggested that agents that would prevent the peripheral metabolism of levodopa by inhibiting the enzyme dopa decarboxylase (aromatic amino acid decarboxylase) might improve the efficacy of levodopa. The major advantages of these agents are the management of side effects due to the formation of active metabolites outside the blood–brain barrier. This often results in a better therapeutic index and better clinical efficacy.

Two such peripheral decarboxylase inhibitors are in use: carbidopa and benseramide. The usefulness of these agents has already been discussed.

Carbidopa comes in two fixed ratios with levodopa: 1/10 and 1/4. The 1/10 is available in two sizes, 10/100 and 25/250, while the 1/4 ratio is available in only one size, 25/100. Most patients require 40 to 80 mg carbidopa/day to block the peripheral decarboxylase sufficiently. Some patients require more inhibitor and do better on the 1/4 ratio preparation. In patients on carbidopa/levodopa, the daily dose of levodopa usually ranges from 300 to 1,250 mg/day with a mean average of about 800 mg/day. This means that the addition of carbidopa decreases the levodopa dosage by about 75%. A reasonable starting dose is 1/2 tablet three times a day with weekly increments. It is often best to start with the 25/100 form to assure complete blockade with even low doses.

Domperidone is a second type of agent being used to treat peripheral side effects of levodopa. It does not appreciably pass the blood–brain barrier *in vivo*. It is used in the specific control of levodopa-related gastrointestinal side effects, is currently under study, and is believed to act as a peripheral receptor site antagonist.

PARKINSONISM AS A POSTSYNAPTIC DISORDER: FAILURE TO RESPOND

Viewed from the perspective of the striatal dopamine receptor sites, parkinsonism in almost all instances is a disorder of presynaptic dopaminergic mechanisms. In both idiopathic and postencephalitic parkinsonism, degeneration of the dopaminergic neurons of the substantia nigra results in decreased dopaminergic activity at striatal dopamine receptors. This decreased dopamine input is believed to be the pathophysiologic basis of the signs and symptoms of parkinsonism. The clinical improvement in parkinsonism resulting from levodopa is presumed to be due to increased dopamine activity at relatively normal dopamine receptors. If parkinsonism is a reflection of altered response of striatal dopamine receptors, parkinsonism could also result from primary dysfunction of the striatal neurons—a form of postsynaptic receptor site dysfunction. Although the clinical manifestations of parkinsonism may be identical in "presynaptic" and "postsynaptic" parkinsonism, the biochemical basis and pharmacologic responses of the two states may be quite different (21,24). Decreased dopaminergic input ("presynaptic dopamine deficiency") should be reflected by biochemical evidence of decreased dopamine turnover as reflected by spinal fluid HVA levels and should respond to increased dopamine turnover as a result of levodopa therapy. Most patients with parkinsonism fall into this category. In most such patients, levodopa results in definite clinical improvement. Some early studies consisting of limited numbers of patients all suggested that patients with higher HVA levels prior to levodopa therapy show less clinical improvement when placed on levodopa and thus raised the possibility that parkinsonism can occur as a result of postsynaptic dysfunction. Parkinsonism in such patients need not be associated with any alteration in CSF HVA. If parkinsonism in such patients is caused by loss of striatal response to dopamine, the efficacy of levodopa may be quite limited. This raises the possibility that some patients may have had postsynaptic striatal dysfunction that could produce clinical parkinsonism not associated with altered CSF HVA, which would be unresponsive to levodopa. It has become clear that several such states do exist.

The first of these is a striatonigral degeneration. This disease is characterized clinically by parkinsonism and pathologically by degeneration of both the substantia nigra and the putamen. Although there are no studies of CSF HVA in such patients, clearly these patients do not respond as well to chronic levodopa therapy as patients with parkinsonism per se.

Postsynaptic striatal dysfunction also results in parkinsonism in the so-called rigid or akinetic form of Huntington's chorea. Although the akinetic form of Huntington's disease usually occurs before the age of 20, the clinical manifestations include parkinson-like akinesia and rigidity. The parkinson-like manifestations of the akinetic form of Huntington's disease are thought to be related to degeneration of striatal neurons and loss of response to dopamine. If the parkinsonian features of this form of Huntington's disease are related to a decreased effect of dopamine, it is reasonable to use levodopa in an attempt to increase the activity of dopamine within the striatum. Akinetic Huntington's disease apparently is associated with normal CSF HVA and a limited response to levodopa.

We recently studied a patient with levodopa-resistant parkinsonism owing to basal ganglia calcification related to surgically induced hypoparathyroidism. The parkinsonism in this patient was associated with normal levels of CSF HVA, and the patient showed no clinical response to levodopa.

A fourth state in which parkinsonism is related to postsynaptic striatal pathology is the Shy-Drager syndrome. Here again, the response to levodopa therapy is poor.

These various observations have several possible implications for the study of the biochemistry and pharmacology of parkinsonism and any other neurologic disorder involving decreased activity of any neurotransmitter:

(a) Presynaptic deficiency and postsynaptic dysfunction in relation to the same amine system can result in identical clinical pictures.

(b) Only the presynaptic deficiency state is associated with detectable alterations in amine metabolites in the CSF.

(c) The two states may well differ in the response to precursor load therapy.

EFFECT OF VITAMIN B_6

A striking reversal of the levodopa effect on parkinsonism often occurs when patients are placed on vitamin B_6. Vitamin B_6 in the form of pyridoxal phosphate has also been shown to potentiate the vasopressor effect of intravenous levodopa. It is believed that this potentiation is due to a B_6-stimulated increase in the peripheral dopa decarboxylase activity. This enzyme decarboxylates dopa to dopamine, and any increase in its activity would increase the rate of dopamine formation from levodopa. An increased rate of dopamine formation would potentiate the peripheral effects of levodopa and, at the same time, would lower levodopa blood levels and decrease the amount of levodopa crossing into the brain to exert an antiparkinson effect.

We have found that doses of B_6 10 to 20 times greater than that necessary to reverse the effect of levodopa in patients on levodopa alone could no longer reverse the effect if the activity of dopa decarboxylase was blocked by a dopa decarboxylase inhibitor (20). This suggests that the B_6 effect involves dopa decarboxylase, which is probably not saturated with B_6 at usual levels of this vitamin.

AMANTADINE

In 1968, a 58-year-old woman with Parkinson's disease who had been on amantadine hydrochloride for protection against A_2 influenza reported marked relief of her parkinsonian symptoms. This led to a prolonged study of the drug by Schwab et al. (36).

Amantadine (1-adamantanamine hydrochloride) is a stable, white, crystalline, 10-carbon-cage amine that is soluble in water. Its use in preventing A_2 influenza virus infection may be based either on its ability to absorb onto cells, or on a direct interference with viral replication.

Schwab et al. (36) have reported on 163 patients treated with amantadine in addition to their usual antiparkinson medications. A significant percentage of these patients showed sustained benefits for 3 to 8 months. However, one-third of those who initially had a striking improvement in symptoms, especially the akinesia and rigidity, showed a steady reduction in benefit after 4 to 8 weeks. This tendency leveled off, leaving them moderately improved. The beneficial effect of amantadine and its decreasing efficacy with time has been confirmed by numerous studies. Interestingly enough, 9 of Schwab's patients who responded well to amantadine also responded well to levodopa. Two who failed to respond well to amantadine likewise did poorly with levodopa.

On the basis of clinical observations that the toxic side effects of amantadine were similar to those of standard antiparkinson agents, Schwab et al. (36) suggested that they might have a similar mechanism of action. Others have concluded that the mechanism of amantadine must be similar to that of levodopa since the range of therapeutic activity is similar in both drugs. A more reasonable hypothesis can be drawn from known pharmacological action to amantadine.

It has been shown that pretreatment with amantadine increases the hypertensive effect of norepinephrine, although amantadine by itself produces no change in blood pressure. Pretreatment with amantadine also decreases the uptake of labeled norepinephrine into the heart. These results demonstrate that amantadine increases the effect of norepinephrine while at the same time decreasing its uptake into peripheral nerves. It is generally believed that amantadine acts as an indirect dopamine agonist. It, itself, has no effect on dopamine receptors but blocks neuronal membrane reuptake of dopamine. This block of dopamine reuptake increases and prolongs the activity of whatever dopamine is being released. Amantadine may also increase the release of dopamine.

Clinical response to amantadine requires both the release of dopamine and the presence of receptor sites in the striatum capable of responding to dopamine. Clinical improvement in parkinsonism owing to amantadine demonstrates that the striatal dopamine receptor sites are still capable of responding to dopamine. According to this concept, patients who respond to amantadine should improve on levodopa unless their improvement is prevented by peripheral or other side effects. It does appear that patients who improve on amantadine also improve on levodopa. This is consistent with the concept that amantadine works through a dopaminergic mechanism and that improvement on amantadine demonstrates that the striatal dopaminergic receptors are still capable of responding to levodopa. Amantadine has also been shown to decrease the amount of levodopa necessary to produce clinical improvement. This is again consistent with the proposed mechanism that it blocks dopamine reuptake and, therefore, accentuates the physiological activity of any dopamine formed from levodopa in the CNS.

Amantadine, perhaps because of a better therapeutic index, is more efficacious than the various anticholinergics and even demonstrates efficacy in relationship to akinesia and loss of postural reflexes. Because of its efficacy against these manifestations of parkinsonism it is particularly useful in the management of patients who respond poorly to levodopa. Most patients derive some benefit from amantadine. Some patients do develop tolerance in weeks to months.

Amantadine is generally given in an initial dose of 100 mg daily, which is doubled after a week if, as is usual, there are no adverse reactions. Since restlessness and insomnia are common, the second dose of amantadine should not be taken late in the day. Occasionally, patients do better on 300 mg/day. Amantadine can also cause dizziness, confusion, hallucinations, mood changes, nausea, abdominal discomfort, headache, edema, pruritus, and, rarely, cardiac arrhythmias. These are all reversible on discontinuation of the drug.

Amantadine is very poorly metabolized so that 80 to 90% of an administered dose is excreted unchanged in the urine. Because of this, amantadine builds up quickly in any patient with impaired renal function. In such patients usual therapeutic doses can easily result in confusion, hallucinations, toxic psychosis, and even coma. Consequently, significantly impaired renal function must be considered to be a relative contraindication to the use of amantadine. Amantadine is only poorly and slowly dialysized, which makes dialysis only a moderately effective treatment for toxicity owing to renal failure.

Amantadine overdose is reported to precipitate convulsions, so amantadine is usually given cautiously in patients with a history of seizures. Many, if not most, patients on amantadine develop livedo reticularis, a condition in which there is an edema and shininess of skin with a livid red appearance and increased prominence of small superficial vessels. This occurs especially on the dorsum of the foot and dorsum of the hands and has no pathologic significance.

DIRECT-ACTING DOPAMINE AGONISTS

If the best pharmacological approach to parkinsonism is to increase the activity of dopamine at selected dopaminergic receptors, it might be possible to find drugs that can act directly at these sites without having to undergo chemical transformation within the brain. An agent of this type could directly cross the blood–brain barrier and act at the dopaminergic receptor sites on the striatal neurons (a direct-acting dopamine agonist). It is quite possible that such a drug might have distinct advantages over levodopa as far as increased efficacy or a better therapeutic index. If a dopaminergic agonist can be found that has a selective action on those striatal receptors that are primarily involved in the pathological processes underlying parkinsonism, such an agonist might have a lower incidence of such side effects as dyskinesias and psychosis.

Apomorphine is the prototype of such agents. The structure of apomorphine and other direct-acting dopamine agonists and their similarities to dopamine are shown in Fig. 3. In the early 1950s, Schwab et al. gave parkinsonian patients subemetic

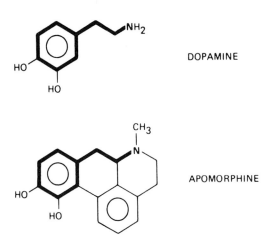

FIG. 3. Structures of dopamine and apomorphine (with dopamine moiety emphasized).

doses of apomorphine subcutaneously (35). This initially produced mild nausea, which was followed by a period of decreased tremor, increased voluntary strength, and reduced rigidity associated with subjective well-being. The short-lived action of the drug (30–180 min) necessitated repeated injections, and the side effects, especially nausea and hypotension, were significant.

More recently, Cotzias et al. reported similar results with subcutaneous apomorphine (10). They were able to alleviate the cardinal symptoms of parkinsonism in 5 of 6 patients. It is of interest that one parkinsonian patient who showed choreoathetoid movements while on levodopa exhibited identical movements after receiving apomorphine. Unfortunately, high oral doses of apomorphine led to pre-renal azotemia, so that this form of therapy was abandoned.

Most recently the search for a better dopamine agonist has centered on ergot alkaloids, many of which are dopaminergic agonists (6). The ergots are now in three groups:

(a) Ergolines, which are substances containing the tetracyclic nucleus of lysergic acid, together with any nonpeptide moiety.

(b) Naturally occurring ergolines.

(c) Ergopeptine, a tetracyclic lysergic acid nucleus combined with a peptide.

Bromocriptine

Bromocriptine (see Fig. 4) is an ergopeptine which is a direct-acting dopamine agonist.

In the initial studies of parkinsonism, small doses of bromocriptine (up to 20 mg daily) showed somewhat controversial results, but more recent studies with higher intake (up to 150 mg daily) demonstrated definite clinical improvement (18,29,33). All the clinical features of parkinsonism improved. The overall extent of the therapeutic response is comparable to that obtained with levodopa, but optimal results

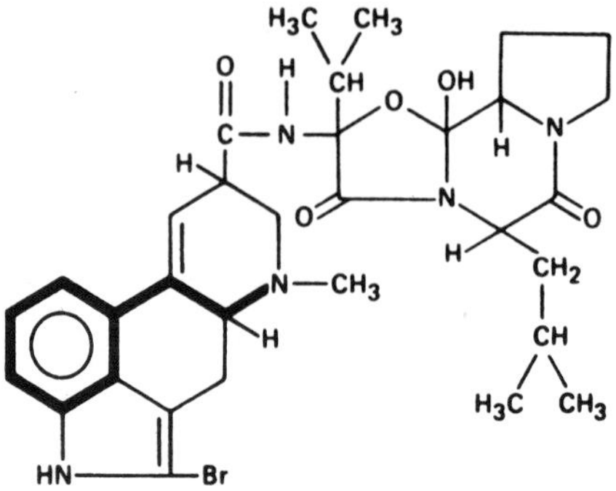

FIG. 4. Structure of bromocriptine (with dopamine moiety emphasized).

are usually achieved by combining submaximal doses of bromocriptine and levodopa (18). One advantage of bromocriptine over levodopa is reduction in the severity and frequency of on–off reactions. There are conflicting reports as to whether patients who have become refractory to levodopa gain any benefit from bromocriptine.

Adverse reactions to bromocriptine are similar to those of levodopa, but there is a tendency for dyskinesia to be less prominent. Unfortunately, psychiatric reactions are more common and more severe with bromocriptine, and in some patients hallucinations and delusions have taken several weeks to clear after treatment has been stopped.

A new problem occasionally encountered with bromocriptine is the induction of erythema, edema, and tenderness of the lower legs, ankles, and feet. This problem can simulate cellulitis or thrombophlebitis. Very rarely, this syndrome is accompanied by livedo reticularis, or polyarthralgia. The entire symptomatology disappears within a few days of stopping bromocriptine. Finally, there have been recent reports of pleural thickening and related pulmonary disorders in patients receiving chronic high-dose bromocriptine therapy. Most of these patients were concurrently receiving levodopa. The frequency and significance of these changes are now being studied.

The most important question relating to bromocriptine therapy is unanswered. If patients treated with bromocriptine without previous or concomitant levodopa treatment will develop the same problems as those associated with prolonged levodopa therapy is still unknown. Only a negative answer to this would justify initiating long-term treatment with bromocriptine.

Lergotrile

Lergotrile is an ergoline that is simpler in structure and easier to synthesize than bromocriptine (Fig. 5). Clinically, lergotrile has an antiparkinsonian efficacy comparable to bromocriptine, but dosage must be started at lower levels, with a slower build-up, because transient hypotension is more common and severe than with

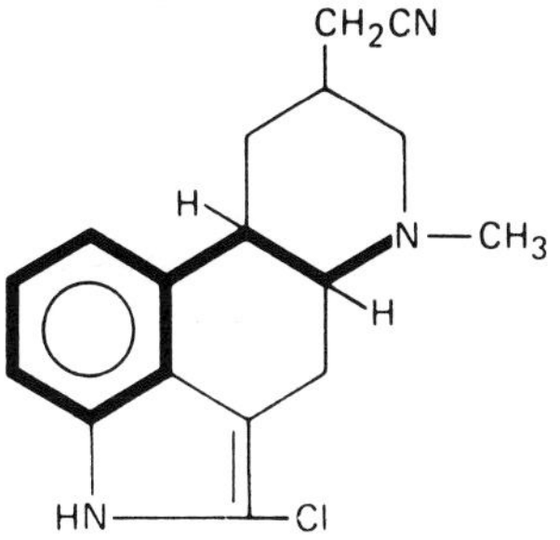

FIG. 5. Structure of lergotrile (with dopamine moiety emphasized).

bromocriptine (6,27,30). Cross-tolerance between lergotrile and bromocriptine has been demonstrated, so patients can be changed rapidly from one drug to the other without prolonged dose titrations. In one controlled study of lergotrile and bromocriptine, it was found that dyskinesia was less marked with lergotrile. Once again on–off effects often improved during lergotrile therapy. Lergotrile may not result in as much psychosis as bromocriptine. Elevation of plasma transaminase levels (SGOT and SGPT) occurs quite frequently with lergotrile in high doses employed for treating parkinsonism (up to 150 mg daily), and these disturbances have been correlated with biopsy evidence of hepatocellular damage. The hepatic changes are reversible on stopping lergotrile therapy, and in some patients the enzyme levels return to normal in spite of continued treatment. Because of the liver involvement, study of this agent has been discontinued.

Pergolide Mesylate

Like lergotrile, pergolide is a synthetic ergoline. It has been shown to be quite long acting and is a potent direct-acting central dopamine agonist with high affinity for dopamine receptors. This drug is 20 times more potent milligram per milligram than bromocriptine or lergotrile. Its half-life is estimated to be over 24 hr, and it suppresses prolactin secretion for up to 40 hr after a single 0.1 mg dose. Like bromocriptine, preliminary reports suggest that pergolide has efficacy in patients having problems with long-term levodopa therapy, especially on–off phenomena. It is still being evaluated in selected centers.

One other direct-acting agonist, lisuride, is also being studied.

SELECTIVE MONOAMINE OXIDASE INHIBITORS

Two forms of the enzyme monoamine oxidase (MAO) have been demonstrated in various animals and termed MAO_A and MAO_B. MAO_A oxidizes norepinephrine, serotonin, and dopamine, whereas MAO_B acts fairly specifically on dopamine. Because of this differential substrate specificity, a specific inhibitor of MAO_B might result in selective elevation of brain dopamine levels. Deprenyl, a selective inhibitor of MAO_B, has been used by Birkmayer in parkinsonism. A definite potentiation of the therapeutic response to levodopa (in combination with an extracerebral decarboxylase inhibitor) was shown when deprenyl was administered intravenously, intramuscularly, or orally. Chronic long-term potentiation has also been reported with oral deprenyl (5). The exact efficacy and role of deprenyl remain to be defined. A recent double-blind study that compared deprenyl with placebo in 11 patients did not demonstrate significant efficacy (13a).

THE PHARMACOLOGY OF DISEASES CLOSELY RELATED TO PARKINSONISM

The marked efficacy of levodopa in the treatment of parkinsonism stimulated attempts to use this agent in other diseases involving the extrapyramidal system. Two of these syndromes, progressive supranuclear palsy (PSP) and olivopontocerebellar degeneration (OPCD), frequently include among their manifestations signs and symptoms of parkinsonism.

Olivopontocerebellar Degeneration

OPCD most often presents as a progressive cerebellar ataxia. However, the substantia nigra is frequently involved in this disease, and this involvement manifests itself as parkinsonism. The parkinsonian manifestations can be mild or can in fact dominate the clinical picture. The combined occurrence of parkinsonism and cerebellar symptoms in an individual patient raises the question as to whether the mixed syndrome is the manifestation of a single pathological entity (OPCD including nigral involvement) or the coincidental occurrence of two separate entities. The fact that progressive parkinsonism with cerebellar dysfunction occurs as a hereditary entity suggests that a single pathological entity is responsible for the combined syndrome.

The results of the use of levodopa in the 2 patients presented by Klawans and Zeitlin support the concept that levodopa acts specifically on symptoms related to lesions of the dopaminergic system (28). The parkinsonian features responded to levodopa but the other features did not. The diagnosis of OPCD implies that there is involvement of the nigrostriatal neurons of the substantia nigra as part of the disease process. This involvement can be identical to the alterations seen in parkinsonism. The assumption that these patients had lesions of the substantia nigra is of practical significance, since the symptoms resulting from such a lesion are usually improved by levodopa.

Progressive Supranuclear Palsy

PSP is a progressive neurological disorder consisting of supranuclear ophthalmoplegia affecting chiefly vertical gaze, pseudobulbar palsy, dysarthria, dystonic rigidity of the neck and upper trunk, mild dementia, and other less constant cerebellar and pyramidal symptoms. In some respects these patients resemble patients with parkinsonism because of their masked faces, marked akinesia, and gait difficulties as well as very poor postural stability. However, patients with PSP have distinct features not seen in parkinsonism. The most obvious of these are the peculiar erect posture with backward retraction of the neck and the marked ophthalmoplegia, especially involving vertical gaze.

Most PSP patients treated with levodopa are reported to have shown improvement in their parkinsonian features (25). As in parkinsonian patients, PSP patients receiving levodopa showed improvement in rigidity, bradykinesia, and postural stability, but still had enough incapacity that their overall functional improvement was poor. This is because the nonparkinsonian features of PSP do not improve significantly on long-term levodopa therapy.

The apparent improvement of the parkinsonian features of PSP on long-term levodopa therapy and the concomitant failure of the nonparkinsonian features to improve suggest that these two types of manifestations may be pathophysiologically quite distinct. This observation is consistent with the proposition that the parkinsonian and nonparkinsonian features of PSP, although etiologically identical, involve different physiologic mechanisms. Such a distinction is important, since the therapy of this condition is directed toward its pathophysiology and not its etiology. Many of the parkinsonian features of PSP, such as akinesia, poor postural stability, and poor vocalization, improve on levodopa. These symptoms may be due to the lesions seen in the substantia nigra and the subsequent dopaminergic denervation of the striatum. Because the pathophysiology of ophthalmoplegia and neck dystonia is not related to dopamine depletion, as are the parkinsonian features, levodopa has little or no efficacy on these manifestations.

More recently it has been claimed that methysergide has a beneficial effect on the specific features of PSP. We unfortunately have used this agent in numerous patients without observing significant benefit.

BIBLIOGRAPHY AND *SELECTED REVIEWS

1. Ahmed, A., and Marshall, P. B. (1962): Relationship between antiacetylcholine and anti-tremor activity in anti-parkinsonian and related drugs. *Br. J. Pharmacology*, 18:247–254.
1a. Barbeau, A. (1962): The pathogenesis of Parkinson's disease. *Can. Med. Assoc. J.*, 87:802–807.
*2. Barbeau, A. (1969): L-Dopa therapy in Parkinson's disease. A critical review of nine years' experience. *Can. Med. Assoc. J.*, 101:59–69.
*3. Barbeau, A. (1976): Six years of high level levodopa therapy in severely akinetic parkinsonian patients. *Arch. Neurol.*, 33:333–338.
4. Barbeau, A., and Gillo-Joffroy, L. (1969): Treatment of Parkinson's disease with L-dopa and RO 4–4602. 9th Int. Congress Neurol., Excerpta Medica Int. Congress Ser. 193:171–183.
5. Birkmayer, W. (1978): Long-term treatment with deprenyl. *J. Neural Transm.*, 43:239–244.
5a. Birkmayer, W., and Hornykiewicz, O. (1962): The L-DOPA effect in Parkinson's syndrome in man. *Arch. Psychiatr. Nervenkr.*, 203:560–574.
*6. Calne, D. B. (1978): Dopaminergic agonists in the treatment of parkinsonism. In: *Clinical Neuropharmacology, Vol. 3*, edited by H. L. Klawans, pp. 153–166. Raven Press, New York.
7. Calne, D. B., Calveria, L. E., and Allen, J. G. (1974): Plasma levodopa and the "on–off" effect. In: *Advances in Neurology, Vol. 5, Second Canadian-American Conference on Parkinson's Disease*, edited by F. McDowell and A. Barbeau, pp. 341–343. Raven Press, New York.
8. Calne, D. B., Reid, J. L., Vokel, S. D., George, C. F., and Rao, S. (1973): Effect of carbidopa and L-DOPA on blood pressure in man. In: *Advances in Neurology, Vol. 2, The Treatment of Parkinsonism*, edited by M. D. Yahr, pp. 149–160. Raven Press, New York.

9. Cotzias, G. C., Lawrence, W. H., Papavasiliou, P. S., Duby, S. E., Ginos, J. Z., and Mena, I. (1972): Apomorphine and parkinsonism. *Trans. Am. Neurol. Assoc.*, 97:156–158.
10. Cotzias, G. C., Van Woert, M. H., and Schiffer, L. M. (1967): Aromatic amino acids and modification of parkinsonism. *N. Engl. J. Med.*, 276:374–378.
11. Coyle, J. T., and Snyder, S. H. (1969): Antiparkinsonism drugs' inhibition of dopamine uptake in the corpus striatum as a possible mechanism of action. *Science*, 166: 899–901.
12. Duvoisin, R. C. (1967): Cholinergic-anticholinergic antagonism in parkinsonism. *Arch. Neurol.*, 17;124–136.
13 Duvoisin, R. C. (1972): Diphenidol for levodopa-induced nausea and vomiting. *J.A.M.A.*, 221:1408.
13a. Eisler, T., Teravainen, M. D., Nelson, R., Krebs, X. X., Weise, V., Lake, C. R., Ebert, M. H., Whetzel, N., Murphy, D. L., Kopin, I. J., and Calne, D. B. (1981): Deprenyl in Parkinson's disease. *Neurology*, 31:19–23.
14. Everett, G. M. (1956): Tremor produced by drugs. *Nature*, 177:1238–1239.
15. Fahn, S. (1974): "On–off" phenomenon with levodopa therapy in parkinsonism. *Neurology (Minneap.)*, 24:431–441.
16. Feldberg, W. (1945): Present views on the mode of action of acetylcholine in the central nervous system. *Physiol. Rev.*, 25:596–642.
17. Hornykiewicz, O. (1966): Dopamine (3-hydroxytyramine) and brain function. *Pharmacol. Rev.*, 18:925–964.
18. Kartzinel, R., Perlow, M., Teychenne, P., Gielin, A. C., Gillespie, M. M., Sadowsky, D. A., and Calne, D. B. (1976): Bromocriptine and levodopa (with or without carbidopa) in parkinsonism. *Lancet*, 2:272–275.
*19. Klawans, H. L. (1968): The pharmacology of parkinsonism. *Dis. Nerv. Syst.*, 29:805–816.
*20. Klawans, H. L. (1973): *The Pharmacology of Extrapyramidal Movement Disorders*. S. Karger, Basel.
21. Klawans, H. L. (1975): Amine precursors in neurologic disorders and the psychoses. In: *Biology of Major Psychoses*, edited by D. X. Freedman, pp. 259–272. Raven Press, New York.
*22. Klawans, H. L., and Bergen, D. (1975): The side effects of levodopa. In: *The Clinical Uses of L-Dopa*, edited by G. Stern, pp. 73–105. Medical and Technical Publishing Co., Oxford.
23. Klawans, H. L., Goetz, C., and Bergen, D. (1975): Levodopa-induced myoclonus. *Arch. Neurol.*, 32:331–334.
24. Klawans, H. L., Lupton, M. D., and Simon, L. (1976): Calcification of the basal ganglia as a cause of levodopa resistant parkinsonism. *Neurology (Minneap.)*, 26:221–225.
25. Klawans, H. L., and Ringel, S. (1971): Observations on the efficacy of L-dopa in progressive supranuclear palsy. *Eur. Neurol.*, 5:107–116.
26. Klawans, H. L., Topel, J. L., and Bergen, D. (1975): Deanol in the treatment of levodopa-induced dyskinesias. *Neurology (Minneap.)*, 25:290–293.
27. Klawans, H. L., Weiner, W. J., Nausieda, P. A., Volkman, P., Goetz, C., and Lupton, M. (1978): Effect of lergotrile in Parkinson's disease. *Neurology (Minneap.)*, 28:699–702.
28. Klawans, H. L., and Zeitlin, E. (1971): L-dopa in parkinsonism associated with cerebellar dysfunction (probably olivopontocerebellar degeneration). *J. Neurol. Neurosurg. Psychiatry*, 23:14–19.
29. Lieberman, A., Kupersmith, M., Estey, E., and Goldstein, M. (1976): Treatment of Parkinson's disease with bromocriptine. *N. Engl. J. Med.*, 295:1400–1404.
30. Lieberman, A., Miyamoto, T., Battista, A. F., and Goldstein, M. (1975): Studies on the antiparkinsonian efficacy of lergotrile. *Neurology*, 25:459–462.
31. Miller, E. (1974): Deanol in the treatment of levodopa-induced dyskinesias. *Neurology (Minneap.)*, 24:116–119.
32. Moskovitz, C., Moses, H., and Klawans, H. L. (1978): Levodopa-induced psychosis: A kindling phenomenon. *Am. J. Psychiatry*, 135:669–675.
33. Parkes, J. D., Marsden, C. D., Donaldson, I., Galea-Debono, A., Walters, J., Kennedy, G., and Asselman, P. (1976): Bromocriptine treatment in Parkinson's disease. *J. Neurol. Neurosurg. Psychiatry*, 39:184–193.
34. Parks, L. C., Watanabe, A. M., and Kopin, I. J. (1970): Prevention or reversal of levodopa-induced cardiac arrhythmias by decarboxylase inhibition. *Lancet*, 2:1014–1015.
35. Schwab, R. S., Amador, L. V., and Lettvin, J. Y. (1951): Apomorphine in Parkinson's disease. *Trans. Am. Neurol. Assoc.*, 76:251–253.

36. Schwab, R. S., England, A. C., Poskanzer, D. C., and Young, R. R. (1969): Amantadine in the treatment of Parkinson's disease. *J.A.M.A.*, 208:1168–1170.
37. Sweet, R. D., and McDowell, R. H. (1974): Plasma dopa concentration and the "on–off" effect after chronic treatment of Parkinson's disease. In: *Advances in Neurology, Vol. 5, Second Canadian-American Conference on Parkinson's Disease*, edited by F. McDowell and A. Barbeau, pp. 953–956. Raven Press, New York.
38. Tarsy, D., Leopold, N., and Sax, D. (1974): Physostigmine in choreiform movement disorders. *Neurology (Minneap.)*, 24:28–34.
39. Yahr, M. D. (1970): Abnormal involuntary movements induced by dopa: Clinical aspects. In: *L-Dopa and Parkinsonism*, edited by A. Barbeau and F. McDowell, pp. 101–108. F. A. Davis, Philadelphia.

Chapter 2

Huntington's Chorea

The word chorea is derived from the Greek word for "dance" and was originally applied to the dance-like gait and continual limb movements seen in acute infectious chorea. The exact meaning of the term has undergone significant alteration so that chorea is now used to describe an entire class of abnormal spontaneous movements. A choreatic movement consists of single, isolated muscle action, producing a short, rapid, uncoordinated jerk of the trunk, limb, or face. The successive occurrence of two or more such isolated movements can result in complex movement patterns, and the superimposition of these movements on normal movements can cause a dance-like gait.

The choreatic syndrome that has the most clearly defined neuropathologic changes is Huntington's chorea. In Huntington's chorea, the major pathologic features are limited to the corpus striatum and cerebral cortex. Striatal atrophy is the most striking change. Although there is particular involvement of the small neurons of the caudate nucleus, it is not unusual to see degeneration in the large caudate neurons as well. Associated with this marked neuronal loss is extensive proliferation of astrocytes. The other striking pathologic feature is diffuse cerebral atrophy. This takes the form of a general reduction in the cortical population, with particularly heavy cell loss in layers 3, 5, and 6. It is generally accepted that the choreiform movements of Huntington's disease are related to striatal pathology and that the mental changes are related to cortical pathology.

In the past, it had been proposed that the striatum functions in part as a filter device for the control of motor activity. Degeneration of the striatum would thus result in the loss of this filter mechanism and produce chorea. According to this theory, as the degeneration of the striatum progressed, one would expect the abnormal involuntary movements to increase proportionally.

Several clinical observations show this to be untrue. First, patients in the terminal phase of Huntington's chorea often manifest less choreatic restlessness than they manifested earlier in the illness. Many patients reach a so-called burned out phase of the illness in which they actually become rigid and akinetic with virtually no abnormal involuntary movements at all. Since the later stages of the disease presumably would coincide with the time of greatest striatal destruction, one would expect the chorea to progress with time if chorea were directly correlated with tissue destruction. A second clinical observation is that some patients who have died in the early stages of Huntington's disease, with marked generalized chorea, have shown no gross changes within the striatum. In fact, even microscopic examination of the striatum sometimes revealed only minimal degenerative changes. In addition, radiologic attempts to correlate the degree of chorea with the degree of striatal atrophy have failed. Because of such observations, it is obvious that the degree of striatal cell loss cannot be accurately related to the degree of chorea observed in Huntington's disease.

DOPAMINERGIC MECHANISMS

Since the degree of striatal degeneration cannot be correlated neuropathologically with the severity of choreiform movements, it is most likely that altered function of these degenerating striatal neurons is the primary step in the production of the abnormal involuntary movements characterized as chorea (10). Following this line of reasoning, we proposed that the pathophysiology of chorea involved an altered response of striatal neurons to one or more neurotransmitters (12,15). Regional biochemical concentration studies have revealed that the striatum contains the highest concentration of dopamine and acetylcholine within the CNS. The striatum also contains a moderate amount of serotonin and gamma-amino-butyric acid (GABA).

In several ways Huntington's chorea can be thought of as the reverse of parkinsonism. The clinical contrast between the akinesia of parkinsonism and the hyperkinesias of Huntington's chorea is striking. In parkinsonism, the most conspicuous and consistent site of neuropathology is the substantia nigra. The dopamine-rich cells of the substantia nigra show marked degenerative changes, whereas the neurons of the striatum are relatively intact. Dopamine is lost from the striatum in parkinsonian patients, and CSF HVA levels are markedly reduced owing to destruction of the nigral neurons, whose axons project to the striatum, and whose terminals contain whatever dopamine is present in the striatum. It is this loss of the dopaminergic input that results in the symptoms of parkinsonism.

In Huntington's chorea the distribution of the pathologic changes is quite different. The dopaminergic cells of the substantia nigra are not particularly altered, but the neurons of the striatum that normally receive the dopamine input are markedly involved. In marked contrast to parkinsonism, in Huntington's chorea the dopamine content of the striatum is normal or near normal, as is the CSF HVA concentration (11). In parkinsonism, the dopamine input to the striatum is abnormal, whereas the cells of the striatum are well preserved. In Huntington's disease, the dopamine input is normal, whereas the striatal cells are abnormal.

If chorea results from altered responsiveness or dysfunction of diseased striatal neurons to normal dopamine concentrations within the striatum, then pharmacologic agents that alter either the concentration of dopamine within the striatum or the ease of access of dopamine in reaching striatal dopamine receptors might conceivably alter the abnormal involuntary movements. Historically, the first agent reported to be of use in the treatment of chorea was reserpine. Reserpine is a rauwolfia alkaloid that is known to deplete the CNS of dopamine. The observation that reserpine both improves chorea and depletes cerebral dopamine is consistent with the concept that altering striatal dopamine concentration affects chorea. Reserpine exerts its pharmacologic effect by blocking the reuptake of biogenic amines into storage granules, so that it produces depletion of serotonin and norepinephrine, as well as dopamine, in the CNS (see Table 1). Under such circumstances it is not possible to make a definitive statement regarding which of these three biologically active agents, when decreased in concentration within the striatum, is responsible for the reserpine-induced decrease in chorea. Tetrabenazine, which has a similar action, has similar efficacy.

The most widely studied agents in Huntington's chorea, aside from reserpine, are the phenothiazine neuroleptics. Of these, chlorpromazine has been used most extensively. Reduction of chorea with chlorpromazine has been reported frequently. Similar beneficial results have been reported with a wide variety of phenothiazine drugs, including perphenazine and trifluoperazine.

The basis of the central activity of chlorpromazine, as well as the other phenothiazines, is thought to be related to blocking of dopamine receptors (23). Although these agents have some effect in blocking acetylcholine and norepinephrine peripherally, the blockade of central dopamine receptors is accepted to be of primary importance in explaining the central activity of these agents. Whereas the effectiveness of reserpine in alleviating chorea could be related to serotonin, norepinephrine, or dopamine, the effectiveness of chlorpromazine could be related only to dopamine. This suggests that dopaminergic mechanisms might well be of primary importance in the initiation of such movements.

Haloperidol, a butyrophenone, has been used in a number of patients with Huntington's chorea, with definite improvement in chorea resulting, and it is perhaps now the most widely used agent in the U.S. The mechanism of action of haloperidol is identical to that of chlorpromazine, that is, central dopamine blockade (23).

Another method of altering the activity of striatal dopamine is the use of α-methyl-p-tyrosine. This agent is an inhibitor of tyrosine hydroxylase. The administration of α-methyl-p-tyrosine to animals results in decreased striatal levels of dopamine and norepinephrine without a change in the striatal concentration of

TABLE 1. *Pharmacology of chorea in Huntington's chorea*

Agent	Effect on chorea	Effect on striatal activity of Dopamine	Norepinephrine	Serotonin
Reserpine	↓	↓	↓	↓
Tetrabenazine	↓	↓	↓	↓
Phenothiazines				
Neuroleptics	↓	↓	Slight ↓ or 0	0
Haloperidol	↓	↓	Slight ↓ or 0	0
α-Methyl-p-tyrosine	↓	↓	↓	0
Methysergide	0	0	0	↓
p-Chlorophenylalanine	0	0	0	↓
Levodopa	↑	↑	0	↓

serotonin. Birkmayer has reported that intravenous use of α-methyl-p-tyrosine in patients with Huntington's chorea results in amelioration of the choreiform movements (6). The effectiveness of α-methyl-p-tyrosine in chorea cannot be related to the influence of striatal serotonin since serotonin remains unaffected by this agent. Methysergide, which blocks serotonin receptors, and p-chlorophenylalanine, which blocks serotonin synthesis, have both been shown to have no effect on chorea.

Taken together, these results suggest that dopamine is of primary importance in the initiation of chorea. Blocking the action of dopamine at the striatal receptors or decreasing the striatal content of dopamine improves chorea despite the fact that the striatal dopamine content is normal in this disease. These observations support the hypothesis that the defect producing chorea may involve dysfunction of the striatal neuron in its response to normal concentrations of dopamine.

Since drugs that decrease the striatal content of dopamine improve chorea, increasing the amount of dopamine that reaches the same receptors should worsen chorea. Levodopa markedly increases the striatal concentration of dopamine, has little effect on the striatal level of norepinephrine, and decreases the cerebral concentration of serotonin. Since levodopa increases striatal dopamine levels, it may increase the amount of dopamine reaching the receptors and thereby heighten chorea. It is now fairly clear that long-term oral levodopa usually increases the hyperkinesia in Huntington's chorea (15).

This review of the role of dopaminergic influences in a diseased striatum suggests that decreasing the concentration of dopamine within the striatum or blocking striatal dopamine receptor sites results in a decrease in choreiform movements, whereas increasing the concentration of dopamine results in increased chorea.

The role of dopamine in chorea may be a bit more complex than this. There are conflicting reports on the effect of bromocriptine on chorea in Huntington's chorea. Some, but not all, reports using low doses claim sustained improvement, whereas all reports employing higher doses report exacerbation of abnormal movements (16). In order to explain these possibly contradictory results, the concept of a dopaminergic presynaptic autoreceptor has been invoked. This type of receptor is located on the axon terminal of the dopaminergic nigrostriatal neuron. When dopamine is released by this cell, some of it reaches and acts on the autoreceptor to decrease the subsequent release of dopamine. This is a form of negative feedback or self inhibition. These observations raise the possibility that low doses of bromocriptine act at autoreceptors to secondarily decrease dopamine activity at postsynaptic sites and that high levels also act directly at the postsynaptic sites. It should be noted that in some reports small doses of bromocriptine have no effect or may even worsen chorea (9). It has also been suggested that low doses of bromocriptine may act as a partial dopamine antagonist (16). In this regard, it should also be noted that apomorphine, when given acutely, can also improve chorea (22). This tends to support the view that the same agonists may (perhaps because of greater affinity) act initially at presynaptic receptors.

A study of the patient population at risk for Huntington's disease provides further support for the thesis that altered striatal neurons responding in an abnormal manner to dopamine result in the production of chorea. It seems a reasonable assumption that in the course of a progressive degenerative disease such as Huntington's chorea, even the most subtle abnormal involuntary movements ought to be preceded by a stage of the disease in which striatal degeneration has begun but there is no overt clinical manifestation. In other words, there may be a preclinical stage of Huntington's disease in which the patient is normal clinically but in which the disease process has already begun within the striatum. If altered responsiveness to dopamine causes chorea, and if this altered responsiveness is an early manifestation of the pathology of chorea, then it might be possible to bring out chorea in presymptomatic Huntington's patients before it would otherwise be evident by means of a trial of levodopa. This hypothesis assumes that levodopa does not induce chorea in normal persons and that in asymptomatic family members two populations can be identified: those in whom levodopa produces chorea and those in whom it does not. Presumably the former would be presymptomatic patients, whereas the latter would be either normal siblings or patients with potential abnormal striatal cells that were not altered sufficiently to respond abnormally to levodopa at the time of administration.

The major levodopa provocation study involved a multicenter investigation of 30 subjects, each at 50% risk of developing Huntington's chorea and 25 control subjects (31). Levodopa was administered orally, and all subjects were examined serially for the appearance of choreic movements. One-third of subjects at risk developed transient and fully reversible chorea while receiving levodopa, whereas no control subject developed abnormal movements. The investigation clearly demonstrated that some subjects at risk have enhanced sensitivity to dopaminergic stimulation. Because of this altered sensitivity, the investigators suggested that this group of patients may carry an increased risk of developing Huntington's disease. The investigators stressed that those at-risk subjects who developed no chorea on levodopa provocation should not be considered likely "escapees," since they may well still carry the gene but not have developed sufficient dopaminergic hypersensitivity to respond abnormally to the administered dose of levodopa. Eight year follow-up data on these patients is presented in Table 2 and demonstrates a clear prognostic difference between the two patient groups (12a). Statistically, the hypothesis that those patients who developed levodopa-related chorea may be at a higher risk for eventual HD appears true. The degree of predictive reliability for this test can only be determined with longer follow-up. This group is still being actively followed, although no new patients are being enrolled in the provocation protocol.

At the present time, neuroleptics are the most widely employed form of therapy of Huntington's chorea, with haloperidol being the most widely used agent. This is usually used in low doses (2–8 mg/day). Improvement in chorea is mild to moderate and is rarely associated with drug-induced parkinsonism. There is no reason to believe that haloperidol is in fact better than other neuroleptics for this disorder. Individual patients often tolerate phenothiazines such as trifluperazine better than haloperidol with less depression and dysphoria. Because of such prob-

TABLE 2. *Effect of levodopa on subjects at risk for Huntington's chorea and controls*

Subjects at risk	Response to Levodopa in 1972		Current diagnosis of Huntington's disease (1980)
	Chorea	No chorea	
9[a]	3		1
		6	0
21[b]	7		4
		14	1
Totals:	10		5
		20	1

Fisher Exact Test performed on the data indicates a significance value of p-0.0088.
[a]University of Montreal.
[b]Rush-Presbyterian-St. Luke's Medical Center and Ohio State University.

lems, reserpine is frequently useful in the control of chorea in Huntington's disease. Reserpine-induced depression can occur but in our experience is infrequent. In the management of patients with Huntington's disease, the physician must keep in mind that both depression and psychosis can be part of the disorder and may respond to appropriate pharmacologic treatment.

CHOLINERGIC MECHANISMS

The concept that a critical striatal balance between acetylcholine and dopamine is essential to normal striatal function and consequently to normal motor control initially received its greatest acceptance in its applicability to Parkinson's disease. The signs of parkinsonism are widely accepted as resulting from imbalance in the dopamine–acetylcholine relationship within the striatum as a result of the loss of striatal dopamine and a consequent imbalance in favor of acetylcholine. The use of levodopa to restore striatal dopamine results in improvement in Parkinson's disease. Parkinsonism is also improved by a wide variety of agents that block the central activity of acetylcholine—anticholinergic agents. This central antagonism of acetylcholine is thought to restore partially the balance between dopamine and acetylcholine.

It has been further demonstrated that the administration of physostigmine, a centrally active anticholinesterase, worsens parkinsonism. Physostigmine has a marked effect in increasing striatal acetylcholine concentration. Presumably, the exacerbation of parkinsonism produced by the administration of physostigmine is a result of further worsening of the imbalance between dopamine and acetylcholine by increasing striatal acetylcholine concentration.

With this background, Klawans and Rubovits studied anticholinergic and cholinergic influences on the abnormal movements seen in Huntington's disease (14).

They demonstrated that the intravenous administration of physostigmine could temporarily reduce chorea. On the other hand, the administration of the anticholinergic agent benztropine resulted in exacerbation of chorea. The physostigmine-induced improvement in chorea could be promptly and effectively reversed by benztropine, and benztropine-induced worsening could be promptly and effectively overcome by the subsequent administration of physostigmine. The benztropine reversal of physostigmine could be annulled by a subsequent second administration of physostigmine. It was postulated that the alteration in cholinergic mechanisms probably affects striatal neuronal function and thereby influences the chorea. Other workers have found that physostigmine improves chorea but the percentage of patients who respond varies from 20 to 80%. These observations have two implications. Anticholinergic agents should be avoided in Huntington's disease patients being treated with neuroleptics since these agents will worsen the chorea. It is also possible that cholinergic agents might sometimes prove to be of value in the treatment of chorea. The acetylcholine precursors choline and lecithin have been used but with very limited efficacy (2).

It is important to note that recent biochemical studies have shown decreased activity of choline acetylase (ChAc) in the basal ganglia of patients dying of Huntington's chorea. It is unlikely that this is the primary defect in such patients, and it seems to be more severe late in the disease (1,15,17). Loss of the ability to synthesize acetylcholine because of decreased ChAc activity in some patients may explain the variability of responsiveness to physostigmine.

DOPAMINERGIC–CHOLINERGIC BALANCE

Since it is postulated that the choreiform movements seen in Huntington's chorea are the result of normal dopaminergic influences acting on altered striatal dopamine receptor sites, the demonstration that increased central activity of acetylcholine can ameliorate the movement disorder, even temporarily, is of great interest. The finding that an increased cholinergic influence can counterbalance the influence of dopamine extends the concept of striatal neurotransmitter balance from its already accepted role in Parkinson's disease to the choreiform disorders. In addition, it suggests and supports the more general theory of a primary neurotransmitter balance between acetylcholine and dopamine as necessary for normal function of the striatum.

The exact cellular mechanism by which dopamine triggers and acetylcholine improves chorea is unclear. Dopamine is usually pictured as an "inhibitory" neurotransmitter that inhibits or hyperpolarizes the neurons of the caudate and putamen. It is of significance, however, that all careful studies of individual striatal neurons have shown that there are at least two cell populations in relation to dopamine. One type has receptors predominantly facilitated by dopamine, whereas the other has receptors predominantly inhibited by dopamine. More recently it has been shown that only one class of dopamine receptors involves dopamine-facilitated adenyl-cyclase. It is of interest that the striatal neurons also include two populations, one that is primarily inhibited and one that is primarily facilitated by acetylcholine. The same neurons that respond to dopamine with inhibition are often facilitated by acetylcholine, and those that are facilitated by dopamine tend to be inhibited by acetylcholine. So each neurotransmitter can have either a facilitatory or an inhibitory effect on a single striatal neuron depending on the receptor type. However, dopamine and acetylcholine are still antagonistic in relation to any one striatal neuron.

By using this concept, the pathophysiology of chorea could be related to an enhanced effect of dopamine on the facilitated neurons of the striatum. These same neurons are inhibited by acetylcholine. Physostigmine improves chorea because it increases the activity of acetylcholine, thus antagonizing the overactivity of dopamine on these striatal neurons, whereas benztropine worsens chorea by inhibiting the effect of acetylcholine on the same neurons.

SEROTONERGIC MECHANISM

The role of serotonin (5-hydroxytryptamine) in choreiform movements is less clear than the role of either dopamine or acetylcholine. The striatum has a relatively high concentration of serotonin, presumably as a result of the many serotonin-containing nerve terminals that synapse in this region. Since the striatum is the region of severe degeneration in Huntington's disease, the possible influence of serotonin on the abnormal involuntary movements seen in this syndrome has been investigated. It has been demonstrated that the administration of 5-hydroxytryptophan, the immediate metabolic precursor of serotonin, results in an exacerbation of the choreiform movements.

If increased serotonin activity exacerbates chorea, it might be possible to ameliorate chorea either by reducing CNS serotonin concentrations or by blocking serotonin activity. Orally administered methysergide, a centrally active serotonin blocking agent, for 1 to 2 months, failed to alter significantly the abnormal involuntary movements (12). Parachlorophenylalanine, which inhibits the hydroxylation of tryptophan to 5-hydroxytryptophan, results in a marked fall in CNS serotonin concentration without significantly affecting the metabolism of the catecholamines. This agent has no significant effect on the degree of the choreiform movements (7). The failure of a centrally active serotonin antagonist to improve chorea, in addition to the failure of a reduction in brain serotonin to improve chorea, suggests that the contribution of serotonin to the pathophysiology of chorea is limited at best.

GABAergic MECHANISMS

A fourth putative neurotransmitter, GABA, has recently been proposed as having an influence in Huntington's chorea. Studies of regional CNS concentration have demonstrated a deficiency in GABA in the substantia nigra, putamen, caudate, and globus pallidus in patients with Huntington's disease as compared to "control" brains (18).

In more recent studies it was shown that the major enzyme involved in the biosynthesis of GABA, glutamic acid decarboxylase (GAD), was reduced by approximately 75% in the basal ganglia of patients dying with Huntington's chorea (5,17). The concentrations were normal in the frontal cortex. Overall, the most consistent biochemical lesion in Huntington's chorea appears to be a loss of GABA synthesizing and containing neurons from the basal ganglia. It has been proposed that the reduced GABA concentration could be explained as being the result of a genetically determined decreased activity of GAD or the result of the loss of a neuronal population that synthesizes GABA as a neurotransmitter.

It is important to note that one patient with Huntington's chorea who had only mild symptomatology when he committed suicide has been studied biochemically. Enzymatic analysis of this patient's striatum revealed normal activities of the pertinent enzymes. The particular finding that GAD activity was normal suggests that there is not a specific alteration in this enzyme characteristic of Huntington's chorea.

The significance of reduced GABA concentrations in the caudate, putamen, substantia nigra, and globus pallidus in Huntington's chorea remains unknown. The finding of a decreased concentration of a neurotransmitter in the striatum in choreatic patients, when viewed from a background of parkinsonism, is of course very seductive. In parkinsonism there is a loss of dopamine, and replacement of dopamine activity by precursor load (levodopa), reuptake blockade (amantadine), or direct-acting agonists (bromocriptine) improves parkinsonism. By analogy, increased GABA activity might ameliorate chorea. Unfortunately this has yet to be definitely demonstrated. A variety of pharmacologic techniques have been employed in this attempt, including:

(a) Precursor load strategy with L-glutamate and pyridoxine. A recent 2-year trial has shown no therapeutic benefit (4).

(b) Treatment with gamma-hydroxybutarate has not been successful.

(c) Possible agonism with baclofen has similarly shown no efficacy (20).

(d) Agonism with muscimol, a direct-acting GABA agonist, has yet to produce significant improvement.

(e) Dipropylacetic acid inhibits GABA transaminase and thereby increases brain GABA levels. It has not been found to improve chorea, however (21).

(f) It has recently been suggested that isoniazid given with pyridoxine will inhibit the breakdown of GABA by blocking GABA transaminase and result in increased brain GABA level. One report of 6 patients who were given this regime chronically found that 1 patient was markedly improved and 2 others less, but still significantly improved (19). This needs to be confirmed.

None of these approaches has yielded reproducible amelioration or prevention of progression. These results, while unfortunate, suggest that the mere demonstration of a biochemical neurotransmitter deficit does not prove that this alteration is of physiologic or pharmacologic significance.

RIGIDITY IN HUNTINGTON'S CHOREA

Patients with Huntington's chorea may manifest rigidity and akinesia, two of the cardinal manifestations of parkinsonism. These signs are seen particularly with juvenile onset of Huntington's disease. Akinesia and rigidity may also be seen late in the course of this syndrome, following the initial choreatic phase. It is generally thought that in parkinsonism rigidity and akinesia are related to loss of dopamine influence on the striatal neurons. If the pathogenesis of rigidity and akinesia in Huntington's chorea is also due to a decreased dopaminergic influence on striatal neurons, then levodopa might also improve rigidity in these patients. Early reports of the use of levodopa in young patients with the rigid form described short-term improvement in the rigidity. This is consistent with the suggestion that decreased dopamine activity may be related to rigidity in Huntington's chorea (12).

It should be noted that levodopa is only of limited efficacy in the treatment of the akinetic form of Huntington's chorea. In our patients, the response has been only moderate and usually quite transient. The fact that the parkinsonian symptoms of Huntington's chorea respond poorly to levodopa compared with the response of these same signs and symptoms in parkinsonism is consistent with considering rigid Huntington's disease as an example of postsynaptic parkinsonism.

BIBLIOGRAPHY AND *SELECTED REVIEWS

1. Aquilonius, S. M. (1972): On the synthesis, release and function of acetylcholine in the central nervous system. Ph.D. dissertation, University of Uppsala.
2. Aquilonius, S. M., and Eckernas, S. A. (1977): Choline therapy in Huntington's chorea. *Neurology*, 27:887–889.
*3. Aquilonius, S. M., and Sjostrom, R. (1971): Cholinergic and dopaminergic mechanisms in Huntington's chorea. *Life Sci.*, 10:405–414.
4. Barr, A. N., Heinze, W., Mendoza, J. E., and Perlik, S. (1978): Long term treatment of Huntington's disease with L-glutamate and pyridoxine. *Neurology*, 28:1280–1282.
5. Bird, E. D., and Iversen, L. L. (1974): Huntington's chorea. *Brain*, 97:457–472.
6. Birkmayer, W. (1969): The alpha-methyl-*p*-tyrosine effect in extrapyramidal disorders. *Wien. Klin. Wochenschr.*, 81:10–12.
7. Chase, T. N., Watanabe, A. M., Brodie, H. K. H., and Donnelly, E. F. (1972): Huntington's chorea: Effect of serotonin depletion. *Arch. Neurol.*, 26:282–284.
*8. Hornykiewicz, O. (1964): Dopamine and brain function. *Pharmacol. Rev.*, 18:925–964.
9. Kartzinel, R., Hunt, R. D., and Calne, D. B. (1976): Bromocriptine in Huntington's chorea. *Arch. Neurol.*, 33:517–519.
*10. Klawans, H. L. (1970): A pharmacologic analysis of Huntington's chorea. *Eur. Neurol.*, 4:148–163.
11. Klawans, H. L. (1971): Cerebrospinal fluid in Huntington's chorea. *J. Neurol. Sci.*, 13:277–281.
*12. Klawans, H. L. (1973): *The Pharmacology of Extrapyramidal Movement Disorders*. S. Karger, Basel.
12a. Klawans, H. L., Goetz, C. G., Perlick, S. (1980): Presymptomatic and early detection in Huntington's disease. *Ann. Neurol.*, 8:343–347.
13. Klawans, H. L., Paulson, G. W., Ringel, S. P., and Barbeau, A. (1972): Use of L-dopa in the detection of presymptomatic Huntington's chorea. *N. Engl. J. Med.*, 286:1332–1334.
14. Klawans, H. L., and Rubovits, R. (1972): Central cholinergic–anticholinergic antagonism in Huntington's chorea. *Neurology*, 22:107–116.
*15. Klawans, H. L., and Weiner, W. J. (1975): The pharmacology of choreatic movement disorders. *Prog. Neurobiol.*, 1–32.
16. Loeb, C., Roccatagaliato, G., Albano, C., and Besio, G. (1979): Bromocriptine and dopaminergic function in Huntington's disease. *Neurology*, 29:730–734.
17. McGeer, P. L., McGeer, E. G., and Fibiger, H. C. (1975): Choline acetylase and glutamic acid decarboxylase in Huntington's chorea. *Neurology*, 23:912–917.
18. Perry, T., Hansen, S., and Kloster, M. (1973): Huntington's chorea: Deficiency of gamma amino butyric acid. *New Engl. J. Med.*, 288:337–342.

19. Perry, T., Wright, J., Hansen, S., and Macloed, P. (1979): Isoniazid therapy of Huntington's disease. *Neurology*, 29:370–375.
20. Shoulson, I., Chase, T. N., and Roberts, E. (1975): Huntington's disease treatment with imidazole-4-acetic acid. *N. Engl. J. Med.*, 293:504–505.
21. Shoulson, I., Kartzinel, R., and Chase, T. N. (1976): Huntington's disease: Treatment with dipropylacetic acid and GABA. *Neurology*, 26:61–63.
22. Tolosa, E. S., and Sparber, S. B. (1974): Apomorphine in Huntington's chorea. *Life Sci.*, 15:1371–1380.
23. van Rossum, J. M. (1966): The significance of dopamine receptor blockade for the action of neuroleptic drugs. In: *Neuro-Psychopharmacology. Proceedings of the 5th International Congress of the Collegium Internationale Neuropsychopharmacologicum, Washington, D. C., March, 1966*, edited by H. Brill, J. O. Cole, P. Deniker, H. Hippius, and P. B. Bradley. International Congress Series No. 129:166.

Chapter 3

Other Choreatic Disorders (Naturally Occurring and Iatrogenic)

Choreatic movements are seen in a variety of disease states other than Huntington's chorea. Phenomenologically, the movements seen in these disorders are similar if not identical to the movements seen in Huntington's chorea. It is therefore reasonable to think of the movements in these other disorders as physiologically and therefore pharmacologically similar to the chorea of Huntington's chorea. In most of these disorders pathological alterations in the striatum are much less striking, but in all, it appears that the pathophysiology of the chorea still is centered on the activity of dopamine at striatal dopamine receptors. It is our belief that the inferences drawn from examination of the effect of striatal neurotransmitters in the manipulation of chorea in Huntington's chorea can be extended to these other choreiform disorders. This implies that increased activity of dopamine at striatal dopamine receptors often resulting from dopamine receptor-site hypersensitivity plays a major role in the pathophysiology of the movements. It also implies that dopamine–acetycholine balance has physiologic significance, so that increasing acetylcholine activity might improve the movements, whereas decreasing this activity would exacerbate them (see Chapter 2).

Table 1 lists those naturally occurring choreatic diseases for which we have some pharmacologic data. These disorders can be divided conveniently into three groups according to the degree of proven striatal pathology (Table 2). The first group of syndromes consists of disease states in which there is definite striatal structural alteration (senile chorea, acquired hepatocerebral degeneration); the second group demonstrates less specific striatal pathology (Sydenham's chorea, systemic lupus

TABLE 1. *Naturally occurring choreatic disorders for which pharmacologic data exist*

Senile chorea
Oral masticatory syndrome
Acquired hepatocerebral degeneration
Sydenham's chorea
Lupus erythematosis
Hyperthyroid chorea

TABLE 2. *Choreatic disorders classified according to degree of proven striatal pathology*

Definite
  Senile chorea
  Acquired hepatocerebral degeneration
  Oral masticatory syndrome
Probable to possible
  Sydenham's chorea
  Systemic lupus erythematosus
No known pathologic alterations
  Hyperthyroid-induced chorea

---

erythematosis); the final syndrome shows no known anatomic alteration of the striatum (chorea associated with hyperthyroidism). The available pharmacologic data are summarized in Table 3.

SENILE CHOREA AND ORAL MASTICATORY SYNDROME OF THE ELDERLY

In senile chorea, there is severe degeneration of neuronal elements in the striatum. The fully developed clinical presentation of senile chorea consists of gradually progressive, generalized, and symmetrical choreiform movements in patients of advanced age with no accompanying evidence of mental deterioration, and it is quite rare. On the other hand, the occurrence of spontaneous lingual–facial–buccal dyskinesia in older persons who do not exhibit any readily identifiable extrapyr-

TABLE 3. *Dopamine–acetylcholine balance in other naturally occurring disorders*

Disorder	DA agent	Effect	ACH agent	Effect
Senile chorea	Antagonist	↓	Blocker	↑
	Reserpine	↓		
	Tetrabenazine	↓		
	Agonist	↑	Agonist	No data
Acquired hepatocerebral degeneration	Blocker	↓	Antagonist	↑
	Reserpine	No data		
	Agonist	No data	Agonist	No data
Systemic lupus erythematosus	Antagonist	↓	Antagonist	No data
	Reserpine	No data		
	Agonist	No data	Agonist	No data
Sydenham's chorea	Antagonist	↓	Antagonist	No data
	Reserpine	↓		
	Agonist	↑	Agonist	No data
Hyperthyroidism	Antagonist	↓	Antagonist	No data
	Reserpine	↓		
	Agonist	No data	Agonist	No data

DA, dopamine; ACH, acetylcholine.

amidal syndrome and who have not been receiving any neuroleptic therapy is fairly common. These lingual–facial–buccal dyskinesias resemble the facial movements of senile chorea. It is quite likely that lingual–facial–buccal dyskinesia in the elderly may be the earliest manifestation of senile degeneration of the striatum.

According to this view, the syndrome of spontaneous lingual–facial–buccal dyskinesia of the elderly (oral masticatory syndrome) is senile chorea, with the initial movements being associated with the initial degeneration of neurons within the striatum related topographically to motor control of the face. This degenerative process can in occasional patients be progressive and eventually involve the entire striatum and result in generalized chorea.

Spontaneous lingual–facial–buccal dyskinesia and senile chorea thus apparently represent the same disease process. Lingual–facial–buccal dyskinesia represents the early stage of the disease for which no specific histopathologic pattern has yet been demonstrated, whereas senile chorea is the full clinical manifestation of the motor disturbance associated with a progressive degenerative process in the corpus striatum. The etiology of this degenerative process remains unknown (34).

If these movements are truly a form of chorea, then spontaneous lingual–facial–buccal dyskinesia in the elderly should be secondary to altered responsiveness of striatal dopamine receptor sites. Pakkenberg and Fog provided supporting evidence for this proposal in a study of 16 elderly patients (age range, 70–90 years) with spontaneous oral lingual–facial–buccal dyskinesias (24). These investigators reported marked decreases in abnormal involuntary movements with either a dopamine-depleting agent (tetrabenazine) or a dopamine receptor-site blocking agent (pimozide), or a combination of both. Haloperidol has also been shown to suppress these movements. The efficacy of these drugs, which have as their basis interference with striatal dopaminergic influences, leads one to speculate that in all probability a pharmacologic agent that could increase central cholinergic influences would also decrease spontaneous lingual–facial–buccal dyskinesia of the elderly. This speculation is reinforced by the observation that anticholinergic agents worsen oral masticatory movements in the elderly. It is also significant that these agents can elicit generalized (i.e., non-lingual–facial–buccal) chorea in such patients (33). This supports the hypothesis that this syndrome is the first manifestation of a more generalized choreatic disorder.

The greatest significance of the syndrome of spontaneous oral masticatory of the elderly may be a medicolegal one. These movements are virtually identical to the movements seen in neuroleptic-induced tardive dyskinesia and may therefore be erroneously attributed to exposure to neuroleptics. The exact incidence of this disorder is unknown, but our experience suggests that it occurs in at least 5% of the population in the eighth decade of life. In older patients with lingual facial buccal movements a diagnosis of tardive dyskinesia should only be made if there is sufficient exposure to account for the production of abnormal movements (see below). Even then the movements may well be idiopathic and not iatrogenic. Withdrawal of neuroleptics may after months improve iatrogenic movements. Withdrawal would only worsen the spontaneous movements and may help, therefore, in differentiating the two.

Oral masticatory movements in older patients usually do not require treatment. If they are so severe as to cause dysphasia, dysarthria, and a threat of aspiration, therapy is mandatory. We use either reserpine or haloperidol to treat such individuals. Both treatment regimes have significant side effects. The use of reserpine is associated with postural hypotension, nasal congestion, drug induced parkinsonism and, especially in patients with a past history of affective disorder, depression. If used, reserpine should be started at low doses (0.1 or 0.2 mg/day) and increased very slowly. Successful therapy often requires doses of 1 to 2 mg/day, and it often takes many months to achieve this level. Haloperidol is probably the treatment of choice in patients with a history of depression. In this age group, the major problems are drug-induced parkinsonism, akathisia, and the possibility of inducing tardive dyskinesia. Again, start with as low a dose as possible (1 to 2 mg/day) and increase the dose slowly.

ACQUIRED HEPATOCEREBRAL DEGENERATION

Acquired hepatocerebral degeneration is the term used to describe the appearance of several chronic neurologic syndromes in association with chronic liver disease. This syndrome usually consists of progressive symptoms including dementia, ataxia, rigidity, tremor, and choreoathetotic movements. It is usually associated with prolonged portal systemic shunting of blood (secondary either to cirrhosis itself or to surgical procedures performed to relieve portal hypertension). Hepatic encephalopathy with asterixis is the most frequent and well known neurological complication of chronic liver disease and is seen intermittently in approximately 80% of all patients with acquired hepatocerebral degeneration. The most consistent pathological finding in acquired hepatocerebral degeneration is widespread, striking proliferation and enlargement of protoplasmic astrocytes. This finding is most impressive in the cerebral cortex and subjacent white matter, but there is also a marked degree of astrocytic proliferation in the striatum (caudate and putamen).

A unique and more distinctive pathological finding in acquired hepatocerebral degeneration is the degeneration of neuronal elements. This is frequently maximal in the cerebral cortex, but it is also present in varying degrees in the putamen and caudate (striatum).

Choreoathetotic movements, especially of the tongue, face, and mouth, have been described frequently in acquired hepatocerebral degeneration. These movements bear no constant relationship to the presence of frank hepatic coma or to the degree of hepatic encephalopathy (as mirrored by the level of consciousness). Once they occur, these movements are usually persistent and are identical to the dyskinesias seen in Huntington's chorea and other choreatic disorders (12). The occurrence of movements in acquired hepatocerebral degeneration identical to those seen in the other choreiform syndromes suggests that the physiology and pharmacology of these movements will be similar.

Since in other syndromes decreasing striatal dopaminergic activity or increasing striatal cholinergic activity has resulted in some amelioration of the movements, it may be that the lingual–facial–buccal dyskinesia of acquired hepatocerebral degeneration can also be influenced in the same way. We have reported a series of 4 patients with acquired hepatocerebral degeneration secondary to advanced post-necrotic cirrhosis whose lingual–facial–buccal dyskinesias were successfully treated with the dopamine blocking agent, haloperidol (23). Three of these 4 patients had CSF HVA analysis prior to the initiation of haloperidol treatment, and the CSF concentration of HVA was normal. This implies that central dopamine turnover is normal. The clinical observation that a dopamine blocking agent ameliorates the dyskinesias in a situation in which the central dopamine turnover is normal suggests that increased dopamine receptor-site sensitivity within the striatum is again involved in the pathogenesis of these movements, as it is in Huntington's chorea.

No data exist on the use of cholinergic agents in this disorder. We have, however, observed anticholinergic worsening and would predict that cholinergic agents might have some efficacy (23).

In our experience, haloperidol has been the best agent for this disorder. Most patients have responded to relatively low doses of 2 to 4 mg/day with significant sustained improvement. Neuroleptic-induced parkinsonism, however, is common in these patients and tends to persist. This later requires the addition of an anti-parkinson agent, either an anticholinergic or amantadine, either of which may partially exacerbate the choreic movements.

SYDENHAM'S CHOREA AND LUPUS ERYTHEMATOSUS

These two disorders represent transitional syndromes in terms of their neuro-pathology. Although in clinical appearance the movements resemble those discussed previously, the neuropathologic alterations in the striatum are not entirely clear. Because of the favorable prognosis of Sydenham's chorea, there have been relatively few postmortem studies. The CNS lesions are usually widespread and nonspecific. They include acute and chronic neuronal degenerative changes as well as vascular and inflammatory lesions. In some instances necrotizing arteritis is found. The brain is often diffusely involved in this process, but most early reports noted a predilection for the striatum. More recent reports have recorded these same lesions of the caudate and putamen but have put more emphasis on the involvement of the cerebral cortex. On the other hand, patients dying from systemic lupus erthematosus with neurologic involvement have both diffuse and focal cerebral degenerative lesions that are secondary to the necrotizing arteritis characteristic of the disease. These lesions usually involve the gray matter. One patient with systemic lupus erythematosus and associated chorea had such a lesion in the striatum. Although specific pathologic changes in the striatum have not been demonstrated in every case of Sydenham's chorea or chorea associated with systemic lupus erythematosus, the widespread CNS pathology in these syndromes often includes the striatum. It is our belief that striatal dysfunction in these disorders underlies the abnormal movements.

Additional support for this concept is derived from the favorable effect that dopamine blocking agents have in these syndromes. Several investigators have reported single patients with systemic lupus erythematosus and recurrent severe chorea. In these patients haloperidol therapy resulted in a marked improvement of abnormal involuntary movements (7,12). The cessation of haloperidol therapy resulted in the resumption of chorea. In one patient we attributed the improvement in chorea to blockade of dopamine receptors because the CSF concentration of HVA rose from 47 ng/ml to 97 ng/ml following haloperidol treatment. This was interpreted as indirect biochemical evidence of dopamine receptor blockade with increased dopamine release as a feedback-related attempt to overcome the haloperidol-induced blockade. As in acquired hepatocerebral degeneration, the normal HVA level before treatment suggested normal dopamine turnover, so that the abnormal movements must be related to an altered effect of dopamine at striatal dopamine receptors. None of the patients developed parkinsonian signs despite the neuroleptic-induced improvement in chorea, which supports the previously discussed concept that chorea and parkinsonism are related to different dopamine receptors. No other pharmacologic data are available.

Sydenham's chorea has been treated over the years with various agents including cortisone, ACTH, salicylate, bromides, and barbiturates, with variable and mainly unsatisfactory results. The first specific, successful form of symptomatic therapy in Sydenham's chorea was the use of chlorpromazine. Other phenothiazines have also been used successfully. Haloperidol has been used for symptomatic relief of acute and residual chorea and may be the drug in widest use today. These investigators also noted no neuroleptic-induced parkinsonism while achieving amelioration of chorea (27). Dopamine depleting agents, such as reserpine, have also been shown to produce amelioration in this disorder, whereas dopamine agonists tend to worsen or exacerbate the disorder (see below).

HYPERTHYROID CHOREA

Chorea associated with hyperthyroidism is a rare clinical entity. However, its occurrence allows further speculation into the pathophysiology of choreiform movements. The association of chorea with hyperthyroidism completes the transition from disorders with proven striatal pathologic findings associated with chorea to a syndrome in which there is chorea but presumably an anatomically normal striatum. In the past, the treatment of hyperthyroid chorea consisted of the treatment of the hyperthyroidism itself. As hyperthyroidism abated there was a parallel amelioration of the chorea. In a single case, rapid improvement in the chorea as well as the hyperthyroidism was produced by a combination of reserpine, propranolol, and propylthiouracil, despite continued hyperthyroidism (6). We have reported a case of severe thyrotoxicosis and severe chorea whose choreiform movements were controlled with haloperidol (12,20). The improvement in chorea following treatment with a dopamine blocking agent alone suggests that dopamine is involved in the production of this movement disorder. After 1 week of haloperidol therapy this neuroleptic was stopped and chorea returned. After treatment of hyperthyroidism with radioactive iodine and the achievement of a euthyroid state, the haloperidol was discontinued without a recurrence of the abnormal involuntary movements.

These observations are consistent with the hypothesis that hyperthyroidism induces a functional alteration in the response of dopamine receptor sites to dopamine. In other words, if receptor-site hypersensitivity results in hyperkinetic, abnormal involuntary movements in the other choreatic syndromes reviewed, then an analogous situation may underlie the chorea associated with hyperthyroidism. Alterations in thyroid function have, in fact, been found to influence the sensitivity of adrenergic and dopaminergic receptors to norepinephrine and dopamine. Preclinical studies shed some light on this problem. Hypothyroid rats are markedly hypoadrenergic and at the same time show increased synthesis of norepinephrine in the heart and brain. Despite the excessive sympathetic activity in hyperthyroid rats, these rats manifest decreased catecholamine turnover in the heart and brain. It has been hypothesized that in hyperthyroid animals the increased sensitivity of the receptors produces an increase in sympathetic response. Through negative feedback mechanisms this leads to a decrease in sympathetic neuronal activity, including catecholamine synthesis. In hypothyroidism, decreased receptor sensitivity leads to a decreased sympathetic response and a consequent increased catecholamine turnover.

If hyperthyroidism increases the sensitivity of receptor sites in the striatum to dopamine, any patient with hyperthyroidism with chorea should have decreased dopamine turnover. In the hyperthyroid patient described above, the CSF HVA concentration was significantly below normal (16 ng/ml). This suggests that dopamine synthesis was decreased in this patient despite the fact that he had a symptom (chorea) which usually reflects increased dopaminergic response (20).

The changes in dopamine sensitivity responsible for hyperthyroid chorea appear to be entirely reversible. This implies functional rather than structural alterations in striatal neurons. The similarity of the clinical movements to other choreiform states, the responsiveness of the abnormal movements to dopamine blocking agents, and the demonstrated effect of hyperthyroidism on dopamine receptor-site sensitivity as reflected by dopamine turnover all support the concept that hyperthyroidism can induce altered striatal function that results in chorea.

IATROGENIC CHOREATIC DISORDERS

A wide variety of iatrogenic or drug-induced choreatic disorders have been reported. The more common of these are listed in Table 4, where they are classified according to the degree of preexisting striatal pathology usually required for the occurrence of each disorder. Levodopa, neuroleptics, and amphetamines (and related agents), when used chronically, can apparently elicit chorea in patients with previously normal basal ganglia. Preexisting striatal pathology is usually a prerequisite for acute amphetamine-induced chorea as well as anticholinergic-induced, birth control pill-induced, and phenytoin-induced chorea. The situation as far as antihistamine-induced chorea is unclear.

TABLE 4. *Drug-induced choreatic disorders*
(iatrogenic chorea)

No preexisting striatal pathology
   Levodopa-induced (see chapter 1)
   TD (neuroleptic-induced)
   Amphetamine-induced (chronic)
Preexisting striatal pathology
   Amphetamine-induced (acute)
   Anticholinergic-induced
   Birth control pill-induced
   Phenytoin-induced
Unclear
   Antihistamine-induced

Neuroleptic-Induced Tardive Dyskinesia

After the introduction of neuroleptics into the practice of psychiatry in France in 1952, reports began to appear in the late 1950s of an extrapyramidal disorder characterized by a persistent dyskinetic disturbance associated with the long-term administration of neuroleptics. The late appearance led Uhrband and Faurbye in 1960 to apply the term "tardive dyskinesia" to this disorder (31). By definition, then, the term tardive dyskinesia (TD) is short for neuroleptic tardive dyskinesia and implies an iatrogenic disease owing to the long-term ingestion of neuroleptics.

The early descriptions of this syndrome stressed abnormal motor movements affecting the face, the so-called bucco-lingual masticating syndrome. These movements consisted of involuntary mouthing, chewing, and sucking movements of the tongue, which frequently darted from the oral cavity. Later, the syndrome was broadened to include a variety of abnormal muscular manifestations, including choreoathetoid-type movements of the fingers, hands, arms, and feet; and ballistic-type movements, particularly of the arms; as well as axial hyperkinesias, and diaphragmatic movement resulting in grunting and difficult breathing. The clinical picture closely resembles levodopa-induced dyskinesias both in the character of the movement abnormalities and in the diversity of their clinical manifestations.

Phenomenologically, then, the movements seen in TD are almost invariably choreatic in nature. It is therefore reasonable to assume that they are related to the activity of dopamine at striatal dopamine receptors. The major questions are the nature of this relationship (pathophysiology) and its cause (pathogenesis).

The observation that TDs are frequently permanent despite discontinuation of neuroleptic therapy has stimulated a search for a permanent structural alteration of the brain for this disorder. However, neuropathological studies following acute or chronic administration of antipsychotic drugs in laboratory animals have not demonstrated specific or localized pathological changes in the brain beyond those produced by the diverse systemic effects of these drugs. There is a single report of reduced neuronal cell count in the basal ganglia of rats chronically receiving phenothiazines, but this is of uncertain significance since neither degenerative changes nor gliosis was observed. In man, postmortem neuropathological changes that have been found after chronic phenothiazine treatment in patients without extrapyramidal syndromes have usually consisted of scattered areas of neuronal degeneration and gliosis without convincing localization. Individual patients with drug-induced parkinsonism or TDs have been reported to have postmortem changes in the globus pallidus and putamen, caudate nucleus, and substantia nigra. Hunter et al. reported no significant neuropathological abnormality in 3 patients with TDs, although 2 of these patients showed, among other lesions, neuronal degeneration of the substantia nigra, possibly consistent with greatly advanced age (10). Christensen et al. reported the presence of neuronal degeneration and gliosis of the substantia nigra in 27 of 28 brains from patients with chronic oral dyskinesias (21 of which were attributed to antipsychotic drugs). Only 7 of 28 control brains, matched for age and psychiatric diagnosis, but without dyskinesia, showed similar changes (4). Although the reported nigral degeneration and gliosis may represent a toxic effect of the drug, their occurrence in some elderly individuals without TD raises the possibility that they may be accompanying events of aging that may predispose to the appearance of TD. It is striking that no consistent changes have been found in the striatum.

The neuroleptics that have been reported to produce TDs after prolonged usage are the same agents that regularly result in drug-induced parkinsonism (13). Van Rossum (1966) has hypothesized that chlorpromazine and other neuroleptics act by blocking dopamine receptors in the CNS (32). The competitive blockade by neuroleptics of dopaminergic receptors has been implicated as the basis of neuroleptic-induced parkinsonism. Neuroleptics, by instituting a blockade of these receptors, may thus produce a "chemical denervation" of the dopamine receptors of the striatum. It is possible that after such prolonged chemical denervation some receptors may develop denervation hypersensitivity and may respond in an abnormal manner to any dopamine that reaches them. It is quite likely that TDs are the overt manifestation of the abnormal response of such neurons (13).

The phenomenon of denervation hypersensitivity is well known in peripheral receptor sites, and the experimental work on the nigrostriatal pathway suggests that an analogous phenomenon may occur centrally. The nigrostriatal dopaminergic pathway is composed of neurons whose cell bodies are the melanin-containing neurons of the substantia nigra and whose axon terminals are spread diffusely throughout the ipsilateral striatum (caudate and putamen). When the nigrostriatal pathway is destroyed, the amount of dopamine available to act at the striatum is markedly diminished. It has been found that when one putamen is dopaminergically denervated by the interruption of the ipsilateral nigrostriatal pathway, the dopaminergically denervated striatum demonstrates an increased behavioral response to dopamine agonism. This same behavioral hypersensitivity can be produced in animals by chronic neuroleptic administration. In such animals the degree of behavioral hypersensitivity is paralleled by increased numbers of striatal dopamine receptors (9).

The fact that neuroleptic-induced dyskinesias often make their first appearance after dose reduction or drug withdrawal may be explained by the assumption that a decrease in the striatal level of the neuroleptic permits more of the dopamine to reach the sensitized dopamine receptors. The occurrence of these movements during neuroleptic therapy suggests that the competitive blockade can sometimes be overcome by endogenous dopamine.

The relationship of dopamine to TD is further exemplified by a patient previously reported by our group (15). The patient was a 73-year-old white female who had been receiving chlorpromazine and haloperidol for a psychiatric illness. She developed lingual–facial–buccal dyskinesias and mild rigidity and akinesia after receiving these drugs for several months, but the dyskinesias persisted, as did the mild parkinsonian features. The patient was then placed on levodopa. After receiving this drug for less than 2 weeks her facial dyskinesias worsened strikingly, and she developed choreatic movements of extremities and dyskinesias of the trunk. The levodopa was discontinued but all involuntary movements persisted for several weeks. At this time, her CSF contained a normal concentration of HVA. The worsening of this patient's movement disorder by the institution of levodopa suggests that dopamine is in some way related to the pathogenesis of the abnormal movements. The normal HVA level implies a normal turnover of dopamine at that time and suggests that the patient's abnormal movements were related to altered sensitivity to dopamine rather than to increased dopamine in the CNS.

An additional example of the exacerbating effect of levodopa on this syndrome is the experience of Hippius and Logemann, who studied a large group of patients with TDs. When given single intravenous injections of 100 mg of levodopa, 12 of their 40 patients developed worsening of the abnormal movements (8). These investigators believed that the enhancement of the hyperkinesias by levodopa was related to the effect of levodopa on the extrapyramidal system. It is most probable that the exacerbation of these movements by small doses of levodopa is related to altered receptor site sensitivity to dopamine.

The hypothesis that denervation hypersensitivity causes TD helps in understanding the paucity of pathologic alterations in the striatum. This would not be surprising if the underlying lesion is degeneration of dopamine receptors in the striatum. Such a lesion could not be seen by light microscopy.

It appears, then, that neuroleptic drugs can produce blockade of dopamine receptors and subsequent alterations of these receptors. It is possible that the changes seen in the substantia nigra may themselves contribute to dopaminergic denervation of the striatum and play a role in either individual predisposition (if preexisting) or actual pathogenesis (if neuroleptic-induced). Degeneration of the substantia nigra would result in some degree of anatomic denervation, which could easily be synergistic with the pharmacologic denervation.

In general, agents that increase the central activity of dopamine exacerbate TDs, and agents that decrease or block the central activity of dopamine ameliorate TDs. Dopaminergic influences in the striatum are also of primary importance in determining the severity of chorea in Huntington's disease. Since other striatal neurotransmitters, particularly acetylcholine, appear to affect abnormal involuntary movements seen in Huntington's chorea, it is possible that acetylcholine affects TD as well. If the pathophysiologic mechanism of TD is similar to that in Huntington's chorea, it would be expected that anticholinergic agents would exacerbate TD just as anticholinergic agents exacerbate the chorea of Huntington's disease. Institution of anticholinergic regimens for patients with TD has indeed been found to worsen the abnormal movements (17).

On the other hand, under experimental conditions it has been demonstrated that intravenous administration of physostigmine, a centrally active cholinergic agent, reduces the abnormal movements seen in TD (12,30). In a more recent study, Klawans and Rubovits have shown that physostigmine improves TD, whereas benztropine worsens TD (17).

The acute administration of anticholinergic agents not only worsens preexisting TD but can elicit movements not previously seen. For instance, a patient with lingual–facial–buccal movements may develop limb chorea. This shows that even patients with focal TD may have more diffuse alterations in striatal physiology. Thus the effects of cholinergic drugs on the abnormal movements of TD parallel the effects of cholinergic drugs on the chorea of Huntington's chorea. This suggests that similar pathophysiologic mechanisms are involved in the production of these two movement disorders.

It is important to recognize the role of the cholinergic system in TD because many patients with disorders of the extrapyramidal system are treated with anticholinergics, although the efficacy of anticholinergic therapy has been demonstrated only in parkinsonian syndromes.

Many patients who are on long-term neuroleptic therapy are also given long-term anticholinergic medications in order to reduce the parkinsonian syndrome induced by neuroleptics. Although anticholinergics may mask drug-induced parkinsonism, they may also increase the intensity and duration of TDs in any patient who is prone to develop these types of abnormal movemets. They also worsen chorea in choreatic patients on neuroleptic therapy. The attempt to relieve one of the neurological complications of neuroleptic therapy may promote the appearance of another, more severe, longer lasting, and less reversible neurological complication.

Besides prolonging and potentiating TDs, there is some evidence to suggest that anticholinergic drugs may alter the threshold for the appearance of TDs. Anticholinergic agents may not only increase the severity of TDs in patients prone to this type of movement disorder but may also increase the incidence of TDs by altering the threshold for the appearance of these movements. This concept suggests that inhibition of the cholinergic system, which normally antagonizes the dopaminergic system, produces a physiologic state in which the amount of dopamine acting at dopaminergic receptors necessary to produce lingual–facial–buccal dyskinesias is decreased. Because of this, amounts of dopamine too small to induce TDs in a patient not on anticholinergics may well be able to induce them in a patient who is receiving anticholinergics.

This suggests that the incidence of TDs should be greater in patients receiving both neuroleptics and anticholinergics than in patients receiving neuroleptics alone. This appears to be true. Crane has tentatively suggested that adjunctive anticholinergic medication increases the risk of development of TDs (3). Because most patients receiving long-term neuroleptic therapy develop a tolerance for neuroleptic-induced parkinsonism, continued anticholinergic treatment is usually not warranted. In fact, the only purpose served may be to increase iatrogenically the incidence and severity of an iatrogenic disorder.

Attempts to prevent or treat TD must be based on an understanding of the risk factors, pathogenesis, pathophysiology, and course of the disease. These are all summarized in Table 5. The pathogenesis is thought to be prolonged dopaminergic receptor-site blockade (denervation), and the pathophysiology is the resulting denervation hypersensitivity. The course in many patients tends to be progressive. This is reflected by the epidemiologic evidence, which shows a direct relationship between the incidence of TD and the duration of neuroleptic therapy. In the individual patient TDs are also progressive, usually beginning as a sign, with assorted lingual–facial–buccal dyskinesias, and later becoming more severe and generalized. As neuroleptic therapy is maintained, there is both an increase in severity of the movements in those areas involved and an increase in the number of areas of the body involved. No patient with TD begins with severe generalized chorea, but patients can and do develop this. The longer the pathogenesis persists, the more the physiology is disrupted. In essence, maintenance of the pathogenetic mechanism results in increased pathophysiologic disruption. Because of this, *standard neuroleptics have no role in the routine treatment of TD*. The only role for neuroleptics in a patient with TD is treatment of the patient's psychosis.

There is no evidence that the pathophysiology progresses when neuroleptics are withdrawn. In fact, the opposite appears to be true. Initially after neuroleptic withdrawal, TD may worsen because of better access of dopamine to striatal receptors. But this is usually only a short-term effect. TDs, in fact, are often reversible and spontaneously remit after neuroleptic withdrawal. The earlier the symptoms are recognized and drugs withdrawn, the better the prognosis for recovery. This is

TABLE 5. *Mechanism of TD*

Etiology, neuroleptic exposure
  Risk factors in individual patients
  Age
  Sex
  Preexisting striatal dysfunction
  Drug-induced parkinsonism
Iatrogenic risk factors
  Dosage
  Duration
  Anticholinergic agents
  Pathogenesis
  Dopaminergic denervation
  Denervation hypersensitivity of striatal dopamine receptors
Course
  A definite potential for progression

consistent with the view that TD is a progressive disorder. The chances of TDs becoming irreversible can be decreased by early detection and neuroleptic withdrawal. Patients should be carefully examined for dyskinesias at frequent intervals. TDs can disappear in some cases within 1 to 2 months of discontinuing treatment. Large series, with prolonged follow-up after discontinuation of antipsychotic drugs, have shown that patients can improve for up to 2 years and that patients with milder (and earlier) movement abnormalities are more likely to lose the abnormal movements completely.

The relationship of age to incidence of TD is most likely a reflection of the progressive neuronal alteration seen in the aging population that makes the striatum more susceptible to the production of denervation-induced changes in physiology. The increased incidence in patients with previous brain damage is probably analogous. The role of sex is not as clear. Females have an increased incidence of TD, which may be related to the role of female sex hormones on chorea (see below), but because the daily mg/kg dosage of neuroleptics is often higher in females, the relation of sex to incidence may be artifactual. The persistence of some signs of drug-induced parkinsonism is correlated with an increased incidence of TD. This may reflect individual susceptibility to neuroleptic blockade, preexisting nigral pathology, or drug-induced changes in the substantia nigra.

Two factors related to neuroleptic therapy itself are correlated with risk of developing TD: duration of therapy and daily dosage. Both are directly related to an increased risk of TD (12,17). It is often suggested that polypharmacy per se is bad. This may be true, but there is no evidence that combining two or more neuroleptics results in a greater risk of TD than the equivalent dose of a single neuroleptic.

The following principles should help to decrease the incidence of TD:

(a) Decrease the numbers of subjects at risk. Neuroleptics should be used only where clearly indicated and continued only when efficacy is clear.

(b) Keep the daily dosage as low as possible.

(c) Avoid chronic coadministration of anticholinergics whenever possible.

(d) Keep the duration of therapy as short as possible. Most schizophrenics are maintained on neuroleptics to control chronic symptoms or to prevent exacerbation. In the latter case it is quite possible that neuroleptics can be withdrawn for at least some period of time without a severe exacerbation (drug holiday). It is possible that such drug holidays might decrease the overall incidence of TDs. Data collected from animal studies suggest that drug-free periods should be at least 2 months long to be effective. The decision to withdraw neuroleptics must be individualized for each patient, and the relative mortality of the abnormal movements must be weighed against the danger of a psychotic exacerbation.

(e) Seek early detection and drug withdrawal when possible.

The biggest problem, of course, is what to do once TD has been detected. If the patient is on anticholinergic agents, these should be tapered and withdrawn. Tapering will decrease the likelihood of reemergence of drug-induced parkinsonism. The neuroleptic agents should also be withdrawn if possible. In many patients, of course, this cannot be done because the patients require neuroleptics to control their psychosis. In such patients we tend to switch to thioridazine. This is based on the following considerations:

(a) There appears to be a relationship between drug-induced parkinsonism and TD. Thioridazine has the lowest propensity to cause drug-induced parkinsonism of those neuroleptics available in the U.S.

(b) In animals thioridazine is a much weaker blocker of striatal dopamine receptors than other neuroleptics. In a variety of animal models, the chronic use of thioridazine causes much less hypersensitivity than the other available neuroleptics. The only neuroleptic that has been shown to improve schizophrenia and not induce hypersensitivity in animals or man (tardive dyskinesia) is clozapine. If this drug were safe in other ways and available, it would be the best antipsychotic to use in this situation. Clozapine has the lowest incidence of parkinsonism, appears to be a more specific blocker of nucleus accumbens dopamine receptors than striatal dopamine receptors, and has been reported to improve TD (28). Unfortunately, other toxicities (agranulocytosis) are seen with this agent.

It has been common to attribute the low incidence of parkinsonism caused by thioridazine and clozapine to the ability of these agents to block central muscarinic receptors. The fact that these agents are both dopaminergic and cholinergic blockers might suggest that they should have the highest likelihood of causing TD. This is certainly not the case. No reports of clozapine-induced TD have yet appeared. From a variety of animal behavior studies it is clear that clozapine and thioridazine are not identical to other neuroleptics (e.g., haloperidol) plus an anticholinergic agent, so that the differences in incidence of parkinsonism may not be due solely to their anticholinergic properties but may reflect differences in their ability to block striatal dopamine receptors.

With the exception of clozapine, the relative incidence of TD with different neuroleptics is not known; thioridazine can cause TD, but we tend to feel safer using thioridazine in patients with TD who require neuroleptics.

In general, we tend to advocate relatively rapid withdrawal of neuroleptics to limit the duration of exposure as quickly as possible. Slow reduction of dosage over months or years has also been advocated.

Once TDs have become established, the therapeutic maneuvers that can be used to decrease the severity of the movements center primarily on manipulation of dopaminergic influences, although there has been some recent interest in therapeutic manipulation of cholinergic influences. Reserpine, a striatal catecholamine depletor (1), has been reported to be of benefit in TD (5,26). Interestingly, reserpine itself does not induce TDs. This can be explained by its mechanism of action. The main action of reserpine is to prevent the storage of dopamine in intraneuronal granules by blocking dopamine uptake into these granules. In this way, reserpine depletes the brain of dopamine and may produce akinesia and rigidity. Because of this depletion, less dopamine is present to act at the receptors and TD tends to be decreased. However, it does not block dopamine receptors. Dopamine synthesis, which is extragranular, persists and some dopamine is still available to act at striatal receptors. Reserpine consequently does not produce "chemical denervation" of the receptors. If "denervation hypersensitivity" is in fact significant in the production of TD, reserpine would not be expected to produce TD. Reserpine given in doses up to 1 to 5 mg/day has been shown to reduce TDs in a number of uncontrolled trials. This we feel is the treatment of choice. Reserpine must be begun with low doses to avoid hypotension and built up gradually. Its antipsychotic effects may also decrease the paranoid symptoms in some patients.

Tetrabenazine, a synthetic benzoquinolone derivative which depletes monamines by a similar mechanism, is more rapid in onset, more selective for the CNS, and has fewer hypotensive effects than reserpine. Tetrabenazine, in doses up to 300 mg/day, reduced or absolved TD in several uncontrolled clinical trials as well as brief controlled trials (2). However, in a chronic study, when tetrabenazine was continued for 18 weeks, a significant reduction in this therapeutic effect was observed (11). In our hands, this loss of efficacy has not been as much of a problem with reserpine (14).

There has been recent interest in the use of cholinergic mechanisms to suppress abnormal movements in TD. The rationale for this mode of therapy arises from the proposal that a critical dopamine–acetylcholine balance within the striatum is essential to normal motor control, and that if there is increased sensitivity within the striatum to dopaminergic influences it might be possible to counteract this or to "reset" the balance by increasing striatal cholinergic activity. Using intravenous physostigmine, we have demonstrated that increased central cholinergic activity will transiently suppress dyskinesia. However, this has no proven practical therapeutic value. It is of interest that most observers feel that physostigmine is more likely to be beneficial in TD than in Huntington's chorea. This may be because of the cholinergic neuronal involvement in the latter disorder.

The following cholinergic approaches have been tried in the treatment of TD:

(a) Dimethylaminoethanol.

(b) Choline.

(c) Lecithin.

In general, all reported studies have been very short-term (a real problem in a chronic disease) and inadequately controlled. In our experience dimethylaminoethanol has little, if any, efficacy. Choline and lecithin are said to increase brain acetylcholine synthesis by increasing the rate of delivery of choline. Of the two, lecithin has fewer side effects and more potential promise.

Two other readily available agents have been said to have some effect on TD:

(a) Baclofen. The use of this agent was probably prompted by the analogy between TD and Huntington's chorea. As discussed in Chapter 2, GABA is markedly decreased in the striatum in the latter condition. Baclofen is a GABA analogue and at one time was thought to be a GABA agonist although this is no longer believed. Baclofen has been shown to have a mild-to-moderate efficacy in patients with TD but this has only been shown in patients who were maintained on neuroleptics (20a). In our hands this efficacy was reproducible and could be maintained in some patients for three or more months. Not all patients responded, in fact, less than half clearly benefited.

(b) Levodopa. It has been claimed that levodopa can improve TD (5a). When given to patients with TD, there is almost always an initial worsening of TD and there may well be an accompanying exacerbation of psychosis. If continued for months, however, some patients may have definite amelioration of their TD without continuing worsening of their psychosis. This has not been our experience and we do not recommend the use of this agent at this time.

Other agents have also been tried but remain unproven:

(a) Lithium. Although some published reports have claimed efficacy, this has not been reproducible. In animal models lithium has not been shown to alter neuroleptic-induced hypersensitivity once it has been induced, but it has been demonstrated that the simultaneous administration of lithium and a neuroleptic will prevent the development of neuroleptic-induced hypersensitivity. These observations raise the possiblity that lithium given to patients concurrently with their neuroleptics might either prevent TD or prevent the progression of TD. This hypothesis remains untested in man.

(b) Clonazepam. The mechanism of such an effect, if any, is unclear.

(c) Hydergine. This compound is a combination of three ergot alkaloids and has been claimed to have some efficacy in TD. The components of Hydergine have been shown to have some weak but definite effects on dopamine receptors, which could explain its value in TD, but its clinical efficacy remains to be proven.

Again these are all short-term studies in small groups of patients. None of these modalities can be recommended at this time.

Chorea as a Manifestation of Chronic Amphetamine Abuse

The production of amphetamine psychosis is one of the most striking results of abuse of this compound. However, patients abusing amphetamine have also been reported to develop choreiform syndromes (25). Amphetamine-induced dyskinesias are most often observed in the facial and masticatory musculature, producing chewing, licking, teeth grinding, and protrusion of the tongue. These movements are strikingly similar to the lingual–facial–buccal dyskinesias observed in TDs, levodopa-induced dyskinesias, Huntington's chorea, and a number of other symptomatic choreatic states. The clinical similarity of these disorders to amphetamine-induced dyskinesias suggests that the latter disorder may share a similar pathophysiology, namely, increased dopamine activity at dopamine receptor sites within the corpus striatum.

A single intravenous dose of 10 mg/kg amphetamine has been shown to be sufficient to exacerbate or uncover chorea in patients with Huntington's disease, Sydenham's chorea, or chorea associated with systemic lupus erythematosus, but not in normal controls (19). Each of these disorders is believed to involve physiologic alterations within the basal ganglia and increased sensitivity to dopamine.

The fact that amphetamine usually causes dyskinesias in normal individuals (i.e., those without prior striatal disease) only after chronic abuse suggests that chronic amphetamine administration itself produces hypersensitivity to dopamine by altering the physiology of the basal ganglia. The term "agonist-induced hypersensitivity" has been used to describe this phenomenon, which may also be related to levodopa-induced dyskinesias (see Chapter 1).

Since amphetamine-induced dyskinesias and amphetamine-induced psychoses are often found in association with one another, a dopaminergic mechanism may underlie both of these symptom complexes. This theory is supported by the fact that a clinical picture similar to that induced by amphetamine, including both psychosis and choreatic movements, has been reported in conjunction with many of the dopamine-releasing drugs, including methamphetamine, phenmetrazine, methylphenidate, and cocaine.

Other Drug-Induced Choreas

In levodopa-induced, neuroleptic-induced, and amphetamine-induced chorea the striatum is usually normal before the chronic administration of the offending agent. Other drug-induced choreas are seen only in patients with preexisting striatal pathology or dysfunction. These include acute amphetamine-induced chorea, anticholinergic-induced chorea, birth control pill-induced chorea, and phenytoin-induced chorea.

The acute intravenous administration of *d*-amphetamine exacerbates the chorea of patients with Huntington's chorea, Sydenham's chorea, and chorea associated with systemic lupus erythematosis, but it does not induce chorea in normal controls (19). In a single patient with systemic lupus erythematosis and hemichorea, *d*-amphetamine exacerbated the movement disorder only on the involved side and elicited no abnormal movements on the uninvolved side. Such agents can also elicit chorea in patients with a past history of Sydenham's chorea but no clinical manifestations. The acute precipitation of chorea by amphetamine and other indirect dopamine agonists such as methylphenidate depends on previous striatal dysfunction and is viewed as owing to increasing dopamine activity at previously altered and already hypersensitive receptors.

Most of the other drug-induced choreas are analogous to amphetamine-induced chorea in that preexisting striatal dysfunction is usually a prerequisite. These include:

(a) Anticholinergic-induced chorea. This is usually seen in elderly patients with oral masticatory syndrome and in patients on neuroleptics (16).

(b) Birth control pill-induced chorea. Most patients have a past history of Sydenham's chorea. It appears that female sex hormones (like thyroid hormones) increase striatal dopamine receptor responsiveness and can cause chorea in patients with previous striatal dysfunction (21).

(c) Phenytoin-induced chorea. Phenytoin can induce chorea in two settings: The first is a part of a generalized encephalopathy owing to drug overdosage. The second is as an isolated syndrome with therapeutic phenytoin levels. The latter is seen virtually only in patients with preexisting striatal dysfunction (22).

(d) Antihistamine-induced chorea. The pathogenesis of antihistamine-induced chorea is unclear. Most patients also have a history of indirect catecholamine agonist

therapy, which may be the primary factor. Many antihistamines are also anticholinergic. This syndrome is rarer than any of the above and less well understood.

BIBLIOGRAPHY AND *SELECTED REVIEWS

1. Bein, J. H. (1956): Pharmacology of rauwolfia. *Pharmacol. Rev.*, 8:435–483.
2. Brandrup, E. (1961): Tetrabenazine treatment in persisting dyskinesia caused by psychopharmaca. *Am. J. Psychiatry*, 118:551–552.
3. Christensen, E., Mollier, J. E., and Faurbye, A. (1970): Neuropathological investigation of 28 brains from patients with dyskinesia. *Acta Psychiatr. Scand.*, 46:14–23.
4. Crane, G. E. (1968): Tardive dyskinesia in patients treated with major neuroleptics. *Am. J. Psychiatry*, 124:40–48.
5. Duvoisin, R. D. (1972): Reserpine for tardive dyskinesia. *N. Engl. J. Med.*, 286:611.
5a. Friedhoff, A. J., Rosengarten, H., and Bonnet, K. (1979): Receptor cell sensitivity modification as a model for tardive dyskinesia. *Psychopharmacol. Bull.*, 14:77–79.
6. Heffran, W., and Eaton, R. P. (1970): Thyrotoxicosis presenting as choreoathetosis. *Ann. Intern. Med.*, 73:425–428.
7. Heilman, K. M., Kohler, W. C., and LeMaster, P. C. (1971): Haloperidol treatment of chorea associated with systemic lupus erythematosus. *Neurology*, 21:963–965.
8. Hippius, V. H., and Logemann, G. (1970): Zur Wirkung von Dioxphenylalanin (L-dopa) auf extrapyramidala-motorische Hyperkinesen nach langfristiger neuroleptischer Therapie. *Arzneim. Forsch.*, 20:894–896.
9. Hitri, A., Weiner, W. J., Borison, R. L., Diamond, B. I., Nausieda, P. A., and Klawans, H. L. (1978): Dopamine receptor site binding in an animal model of tardive dyskinesia. *Ann. Neurol.*, 3:134–140.
10. Hunter, R., Blackwood, W., Smith, M. C., and Cummings, J. N. (1968): Neuropathological finding in three cases of persistent dyskinesia following phenothiazine medication. *J. Neurol. Sci.*, 7:263–273.
11. Kazamatsuri, H., Chien, C., and Cole, J. O. (1973): Long-term treatment of tardive dyskinesia with haloperidol and tetrabenazine. *Am. J. Psychiatry*, 130:479–483.
*12. Klawans, H. L. (1973): *The Pharmacology of Extrapyramidal Movement Disorders.* S. Karger, Basel.
*13. Klawans, H. L. (1973): The pharmacology of tardive dyskinesias. *Am. J. Psychiatry*, 130:82–86.
*14. Klawans, H. L. (1976): Therapeutic approaches to neuroleptic induced tardive dyskinesias. In: *The Basal Ganglia*, edited by M. D. Yahr, pp. 447–457. Raven Press, New York.
15. Klawans, H. L., and McKendall, R. R. (1971): Observations on the effect of levodopa on tardive lingual–facial–buccal dyskinesia. *J. Neurol. Sci.*, 14:189–192.
16. Klawans, H. L., and Moskovitz, C. (1977): Cyclizine induced chorea. *J. Neurol. Sci.*, 31:237–244.
17. Klawans, H. L., and Rubovits, R. (1974): The effect of cholinergic and anticholinergic agents on tardive dyskinesias. *J. Neurol. Neurosurg. Psychiatr.*, 37:941–947.
*18. Klawans, H. L., and Weiner, W. J. (1975): The pharmacology of choreatic movement disorders. *Prog. Neurobiol.*, 5:1–32.
19. Klawans, H. L., and Weiner, W. J. (1974b): The effect of *d*-amphetamine on choreiform movement disorders. *Neurology (Minneap.)*, 24:312–318.
20. Klawans, H. L., Shenker, D. M., and Weiner, W. J. (1973): Observations on the dopaminergic nature of chorea. In: *Advances in Neurology, Vol. 1*, edited by A. Barbeau, T. N. Chase, and G. W. Paulson, pp. 543–549. Raven Press, New York.
20a. Kornsgaard, S. (1976): Baclofen in the treatment of neuroleptic induced tardive dyskinesia. *Acta. Psychiatr. Scand.*, 54:17–24.
21. Nausieda, P. A., Koller, W. C., Weiner, W. J., and Klawans, H. L. (1981): Oral contraceptive induced chorea. *Neurology*, 29:1605–1609.
22. Nausieda, P. A., Weiner, W. J., and Klawans, H. L. (1981): Phenytoin induced chorea. *J. Neural. Transm. Neurology*, 45:291–305.
23. O'Neil, D. P., Holmes, A. W., and Klawans, H. L. (1971): Treatment of choreoathetotic movements in chronic liver disease with a dopaminergic blocking agent. *Conf. Neurol.*, 33:258–270.
24. Pakkenberg, H., and Fog, R. (1974): Spontaneous oral dyskinesia. *Arch. Neurol.*, 31:352–353.
25. Rylander, G. (1972): Psychoses and the punding and choreiform syndromes in addition to central stimulant drugs. *Psychiatr. Neurol. Neurochir.*, 75:203–213.

26. Sato, S., Daly, R., and Peters, H. (1971): Reserpine therapy of phenothiazine induced dyskinesia. *Dis. Nerv. Syst.*, 32:680–685.

27. Shenker, D. M., Grossman, H., and Klawans, H. L. (1973): Treatment of Sydenham's chorea with haloperidol. *Dev. Med. Child. Neurol.*, 15:19–24.

28. Simpson, G. M., Lee, J. H., and Shrivastava, R. K. (1978): Clozapine in tardive dyskinesia. *Psychopharmacology*, 56:75–80.

*29. Tarsy, D., and Baldessarini, R. J. (1976): The tardive dyskinesia syndrome. In: *Clinical Neuropharmacology*, edited by H. L. Klawans, pp. 29–61. Raven Press, New York.

30. Tarsy, D., Leopold, N., and Sax, D. (1973): Physostigmine in choreiform movement disorders. *Neurology (Minneap.)*, 23:392.

31. Uhrband, L., and Faurbye, A. (1960): Reversible and irreversible dyskinesias after treatment with perphenazine, chlorpromazine, reserpine and electroconvulsive therapy. *Psychopharmacologia*, 5:408–417.

32. van Rossum, J. M. (1966): The significance of dopamine receptor blockade for mechanism of action of neuroleptic drugs. *Arch. Int. Pharmacodyn. Ther.*, 160:492–494.

33. Weiner, W. J., and Klawans, H. L. (1973): Lingual–facial–buccal movements in the elderly. I. Pathophysiology and treatment. *J. Am. Geriatr. Soc.*, 21:314–317.

34. Weiner, W. J., and Klawans, H. L. (1973): Lingual–facial–buccal movements in the elderly. II. Pathogenesis and relationship to senile chorea. *J. Am. Geriatr. Soc.*, 21:318–320.

Chapter 4

Hemiballismus

Hemiballismus consists of constant, repetitive, nonpurposeful movements of a flinging character and has long been recognized as a distinct form of extrapyramidal disorder. Most reported cases have resulted from acute vascular lesions of the subthalamic nucleus (corpus luysi) or its connections. Acute hemiballismus resulting from such cerebrovascular lesions is generally believed to have a grave prognosis. Death from "exhaustion," pneumonia, or congestive heart failure has been reported to occur in up to 60% of patients, usually within the first 4 to 6 weeks. Severe persistent abnormal movements lasting up to several years have been described in many of those who survive these initial weeks (3).

Since hemiballismus has received very little attention in the last 20 years, many of our views of this disorder are based on scattered reports in an era of markedly different medical care. Futhermore, most of the reports in the literature consist of pathologically proven cases. This is true in much of neurology and always pre-judices the sample toward severe, fatal instances of a disorder. Our experience, as well as other recent series, suggests that the prognosis is not as grave as previously reported and raises the possibility that treatment with dopaminergic antagonists such as haloperidol may improve the prognosis of this disorder.

Because of the apparently grave prognosis, a wide variety of medical and surgical approaches has been advocated. Pharmacologic measures have included hypnotics, which were only effective in anesthetic doses; neuroleptics; reserpine; tetrabenazine; atropine; and curare (4). Of these only the neuroleptics and tetrabenazine have produced consistent improvement. Because the neuroleptics used are all striatal dopamine receptor-site blockers, and tetrabenazine decreases striatal dopamine content, the efficacy of these agents in hemiballismus suggests that dopamine may be involved in the pathophysiology of the ballistic movements.

Our personal experience in 12 patients is presented in Table 1 (3,4). All 12 of our patients received neuroleptic therapy. Chlorpromazine was used in 3 patients with the dosage varying from 150 to 200 mg daily, and haloperidol was used in 9 with the dosage varying from 3 to 12 mg daily. All patients demonstrated prompt and dramatic reduction in adventitious movements. This usually occurred within 1 to 2 days and was always seen within the first week. In several cases reduction of dose in the weeks following the initial event resulted in worsening of symptoms. Reinstitution of the previous dosage invariably resulted in improvement of the movements to the previous level. The duration of the treatment varied from 3

TABLE 1. *Prognosis of treated hemiballismus*

Patient number	Drug	Maximum dose (mg/day)	Maintenance dose (mg/day)	Duration	Prognosis
1	Chlorpromazine	200	100	> 1 yr	Drug withdrawn at 6 and 12 mo with recurrence of hemichorea, but milder than when acute
2	Chlorpromazine	150	150	6 mo	No movements
3	Chlorpromazine	200	150	3 mo	No movements
4	Haloperidol	6	6	> 1 yr	Drug withdrawn at 6 and 12 mo with recurrence of hemichorea, but milder than when acute
5	Haloperidol	3	3	6 mo	Occasional lingual–facial–buccal dyskinesias; no other chorea
6	Haloperidol	4	4	5 mo	Minimal hemichorea on neuroleptics; patient denies any movements
7	Haloperidol	6	6	4 mo	No movements
8	Haloperidol	12	8	> 1 yr	Mild chorea on medication, worse on withdrawal; moderately severe chorea
9	Haloperidol	6	6	6 mo	No movements
10	Haloperidol	8	6	6 mo	Minimal hemichorea on neuroleptics alone
11	Haloperidol	6	3	3 mo	Mild hemichorea especially on stress
12	Haloperidol	8	8	6 mo	No movements

months to more than 1 year. Only 3 of the 12 patients required treatment of more than 6 months. The decision to continue treatment was based on either of two clinical findings. The observation of significant hemiballismus or hemichorea on clinical outpatient follow-up automatically resulted in continuation of neuroleptic therapy. If no movements were noted, attempts were made to withdraw the medication. Any reappearance of movements then resulted in reinstitution of therapy. In 3 patients, withdrawal of haloperidol after 6 months of treatment resulted in prompt return of hemichorea, and maintenance neuroleptic therapy was continued.

The prognosis of treated hemiballismus is also summarized in Table 1. Five of the 12 patients were completely free of abnormal movements when evaluated off all medications 4 to 6 months after the initial onset of hemiballismus. Four other patients had minimal residual movements after the discontinuation of the neuroleptics. One patient had minimal oral–facial dyskinesias when stressed but was free of chorea. Three patients had minimal hemichorea that was evident on examination but not a problem in daily living. Three patients, however, experienced continual adventitious movements whenever dose was tapered, as mentioned above. In summary, 9 of 12 patients experienced complete disappearance of all movements or only minor dyskinesias after neuroleptic treatment, whereas 3 required maintenance therapy. All were able to return to essentially the same level of activity that they had before the onset of hemiballismus.

The occurrence of hemichorea in these patients is of both practical and theoretical interest. The purity of hemiballismus as distinct from hemichorea is somewhat controversial. It has been suggested that, although proximal, flinging movements are the *sine qua non* of ballismus, that patients with ballistic movements often have some element of distal choreatic movements, and that there is a continuum between proximal ballismus and distal chorea. Six of the 12 patients we have seen had clear hemiballismus with pronounced proximal and violent flinging motion associated with chorea. Two had pure hemichorea of distal muscles without proximal activity. Four patients displayed both ballistic and choreatic components. In the latter patients it was common to observe continuous choreatic activity with paroxysms of more violent proximal ballismus. In patients with both ballistic and choreatic movements, the ballistic movements invariably improved first on neuroleptic therapy. In patients with pure hemiballismus, amelioration of the ballistic movements with neuroleptics was often associated with the development of milder choreatic movements. The reverse evolution from chorea to ballismus was never observed. These observations lend support to the notion that hemiballismus and hemichorea are not distinct entities. Patients with pure hemiballismus, pure hemichorea, and mixed hemichorea–hemiballismus all improved on neuroleptics.

The prognosis of the patients reported here was strikingly better than the prevailing pessimistic views in terms of both survival and residual movement disorder. Because all of our patients were treated with neuroleptics that definitely improved their normal movements, they in all probability experienced less exhaustion, and this might have been a factor in their more optimistic prognosis.

At the present time, we recommend that all patients with the sudden onset of hemiballismus or hemichorea owing to an acute vascular lesion be started on neuroleptic therapy. We use haloperidol beginning with 1 mg twice a day and increase to higher doses as required. Other neuroleptics such as prochlorperazine and chlorpromazine have also been shown to be effective. Most recently Johnson and Fahn have published a large series on patients treated with perphenazine with excellent results (2). There is a report of 8 patients with hemiballismus treated with tetrabenazine (1). Seven of these patients did quite well, suggesting that, if available, this is a reasonable form of therapy. Reserpine has also been used successfully in a single patient (5).

Because, as mentioned above, these agents all share the ability to decrease the activity of dopamine at striatal dopamine receptors, it is probable that dopamine plays a major role in the pathophysiology of hemiballismus and hemichorea. In order to investigate dopamine metabolism, we have obtained CSF HVA levels in 3 of our patients (see Table 2). In contrast to the biochemical information available on patients with Huntington's chorea, our preliminary data suggest that dopamine turnover may be increased in hemiballismus. The 3 patients studied had grossly increased levels of CSF HVA, consistent with the occurrence of increased dopamine synthesis and degradation.

The control of dopamine synthesis appears to involve both the striatal cells and the nigral neurons. It is widely believed that striatal dopamine synthesis is controlled by a negative feedback mechanism. It is generally accepted that the activity of dopamine at striatal dopamine receptors inhibits nigrostriatal dopamine synthesis. The synaptic relationships and fiber pathway of this system are poorly defined and controversial.

Lesions interrupting such a system could be responsible for increased dopamine synthesis via interruption of these normal feedback relationships. Hemiballismus could then result from increased presynaptic synthesis and release of dopamine, in contrast to Huntington's chorea, which appears to result from increased receptor-site response to normal dopamine levels. The result of both is a net preponderance of dopaminergic effect, resulting in abnormal movements. Neuroleptics and tetrabenazine would both interrupt the sequence, the former by blocking dopamine receptors and the latter by inhibiting dopamine storage.

TABLE 2. *CSF HVA in hemiballismus*

Patient no.	CSF HVA μg/ml
1	146
2	114
3	96
Mean	119
Normal range	30–75

The long-term administration of neuroleptics has itself been associated with the occurrence of abnormal involuntary movements (TDs). The incidence of these choreatic movements is related to both the duration of neuroleptic therapy and the dosage. In an attempt to prevent the occurrence of TD, we try to keep both the daily dosage and the duration of therapy to a minimum. Each time a patient is seen for follow-up, the possibility of lowering or discontinuing neuroleptic therapy is considered. The only indication for prolonged therapy is the continued occurrence of disabling movements when therapy is lowered or stopped.

BIBLIOGRAPHY AND *SELECTED REVIEW

1. Dalby, M. A. (1969): Effect of tetrabenazine on extrapyramidal movement disorders. *Br. Med. J.*, 2:422–423.
2. Johnson, W. G., and Fahn, S. (1977): Treatment of vascular hemiballismus and hemichorea. *Neurology*, 27:634–636.
3. Klawans, H. L., Moses, H., Nausieda, P. A., Bergan, D., and Weiner, W. J. (1976): Treatment and prognosis of hemiballismus. *New Engl. J. Med.*, 295:1348–1350.
*4. Koller, W. C., Weiner, W. J., Nausieda, P. A., and Klawans, H. L. (1979): The pharmacology of ballismus. In: *Clinical Neuropharmacology, Vol. 5*, edited by H. L. Klawans. Raven Press, New York, 157–174.
5. Obeso, J. A., Marti-Masso, J. F., Astudillo, W., de la Puenta, E., and Carrera, N. (1979): Treatment of hemiballismus with reserpine. *Ann. Neurol.*, 7:581–582.

Chapter 5

Dystonia

The term "dystonia" is used to describe a class of abnormal involuntary movements that are relatively slow and long sustained. It is the maintenance of an abnormal or altered posture that is the *sine qua non* of dystonia. These contorting, nonpatterned, and powerful dystonic movements can involve both axial and appendicular musculature and commonly are more proximal than distal. Because of the nature of the dystonic postures and their associated alterations in muscle tonus, the term torsion spasm has also been used. The distribution of involvement may be generalized as in dystonia musculorum deformans (DMD) or may remain segmental as in spasmodic torticollis. As with most disorders of the extrapyramidal system, dystonia appears to be aggravated by emotional stress. Frequently, dystonic movements and postures revert to normal during periods of relaxation, especially sleep.

Dystonia is most commonly seen as the sole manifestation of a number of neurologic disorders that are called primary dystonias. These diseases are listed in Table 1. The dystonia in such disorders can be either generalized or localized (partial). Since there are no known pathologic alterations in the brain of patients dying with primary dystonias or any known biochemical alterations, the pathophysiology of dystonia remains unknown. The pathophysiology is assumed to be similar in all dystonic disorders and is assumed to involve the basal ganglia, since dystonia is seen at times as a symptom of diseases known to be associated with pathologic changes in the basal ganglia. These disorders are often referred to as symptomatic dystonias. Neuroleptic agents including both phenothiazines and haloperidol can elicit either generalized or, more frequently, partial dystonias. Because of this, dopamine is thought to be involved in the pathophysiology of dystonia.

DMD (idiopathic torsion dystonia) is a genetically determined disease characterized by the typical involuntary motor manifestations of dystonia. The most common initial symptom of DMD is an action dystonia of the leg. An action dystonia is a dystonic movement superimposed upon a volitional movement. A child with DMD might present with an involuntary flexion inversion of the leg while walking. If both legs are affected by the hypertonic manifestation of dystonia, the gait may appear spastic or scissorlike. Facial grimacing may be mistaken for a behaviorally related problem. The initial period of the disease, manifested by a single extremity or neck involvement, may last for a few weeks or a few years. Depending on the age of onset, the pattern of dystonia may remain segmental but more likely will

TABLE 1. *Classification of major dystonic disorders*

Primary dystonias
  Generalized
    DMD (torsion spasm, torsion dystonia)
  Partial
    Spasmodic torticollis, neck
    Retrocollis, neck
    Meigs' syndrome, blepharospasm
    Breugel's syndrome, blepharospasm and lower
    face
    Writers' cramp, hand
  Reflex
    Kinesigenic choreoathetosis, variable
Symptomatic dystonias
  Perinatal injury (status marmoratus)
  Wilson's disease
  Encephalitis lethargica
  Hallervorden Spatz disease
  Manganese intoxication
  Basal ganglia destructive lesions including
  infections, surgical insults, etc.
Drug-induced dystonia

become generalized. When the disease presents before the age of 20, more than 50% of patients will present with dystonic spasms in the legs, approximately 25% in the arm, and almost 10% in the axial musculature.

Partial dystonias comprise a curious set of disorders of motor system function. Although said to occupy a gray area between neurology and psychiatry, the segmental dystonias are now generally considered abnormalities of motor system function. In support of this view, it has been shown that these entities occur as the only manifestation of inherited dystonia. Other factors favoring a neurologic origin of these disorders are their appearance in known disorders of the basal ganglia, their induction by various neuroleptic agents, the occasional spread of the dystonic features to other parts of the body, and the infrequent association of psychiatric disability.

The most common partial dystonia is spasmodic torticollis. Frequently known as wryneck, spasmodic torticollis may be defined as an abnormal involuntary contraction of neck muscles resulting in relatively sustained movement or posture of the head. The muscles known to be involved in the production of spasmodic torticollis are the sternocleidomastoids, the trapezius, and the splenius. Although a unilateral pattern is often seen, bilateral involuntary movements of the neck are present in most patients with spasmodic torticollis.

Retrocollis is a posterior flexion of the head on the neck, secondary to increased tonus of the posterior neck muscles. A rare isolated dystonia, retrocollis is most often seen as part of spasmodic torticollis. The movement disorder is commonly seen in association with acute dystonia secondary to neuroleptic antipsychotic drug therapy.

Writer's cramp is a segmental dystonia caused by spasms of the muscles of the forearm and hand. As writer's cramp is usually provoked by the performance of fine movements of the distal upper extremity, it is considered to be a form of action dystonia. Frequently, the patient will complain of pain in the forearm and hand in connection with writing or using hand utensils. As is the case with most dystonias, writer's cramp has been felt to be of psychogenic origin, as it is frequently occupationally related and may lead to significant disability on the job. This segmental dystonia has been seen, however, as part of DMD, and an organic substrate for the production of this entity is now generally accepted.

Neurologic evaluation of the patient with writer's cramp may at times reveal increased muscle tone in asymptomatic extremities, and occasionally subtle torsion spasms of the face, neck, or lower extremity may be seen.

Another example of adult-onset focal dystonia is Meige or Bruegel's syndrome. This appears to be a variant of adult-onset torsion dystonia and consists of oromandibular dystonia in conjunction with blepharospasm. The movements are distinct from the lingual-facial-buccal choreiform dyskinesias and are characterized by prolonged contraction of the muscles of the mouth and jaw. The dystonic movements may last a minute or two and are often repetitive but irregular in timing.

The syndrome may present as blepharospasm alone with the dystonic movements of the orofacial musculature following at a variable interval. Patients with Meige syndrome often have some degree of dysphagia resulting from involvement of hypopharyngeal musculature.

DRUG-INDUCED DYSTONIA

Acute neuroleptic-induced dystonias are seen early in the course of chronic neuroleptic therapy with either phenothiazines or haloperidol. These often occur following a single, frequently parenteral, administration of a neuroleptic. The manifestations can be quite diverse and are listed in Table 2. The most common clinical manifestations involve the eyes and neck.

Patients with oculogyric crisis often complain of inability to move their eyes in the vertical plane, as well as double vision, blurred vision, and, rarely, pain on attempted gaze. Most often the eyes maintain a sustained upward gaze. The severe dystonic displacement of the eyes may itself be painful, as may other severe acute contorting dystonias. The abnormal posture of the head and neck including opisthotonus, in which the head and neck are in a retrocollic position, give the patient a most bizarre appearance. Other muscles may be involved in the acute drug-induced dystonia, but this is much less common.

The incidence of dystonia with different neuroleptics seems to parallel the differential incidence of drug-induced parkinsonism (1). Agents with a high incidence of parkinsonism have a high incidence of drug-induced dystonia, whereas those with a low incidence of parkinsonism have a low incidence of dystonia. Hence,

TABLE 2. *Manifestations of neuroleptic-induced dystonia*

Generalized
   Torsion dystonia
   Opisthotonus
Partial
   Torticollis
   Retrocollis
   Oculogyric crises
   Trismus
   Involvement of one limb

piperazine phenothiazines and haloperidol have the highest incidence of drug-induced dystonia, followed by the alaphatic group. The group least likely to induce dystonia are the piperidine phenothiazines. The simultaneous administration of anticholinergic agents is thought to decrease the incidence of neuroleptic-induced dystonia, and the acute administration of anticholinergic agents almost invariably reverses these dystonias. Physiologically acute neuroleptic-induced dystonia is believed to represent an acute disruption of basal ganglia function in some way related to dopamine. This alteration is most probably acute dopaminergic receptor blockade, since all offending agents are capable of blocking striatal dopamine receptors. The ability of anticholinergic agents to prevent and ameliorate these dystonias suggests that dopamine–acetylcholine balance is involved in these events.

Acute neuroleptic-induced dystonia is more common in younger patients, especially children or adolescents given prochlorperazine for vomiting, and young adults (especially between the ages of 20 and 40) being started on chronic neuroleptic therapy. The dystonia often appears within hours of the first parenteral dose or within 1 to 3 weeks of the initiation of daily therapy. The dystonias are always self-limited and will revert spontaneously, usually within 24 hr after withdrawal of the offending agent. If they are distressing, they usually respond rapidly to the intravenous administration of either diphenylhydramine or benztropine. These agents will almost always produce relief of symptoms within minutes, and the amelioration may persist or the patient may require oral doses of anticholinergic agents over the ensuing 24 to 48 hr. If the patient's psychosis requires continued neuroleptic therapy, he should be placed on maintenance anticholinergic therapy for several weeks or switched to another neuroleptic with a lower propensity to cause dystonia (e.g., thioridazine).

The ability of neuroleptics to elicit dystonia disappears to a great extent as the duration of therapy is extended. New dystonias are rare after the first few weeks, and dystonias that occur in the acute phase are usually no longer present after months of therapy. As a result, the anticholinergic agents used to treat and/or prevent dystonia can be decreased and withdrawn in most patients after 1 to 2 months of use. An occasional patient will continue to have dystonia for longer and require a longer duration of maintenance anticholinergic therapy. In our experience such persistence is most likely to involve oculogyric crises. But even most of these patients can be slowly withdrawn from anticholinergics.

Metoclopromide is a relatively new antiemetic, which is not known to have neuroleptic properties and is not chemically related to the phenothiazines or butyrophenones. Its use, especially in children, has been associated with the occurrence of acute dystonic reactions that resemble those seen with acute neuroleptic administration. The most prominent manifestations include retrocollis, torticollis, and oculogyric crises, which are often both quite alarming and distressing. These reactions are always self-limited and usually disappear within hours of discontinuing the drug (2). Parenteral diphenylhydramine has been found to relieve these dystonias. Like neuroleptic-induced dystonias, these reactions are probably related to acute dopamine receptor-site blockade.

TREATMENT OF IDIOPATHIC DYSTONIA

Since the physiologic basis of dystonia is unknown, there is no true pharmacology. Unfortunately it often seems that there is no true therapeutics either. As shown in Table 3, a wide variety of agents has been used for the various dystonias. The true efficacy of these drugs remains unclear. These agents have rarely been studied with adequate, double-blind, placebo-controlled clinical trials. Moreover, the diversity of dystonic disorders complicates the interpretation of all the data. In Table 3 the various classes of agents are listed in order of the efficacy we have personally observed.

The combination of scopolamine plus morphine was advocated for the treatment of torsion dystonia nearly half a century ago. Although narcotics are of course no longer advocated, anticholinergic agents still have a role, especially in the treatment of spasmodic torticollis and other partial dystonias. The efficacy of these agents is limited both because of their low therapeutic index (relief of dystonia versus central anticholinergic intoxication) and because of the limited duration of their efficacy. Most, but not all, adults will become tolerant after several months of

TABLE 3. *Therapeutics of dystonia*

Anticholinergic agents
Baclofen
Dopamine antagonists, especially haloperidol
Tetrabenazine or reserpine
Dopaminergic agents
  Levodopa
  Amantadine
Anticonvulsants, especially carbamazepine
For symptomatic relief
  Diazepam
  Muscle relaxants

---

therapy. In a recent, acute study we demonstrated that acute intravenous administration of physostigmine markedly and reproducibly exacerbated torticollis, whereas the subsequent administration of benztropine consistently reversed this effect (12). This study demonstrates that acetylcholine plays some role in the pathophysiology of torticollis. It is our practice to use trihexyphenidyl as the first agent of choice in all partial dystonias. Children with DMD, for unknown reasons, often tolerate remarkably high doses of anticholinergic agents and may show a remarkable degree of improvement with relatively little tolerance.

The efficacy of anticholinergic agents in an extrapyramidal disorder, of course, raises the possibility that dopamine–acetylcholine balance could be significant in dystonia. Unfortunately the situation is not this straightforward, as both neuroleptics and levodopa have been claimed to have efficacy in various dystonias. A variety of neuroleptics, especially haloperidol, is widely used for the symptomatic relief of dystonia. A review of the literature suggests that neuroleptics are the most effective agents used for the amelioration of dystonia. Unfortunately, beneficial results are often proportional to the degree of drug-induced parkinsonism (3,7). We have been less impressed with haloperidol or other neuroleptics than the literature would suggest. We have found that prolonged (i.e., duration of more than a few months) symptomatic relief is unusual if not rare. The therapeutic index is low not because of parkinsonism but because of sedation, akathisia, and drug-induced dysphoria. Furthermore, the efficacy is limited and the duration is often short (several months). Once again, greater efficacy is seen with partial rather than generalized dystonia.

We have found that some patients with torticollis and occasionally other partial and generalized dystonias may improve remarkably on baclofen. The mechanism behind this is unknown. If a patient does respond, rapid development of tolerance has not been as much of a problem as it is with either anticholinergics or antipsychotics. In most patients a combination of baclofen and an anticholinergic agent bring about the greatest degree of improvement. The one form of partial dystonia in which we have personally observed prolonged, sustained efficacy with haloperidol is writer's cramp.

Occasional patients with either partial or generalized dystonia respond to reserpine or tetrabenazine and may not develop tolerance (11).

Amantadine has been reported to benefit some individuals with spasmodic torticollis but this has not been our experience. A rare patient with DMD (but not partial dystonia) may do better on levodopa (4). One patient with blepharospasm has been reported to improve on clonazepam, but the movements in this patient were more myoclonic than dystonic (10).

Patients with paroxysmal kinesigenic choreoathetosis (the movement of which often appears to be dystonic in nature) are usually substantially improved by anticonvulsants, such as phenytoin, phenobarbitol, and carbamazepine (8). These results have prompted clinical trials of carbamazepine in other forms of dystonia. Although the initial studies of carbamazepine in both DMD and symptomatic dystonia were very enthusiastic, subsequent reports as well as our experience have usually been disappointing. Rare patients with DMD do improve on carbamazepine, and this improvement can be sustained for 6 or more months (5,6).

A variety of muscle relaxants, including orphenadrine and chlorzoxazone, has been reported to improve patients with dystonia. The improvement is usually only slight and rarely decreases disability significantly, although pain and discomfort may be decreased. The adverse effects of this group are generally mild but may include apathy, lethargy, and weakness, and there is a marked tendency for tolerance to the limited efficacy.

Diazepam is widely used in patients with dystonia and produces some improvement in many dystonic patients, although almost all remain severely disabled (9). The effect of diazepam seems to be similar to that of muscle relaxants, i.e., decrease in symptoms (pain and discomfort) without alteration in the dystonia itself. In this regard, diazepam appears to be more reliable than the muscle relaxants and less susceptible to tolerance.

BIBLIOGRAPHY AND *SELECTED REVIEWS

1. Ayd, F. J. (1961): Neuroleptics and extrapyramidal reactions in psychiatric patients. *Rev. Can. Biol.*, 20:451–459.
2. Casteels-Van Daele, M., Jaeken, J., Van Der Schuren, P., Zimmerman, A., and Van Den Bon, P. (1970): Dystonic reaction in children caused by metoclopromide. *Arch. Dis. Child*, 45:130–134.
3. Couch, J. R. (1976): Dystonia and tremor in spasmodic torticollis. In: *Advances in Neurology, Vol. 14, Dystonia*, edited by R. Eldridge and S. Fahn, pp. 245–258. Raven Press, New York.
4. Eldridge, R., Kanter, W., and Koerber, T. (1973): Levodopa in dystonia. *Lancet*, II:1027–1028.
5. Geller, M., Kaplan, B., and Christoff, N. (1976): Treatment of dystonic symptoms with carbamazepine. In: *Advances in Neurology, Vol. 14, Dystonia*, edited by R. Eldridge and S. Fahn, pp. 403–410. Raven Press, New York.
6. Isgreen, W. P., Fahn, S., Barrett, R. E., Snider, S. R., and Chutorian, A. M. (1976): Carbamazepine in torsion dystonia. In: *Advances in Neurology, Vol. 14, Dystonia*, edited by R. Eldridge and S. Fahn, pp. 411–416. Raven Press, New York.
*7. Kartzinel, R., and Chase, T. N. (1977): Pharmacology of dystonia. In: *Clinical Neuropharmacology, Vol. 2*, edited by H. Klawans, pp. 43–53. Raven Press, New York.
8. Kato, M., and Arki, S. (1969): Paroxysmal kinesigesic choreoathetosis. Report of a case relieved by carbamazine. *Arch. Neurol.*, 20:508–513.
*9. Marsden, C. B., and Harrison, M. G. (1974): Idiopathic dystonia musculorum deformans. A review of 42 patients. *Brain*, 97:793–810.
10. Merikangas, J. R., and Reynolds, C. F. (1979): Blepharospasm: Successful treatment with clonazepam. *Ann. Neurol.*, 5:401–402.
11. Swash, M., Roberts, A. H., Zakko, H., and Heathfield, K. W. G. (1972): Treatment of involuntary movement disorders with tetrabenazine. *J. Neurol. Neurosurg. Psychiatry*, 35:186–191.
12. Tanner, C. M., Goetz, C. G., and Klawans, H. L. (1979): Cholinergic mechanisms in movement disorders: Result of physostigmine and scopolamine administration. In: *Nutrition and the Brain, Volume 5*, edited by A. Barbeau, J. Growdon, and R. J. Wurtman, pp. 217–228. Raven Press, New York.

Chapter 6

Gilles de la Tourette Syndrome (Chronic Multiple Tic Syndrome)

The term "tic" is applied to a group of abnormal involuntary movements that are rapid, spasmodic, and purposeless, and tend to repeat themselves in a stereotyped manner. Tics occur primarily during childhood but may persist into adult life, and at times they include such manifestations as involuntary noises or words. Tics usually decrease when the individual is relaxed or involved in nonanxiety-related activity, tend to increase with tension, and invariably disappear during sleep. Although tics can often be voluntarily suppressed for variable periods of time, such suppression is often followed by a period of increased tics. The diagnostic criteria for Gilles de la Tourette syndrome are shown in Table 1 (8). Persistence until adulthood is a requirement for the diagnosis. This is important to recognize since some children with multifocal tics will undergo spontaneous remission. Coprolalia in childhood virtually assures the diagnosis of GTS, and significant degrees of other vocalizations, respiratory tics, and noises are bad prognostic signs. This disorder begins with a single or simple tic in approximately half the patients and with multiple tics in the others. All patients ultimately develop multiple types of involuntary muscular movements and noises, but only 60% develop coprolalia.

TABLE 1. *Diagnostic criteria for Gilles de la Tourette syndrome*

Required for the diagnosis
Age of onset between 2 and 15 years
Multiple involuntary muscular and verbal tics
Tic severity and frequency wax and wane
Slow change in type of tics, usually over a 3-month period
An old tic may disappear or a new tic may replace or be added to preexisting tics
Chronic lifelong illness
Confirmatory, but not essential for the diagnosis
Coprolalia (involuntary swearing)
Copropraxia (involuntary obscene gesturing)
Echolalia (involuntary repetition of words or sounds of others)
Echopraxia (involuntary imitation of the movements of others)
Palilalia (involuntary repetition of one's own words or sounds)

Adapted from Sweet et al. (7).

Haloperidol is widely and often successfully used in the treatment of Gilles de la Tourette syndrome. Despite this therapeutic efficacy, neither the pathophysiology nor the pharmacology of Gilles de la Tourette syndrome is well understood. Shortly after their introduction into psychiatry, several phenothiazine neuroleptics were used in the treatment of Gilles de la Tourette syndrome, most likely because of the concept that the tics represented some form of psychopathology. Although the tics were partially suppressed, there was no dramatic amelioration. In contrast, haloperidol, first used by Seignot in 1960, was reported to have a marked effect on tics (5). These results were soon confirmed by other investigators (6). The efficacy of this dopamine antagonist raises the possibility that dopamine plays a significant role in the pathophysiology of tics seen in Gilles de la Tourette syndrome.

The response of patients with Gilles de la Tourette syndrome to haloperidol is quite variable. Some patients respond to very low doses of 2 to 4 mg/day, whereas others require heroic doses (up to 100 mg/day or more) for at least some periods of time (7). Haloperidol is usually started with a low dose, which is slowly increased until a therapeutic or adverse effect is obtained. The preferred rate of increase is not entirely clear. Some investigators such as Sweet et al. tend to increase dosage fairly rapidly, in increments of 2 to 10 mg/day or week, and later decrease the dosage (8). We tend to increase dosages much more slowly, especially in school-age children and adolescents.

Adverse effects such as akinesia and akathisia may be prominent early in the course of haloperidol administration. Sweet et al. believe that these often regress after tics have been suppressed and the dosage of haloperidol has been gradually decreased over a period of weeks (8). In patients whose dosage is increased in small increments, tolerance to this effect also occurs with time. Anticholinergic agents can of course be given to ameliorate akinesia and, to a lesser extent, the akathisia.

The best long-term study of the efficacy of haloperidol in Gilles de la Tourette syndrome is that of Shapiro's group, which studied 78 Gilles de la Tourette syndrome patients seen over an 8-year period (8). Four of the patients had sustained spontaneous remission of their tics. Fifty-nine patients remained on chronic haloperidol with an average improvement in tics of 79%. The other patients on no medication, or medication other than haloperidol, had an average improvement of only 25%. The pretreatment degree of severity of tics did not correlate with the response to treatment. The degree of improvement increased with the duration of therapy. Patients who had taken haloperidol for 2 years or less showed an average improvement of 74%. Those treated between 2 and 4 years had an average improvement of 80%, and those treated for more than 4 years had an average improvement of 94%. Adverse effects reported by patients were akinesia in 51%, drowsiness in 40%, depression in 28%, blurred vision in 21%, akathisia in 26%, and dyskinesia in 9%. Other effects were inability to concentrate, forgetfulness, fatigue, insomnia, dizziness, slurred speech, and nausea. Not all of the manifestations of GTS respond equally well to treatment with haloperidol (or other neuroleptics). Vocalizations and coprolalia respond least well whereas other respiratory tics and noises also do not improve as much as most bodily and head and facial tics. It is becoming increasingly clear that the efficacy of haloperidol is not as specific as it was once thought to be. Several phenothiazine neuroleptics have been shown to have definite efficacy in Gilles de la Tourette syndrome (3). The most effective of these compounds have been those with a piperazine side chain such as fluphenazine and perphenazine. We find these agents particularly useful in patients who cannot tolerate haloperidol because of sedation. Like haloperidol, these agents have a very high incidence of acute dyskinetic responses and drug-induced parkinsonism. This further supports the concept that haloperidol improves Gilles de la Tourette syndrome by decreasing the activity of dopamine at dopamine receptors, perhaps in the striatum (10).

Other pharmacologic studies support the role of dopamine in Gilles de la Tourette syndrome. These include:

(a) Occasionally worsening of tics in patients with Gilles de la Tourette syndrome who are given levodopa;

(b) Mild increases in tic frequency in patients with Gilles de la Tourette syndrome who are given apomorphine (8);

(c) Exacerbation of tics in patients with Gilles de la Tourette syndrome by amphetamine (4);

(d) Precipitation of Gilles de la Tourette syndrome following treatment of minimal brain damage with methylphenidate (2);

(e) Improvement of Gilles de la Tourette syndrome following treatment with α-methyl-*p*-tyrosine, which inhibits tyrosine hydroxylase and blocks dopamine and norepinephrine synthesis (7);

(f) Improvement of Gilles de la Tourette syndrome following treatment with tetrabenzamine, which blocks storage catecholamines in the brain (8).

If dopamine does play a role in the pathophysiology of Gilles de la Tourette syndrome, then it is possible that acetylcholine–dopamine balance may be significant in this disorder. In order to examine the role of the cholinergic system in Tourette syndrome, we administered intramuscular physostigmine and scopolamine to 10 patients with attention to drug effects on both motor tics and involuntary vocalizations (9). Patients showed a consistent abatement of motor tics after scopolamine injection with reversal of scopolamine effect after physostigmine. In one case physostigmine aggravated the tics to a level that was worse than baseline. The fact that scopolamine had a moderate sedative effect and at the same time abated the tics is particularly surprising since patients consistently report that when they are fatigued and less alert, their tics become more pronounced. Vocalizations were less affected by drugs than motor tics. Since it has previously been reported that neuroleptic drugs also are less effective in abating vocalization, the pharmacology of motor tics and abnormal vocalization in Tourette syndrome may be different. The findings suggest that at some levels of the nervous system dopamine and acetylcholine may act synergistically and not as antagonists as seen at the striatum. Furthermore, anticholinergic drugs or neuroleptics with anticholinergic activity may offer future therapeutic potential in the treatment of Tourette syndrome. Chonic drug trials with anticholinergic drugs in Tourette syndrome have not been reported.

Acute intravenous administration of benztropine or physostigmine had no consistent effect on tic frequency (8).

From the available data, it appears that haloperidol is presently the best drug available for the treatment of Gilles de la Tourette syndrome. Patients taking this medication have an average of 75% improvement in symptoms. The effectiveness of haloperidol is frequently limited by significant side effects that often force patients to reach a balance between relief of symptoms and discomfort from adverse effects. The dosage of haloperidol must be continuously adjusted, especially during the early months of therapy. All adjustments should be made in small increments and infrequently enough (once per week if possible) that it is possible to observe the effect of the alteration.

Over the last few years, we have been impressed that, for reasons which are unclear, many children with multifocal tics or GTS tolerate fluphenazine better than they tolerate haloperidol. Certainly any patient who has difficulty with haloperidol (sedation, depression, inability to concentrate, akathesia) should be switched to another neuroleptic, and we suggest fluphenazine. Often we even initiate treatment with fluphenazine. Several other agents have been tried and reported to have efficacy in patients for short periods of time. None of these have been shown to produce sustained, long-term benefits in the majority of patients with GTS but may be worth a trial in a severely affected patient who does not respond to neuroleptics. These include:

(a) Clonazepam. We have observed some improvement with this agent.

(b) Lithium. We have had no experience with this agent.

(c) Clonidine. We have used this agent in numerous patients without observing any efficacy.

We do not recommend any of these agents unless neuroleptics have definitely failed and the patient is severely disabled.

Treatment in GTS is directed at decreasing the social and secondary psychiatric disability caused by the tics and not merely suppression of the tics themselves. The severity of the movements as seen by the doctor in his office is nowhere near as reliable as a good history in evaluating either the need for or efficacy of treatment. Whereas numerous forms of behavioral modification techniques and psychotherapy have been tried, none of these has been shown to ameliorate the tics themselves. Obviously patients with GTS may have psychiatric problems that could benefit from psychotherapy. But the therapist must never confuse his goal and the attempt to use the tics and their severity as the measure of psychological well being. Tics may often be influenced by psychological states but they remain primarily a manifestation of neurologic disorder.

There is one situation in which there is a clear-cut neurologic indication for control of the tics per se. This is the occurrence of a compressive neuropathy or radiculopathy secondary to severe uncontrolled tics (1).

BIBLIOGRAPHY AND *SELECTED REVIEWS

1. Goetz, C. G., Klawans, H. L. (1980): Tourette syndrome and compressive neuropathies. *Ann. Neurol.*, 8:453.

2. Golden, G. S. (1974): Gilles de la Tourette's syndrome following methylphenidate administration. *Dev. Med. Child. Neurol.*, 16:76–78.
3. Levy, B. S., and Ascher, E. (1968): Phenothiazines in the treatment of Gilles de la Tourette's disease. *J. Nerv. Ment. Dis.*, 146:36–40.
4. Meyerhoff, J. L., and Snyder, S. H. (1973): Gilles de la Tourette's disease and minimal brain dysfunction: Amphetamine isomers reveal catecholamine correlates in an affected patient. *Psychopharmacologia*, 29:211–220.
5. Seignot, M. J. N. (1961): A case of the syndrome of tics of Gilles de la Tourette controlled by R 1625. *Am. Med. Psychol.*, 119:578–579.
6. Shapiro, A. K., Shapiro, E., and Wayne, H. (1973): Treatment of Tourette's syndrome with haloperidol: Review of 34 cases. *Arch. Gen. Psychiatry*, 28:92–97.
7. Sweet, R. D., Bruun, R., Shapiro, E., and Shapiro, A. K. (1974): Presynaptic catecholamine antagonists as treatment for Tourette's syndrome. *Arch. Gen. Psychiatry*, 31:857–861.
*8. Sweet, R. D., Bruun, R. D., Shapiro, A. K., and Shapiro, E. (1976): The pharmacology of Gilles de la Tourette's syndrome. In: *Clinical Neuropharmacology, Vol. 1*, edited by H. L. Klawans, pp. 81–105. Raven Press, New York.
9. Tanner, C. M., Goetz, C. G., Klawans, H. L. (1980): Cholinergic and anticholinergic effects in Tourette syndrome. *Neurology*, 30:384.
10. van Rossum, J. M. (1966): The significance of dopamine receptor blockade for mechanism of action of neuroleptic drugs. *Arch. Int. Pharmacodyn. Ther.*, 160:492–494.

Chapter 7

Wilson's Disease

Although the pharmacology of Wilson's disease could be discussed within Chapter 8, which deals with chelating agents in neurologic dysfunctions, Wilson's disease has been and continues to be of such interest that a separate discussion is warranted. This disease is inherited in an autosomal recessive manner and is always characterized by excess deposition of copper in many organ systems, the most prominent pathological involvement being in those tissues where the copper deposition is greatest: the brain, liver, cornea, and kidneys. The neurologic symptomatology, which results primarily from basal ganglia dysfunction, can produce an extraordinarily wide range of symptoms and signs including resting and action tremors, rigidity, loss of postural reflexes, bradykinesia, chorea, athetosis, ballistic movements, and dystonia. Dysarthria, dysphagia, and a fixed grimace-like smile are also seen. The variations in the symptomatology make it necessary to consider Wilson's disease as part of the differential diagnosis in any patient under the age of 40 who presents with extrapyramidal signs. The neurologic syndrome tends to be progressive, and the most common age of onset is 18.9 years according to Walshe (16). Although there are no pathognomonic neurologic symptoms, there is a pathognomonic physical sign that was even overlooked by Wilson in the original description of the syndrome. This is the Kayser-Fleischer ring, which is seen as the brownish or green-brown ring in the cornea. The ring is the result of copper deposition in Decemet's membrane.

The association of hepatic dysfunction with the CNS involvement in Wilson's disease is universal. The degree of liver involvement may vary from an asymptomatic cirrhosis in a patient with primary involvement of the brain to a fulminating hepatic necrosis in a patient otherwise asymptomatic. It is important to recognize that liver disease alone is the presenting symptom in almost half the patients with Wilson's disease. The average age of onset for the primarily hepatic presentation is 11.4 years. In fact, biopsy-demonstrated "chronic hepatitis" in neurologically normal patients has later been shown to be secondary to Wilson's disease. It is important to remember this nonneurological presentation of this disease, since the chronic hepatitis associated with Wilson's disease is the only form of chronic hepatitis for which there is a specific and definitive treatment (12).

The clinical biochemical profile seen in untreated Wilson's disease includes low serum copper, increased urinary copper excretion, increased copper concentration in the liver, and low serum ceruloplasmin. Serum copper in Wilson's disease may be severely depressed or almost normal in different patients. Elevated serum copper is seen in pregnancy, estrogen therapy, chronic infection, and chronic liver disease. The increased 24-hour urinary excretion of copper and the increased copper concentration in liver biopsy specimens are universal findings. Although ceruloplasmin levels tend to be absent or low, there are families in which the ceruloplasmin falls just below the normal range or actually falls within normal limits. There may, of course, be other biochemical evidence of hepatic dysfunction present including elevated SGOT and LDH. Renal dysfunction may also be present in the form of glycosuria, phosphaturia, uricosuria, and amino aciduria. However, this latter evidence of hepatic and renal dysfunction by itself is not enough evidence to establish the diagnosis of Wilson's disease. In fact, because of the variations in serum copper, urinary excretion of copper, and serum ceruloplasmin levels seen in patients with Wilson's disease, there is no single, noninvasive, definitive biochemical test that establishes the diagnosis.

It is well established that it is a disturbance of copper balance that underlies the pathogenesis of Wilson's disease. Those tissues which have the greatest degree of abnormal copper deposition have the greatest degree of clinical dysfunction. The establishment of a negative copper balance with the use of chelating agents will result in clinical recovery in an extraordinarily high percentage of patients. How the abnormal physiology of copper, including its storage, transport, and excretion, as well as its normal function as a trace element, translates into the varying symptomatology seen in Wilson's disease is not as clear as might be assumed. Copper is usually absorbed from the gastrointestinal tract and sequestered in the liver. The majority of this copper is bound to the storage protein metallothionum, and the remainder is incorporated into ceruloplasmin, cytochrome oxidase, and superoxide dimutase. Copper is excreted into the biliary system, and very little normally appears in the urine. Although copper is an essential trace element, the only two copper-containing enzymes of known function include cytochrome C oxidase, which plays a fundamental role in the reduction of molecular oxygen, and tyrosinase, which oxidizes tyrosine to dopa quinone, an intermediary in the synthesis of melanin. There are many other copper-containing proteins that are involved in erythropoiesis, connective tissue metabolism, and bone development. One of these remaining copper-containing proteins is ceruloplasmin. Although it is known that ceruloplasmin carries copper in the serum, its function as a copper transport protein has been questioned and its potential enzymatic properties have been downplayed (2). In short, the physiologic role of ceruloplasmin in healthy individuals is not known.

The accumulation of copper in the tissues in Wilson's disease must in the end be explained by either increased absorption of copper or decreased excretion of copper. On the basis of recent clinical experimental studies, it would appear that the problem in Wilson's disease is based not on increased gastrointestinal absorption or heightened copper protein binding, but on failure of excretion of copper into the biliary system. Presumably after the liver's copper binding capacity is exceeded, nonceruloplasmin copper reaches the circulation and is deposited in the various tissues. Although it is the copper excess in the tissues which is presumably toxic and which causes cellular dysfunction, two copper-containing enzymes, tyrosinase and cytochrome C oxidase, function normally in Wilson's disease. On the other hand, the dramatic reversal in symptomatology when negative copper balance is achieved makes it difficult not to believe that copper toxicity is directly related to cellular dysfunction.

As already pointed out, the role of ceruloplasmin in normal individuals is unknown and its role in Wilson's disease is equally unclear. Although a large percentage of patients with Wilson's disease have decreased ceruloplasmin, there are a significant number of patients with Wilson's disease who have normal or near normal ceruloplasmin concentrations. In addition, there are asymptomatic heterozygotes who have very low ceruloplasmin levels. Cartwright et al. (4) have demonstrated that there is no correlation between ceruloplasmin levels and onset or severity of symptoms. Attempts to use ceruloplasmin as a therapeutic agent have also failed. The role of ceruloplasmin, if any, in the pathogenesis of Wilson's disease is unknown.

The general biochemical and pharmacological aspects of the chelating agents used in the treatment of Wilson's disease will be discussed in Chapter 8. Here we shall limit ourselves to the use of British Anti-Lewisite (BAL) and penicillamine in the treatment of Wilson's disease.

BAL was first advocated as a means of removing excess copper in Wilson's disease in 1948. The initial trials were partially successful, and BAL became the first available chelating agent to be used in Wilson's disease. However, because BAL is not water soluble it must be administered in oil as an i.m. injection. This necessitated repeated i.m. injections, which were painful and which were associated with toxic reactions. In addition, although there were some definite therapeutic successes with BAL in Wilson's disease, the effect was often not sustained.

The real advance in the treatment of Wilson's disease came when Walshe demonstrated that penicillamine could increase urinary copper excretion in both normals and patients (14). Penicillamine chelates plasma copper and renders it available for renal filtration and excretion. This reduction in plasma copper alters the copper distribution equilibrium between serum and tissues and begins the reverse flow of copper from tissue to serum. The advantages of penicillamine over BAL became apparent because penicillamine was an effective copper chelating agent and it could be administered orally with fewer toxic effects. There are certainly toxic side effects associated with institution of penicillamine therapy. These include urticaria, fever, oral ulcers, purpura, and eosinophilia. The reactions are, for the most part, tolerated with a certain degree of anxiety by both patient and physician. The need to terminate therapy rarely arises. When penicillamine treatment is successful the neurologic symptomatology responds slowly, and it may take up to 6 to 12 months to observe improvement. In addition, it has been noted that shortly after initiating therapy neurologic symptomatology may become transiently worse. There was initial concern related to whether or not long-term penicillamine therapy would remain effective. However, Goldstein and Gross (6) have recently reported that patients followed for 10 to 17 years have continued to do well.

A second approach to altering the positive copper balance in Wilson's disease is to affect copper intake and absorption. Restriction of foods high in copper content can reduce the daily intake of dietary copper from approximately 5 mg/day to 1 to 2 mg/day. This can be done without the dietary restriction becoming socially restrictive (Table 1). In addition, some have advocated the use of potassium sulfide or carbacrylamine resins to precipitate dietary copper in the gut and prevent absorption. However, patient acceptance of these methods was not achieved because of both their terrible taste and the peculiar odor produced. An additional adjunct to altering copper balance in Wilson's disease is the use of orally administered zinc sulfate. Zinc interferes with the gastrointestinal absorption of copper. A report of the use of zinc sulfate in the treatment of Wilson's disease has been published (7). The patient is a 13-year-old male with neurologic symptomatology who was treated for 3 months with zinc sulfate (200 mg t.i.d.) with no improvement. This was followed by 3 months of penicillamine alone, which also did not result in improvement. Combined therapy with both penicillamine and zinc eventually resulted in improvement in his neurologic signs. The authors concluded that the additional use of zinc contributed to the establishment of a negative copper balance. Side effects reported with the use of oral zinc included gastrointestinal irritation, hematemesis, and melena. Long-term side effects are unknown at this time.

The recognition of the biochemical problems in patients with Wilson's disease has led to the detection among their siblings of presymptomatic, biochemically identifiable patients. Although lifetime therapy with a potentially toxic agent like penicillamine is not to be undertaken lightly, Sternlieb and Scheinberg (11) have demonstrated that presymptomatic patients can be prevented from developing overt Wilson's disease by institution of chelation therapy. Treatment of presymptomatic patients should be undertaken (3).

Long-term toxicity associated with penicillamine administration has been related to penicillamine–pyridoxine interactions with the potential for peripheral neuropathy or seizures occurring. Penicillamine can form a stable thiozolidine compound with pyridoxal-5-phosphate, and this is believed to be the basis for its action as an antipyridoxine agent. Although pyridoxine deficiency can produce peripheral neuropathy, there is no good clinical evidence of this occurring with penicillamine

TABLE 1. *Foods high in copper*

Shellfish
Liver
Nuts
Mushrooms
Broccoli
Dried fruit
Chocolate
Cocoa
Whiskey (copper stills)

therapy in Wilson's disease. The antipyridoxine effect on GABA synthesis has been related to seizures occurring in Wilson's disease. However, seizures can also occur in untreated Wilson's disease, and whether or not the potential effect on GABA synthesis has meaningful clinical correlations is unknown. However, common clinical practice is to administer pyridoxine to patients on long-term penicillamine therapy.

Successful therapy in Wilson's disease has led to the question of penicillamine treatment during pregnancy. This has been raised with particular urgency since a child was delivered with a generalized connective tissue disorder after the mother received penicillamine during gestation. Penicillamine interferes with collagen synthesis and results in the accumulation of poorly cross-linked soluble collagens. This case report involved not Wilson's disease but penicillamine therapy in cystinuria. However, the issue has been examined in Wilson's disease by Scheinberg and Sternlieb (10). There is no evidence that penicillamine therapy during pregnancy adversely affects fetal outcome. Copper chelation of the fetus is no substitute for penicillamine.

Other neurologic syndromes associated with chronic penicillamine use include polymyositis and myasthenia gravis. The pharmacologic mechanisms responsible for these rare complications of therapy are unclear. However, it should be noted that many of these complications have occurred in patients being treated for illnesses other than Wilson's disease. In fact, the most common therapeutic use of penicillamine today is in the treatment of rheumatoid arthritis (9).

The role of excess copper deposition in producing pathologic alterations in the CNS that result in the previously described wide range of movement disorders seen in Wilson's disease is established. Surprisingly, investigation of central neurotransmitters (dopamine, acetylcholine, serotonin, GABA), which are thought to be involved in a variety of movement disorders, has not received vigorous attention in Wilson's disease. Recently Tarsy et al. (13) investigated the role of cholinergic mechanisms in a 21-year-old male patient with Wilson's disease. This patient received physostigmine (1 mg i.v.), a centrally acting anticholinesterase, and a fine postural tremor of the upper extremities was dramatically changed to a "classic" wing beating tremor. In addition, the patient's trunkal flexion posture and facial masking increased. These exacerbations of symptoms lasted 15 min and resolved. This dramatic increase in symptomatology suggested to the investigators that there might be a relative striatal dopaminergic deficiency (analogous to the situation in Parkinson's disease) that was being exacerbated by the transient increase in central cholinergic activity. In this patient CSF HVA levels were normal, and the administration of levodopa did not alter the motor symptomatology. Previous investigators have reported some benefit to the administration of levodopa in Wilson's disease (1,5). Another investigation of central neurotransmitter activity in Wilson's disease involved the study of two sisters with this disorder. The 21-year-old had CNS involvement, and examination of her CSF revealed extremely low concentrations of HVA and 5HIAA, whereas her 19-year-old sister without CNS involvement had normal CSF HVA and 5HIAA concentrations. After penicillamine treatment the

21-year-old patient's central symptoms improved but there was very little change in her CSF concentration of HVA and 5HIAA. These investigators concluded that the central damage to dopaminergic and serotonergic neurons might be only partially reversible (8).

BIBLIOGRAPHY AND *SELECTED REVIEWS

1. Berio, A., Ventor, R., and Di Stefano, A. (1973): Favorevoli resultati dell'associazione delle L-Dopa e della amantadina alla penicillamina nella terapia del morbo di Wilson. *Minerva Pediatr.*, 25:807–813.
2. Broman, L.: Chromatographic and magnetic studies of human ceruloplasmin. *Acta Soc. Med. Upsala*, 64 (Suppl. 7).
3. Cartwright, G. E. (1978): Diagnosis of treatable Wilson disease. *N. Engl. J. Med.*, 298:2347–2350.
4. Cartwright, G. E., Markowitz, H., Shields, G. S., and Wintrobe, M. M. (1960): Studies on copper metabolism. XXIX. A critical analysis of serum copper and ceruloplasmin concentrations in normal subjects, patients with Wilson's disease and relatives of patients with Wilson's disease. *Am. J. Med.*, 28:555–563.
5. Gelmers, H. J., Troost, J., and Wallense, J. (1973): Wilson disease: Modification by L-dopa. *Neuropaediatrie*, 4:453.
*6. Goldstein, N. P., and Gross, J. B. (1976): Treatment of Wilson disease. In: *Clinical Neuropharmacology*, Vol. 2, edited by H. L. Klawans, pp. 94–112. Raven Press, New York.
7. Hoogenraad, T. U., Van Den Homer, C. J., Koevoet, R., and De Ruyter Korver, E. G. (1978): Oral zinc in Wilson's disease. *Lancet*, 2:1262.
8. Nijeholt, J. L., and Korf, J. (1978): Wilson disease and monoamines. *Arch. Neurol.*, 35:617–618.
9. Russell, A. S., and Lindstrom, J. M. (1978): Penicillamine-induced myasthenia gravis associated with antibodies to acetylcholine receptor. *Neurology*, 28:847–849.
10. Scheinberg, I., and Sternlieb, I. (1975): Pregnancy in penicillamine treated patients with Wilson disease. *N. Engl. J. Med.*, 293:1298–1302.
11. Sternlieb, I., and Scheinberg, I. (1968): Prevention of Wilson's disease in asymptomatic patients. *N. Engl. J. Med.*, 278:352–359.
12. Sternlieb, I., and Scheinberg, I. (1972): Chronic hepatitis as a first manifestation of Wilson's disease. *Ann. Intern. Med.*, 76:59–64.
13. Tarsy, D., Mahoney, J. F., and Cummings, J. L. (1978): Physostigmine in Wilson disease. *Ann. Neurol.*, 3:372–373.
14. Walshe, J. M. (1956): Penicillamine, a new oral therapy for Wilson's disease. *Am. J. Med.*, 21:487–495.
15. Walshe, J. M. (1967): The physiology of copper in man and its relation to Wilson's disease. *Brain*, 90:149–176.
*16. Walshe, J. M. (1976): Wilson's disease: Diagnosis, pathogenesis, management. In: *Handbook of Clinical Neurology, Vol. 27*, edited by P. J. Vinken and G. W. Bruyn, pp. 379–414. North-Holland Pub., Amsterdam.

Chapter 8

Heavy Metal Intoxication (Chelating Agents)

Chelating agents are the major pharmacological modalities used in the therapy of heavy metal intoxication (1,2,3). Chelation in therapeutics began during World War II when BAL was developed as an antidote to arsenical mustard gas; the other two major clinically available chelators, ethylenediaminetetraacetate (EDTA) and penicillamine, were introduced in 1951 and 1956. The word chelation, from the Greek *chele* for claw, describes the interaction between a heavy metal and the chelator as the chelator binding entraps and holds the metallic ions. In aqueous solutions metal ions exist in their hydrated forms. The replacement of the water molecules attached to the metal ions by other molecules leads to the formation of metal complexes. The replacement molecule in a specific reaction is designated the ligand. In this chapter, it will become apparent that treatment in heavy metal intoxication is based on the reaction between metallic ions and ligands. This reaction can be simply described as:

$$\text{metal} + \text{ligand} \rightleftarrows \text{metal–ligand complex}$$

and the stability of the chelate formed, which itself is crucial in removing excessive metallic ions from the body, can be described as:

$$K = \frac{(\text{metal–ligand complex})}{(\text{metal}) \, (\text{ligand})}$$

Although the principal aim of chelation therapy is the acceleration of the excretion of toxic metals from the organism in order to stop, prevent, and, one hopes, reverse the toxicity caused by the metal in question, it should not be overlooked that the process of chelation is widespread *in vivo* and plays an essential biological role. The chelation of many trace elements to enzyme systems and other functional proteins (e.g., iron – hemoglobin, copper and iron – cytochrome oxidase, cobalt – vitamin B_{12}) is essential to the life of the organism. The fact that these endogenous chelators exist represents both a theoretical and a practical element that must be considered when therapeutic chelating agents are administered. Chelating agents do not react only with the specific metallic ions that happen to be toxic in a given instance, but with all endogenous metals. If a chelating agent's affinity for any given metal is higher than its affinity for the metallic ion in question, then the chelating agent will complex with the endogenous metal and result in its removal. Since the endogenous chelators are involved in vital biological systems, their disruption can result in further toxicity. In fact, it is the disruption of these endogenous chelators by exogenous metals that forms the basis of the metal toxicity. The metal ion enters into stable complexes with these proteins and prevents them from performing their physiologic function.

Although a chelating agent may produce enhanced excretion of the metallic ion in question, this alone is not sufficient evidence of therapeutic efficacy. Enhanced excretion must be accompanied by a decrease in the toxic metal's concentration in the affected organ of the body. In addition, the chelating agent must not cause a shift in concentration of the metal to the observed affected organ, which would, of course, increase toxicity and not decrease it. Other general requirements for a successful chelator include resistance to metabolic degradation, water solubility, accessibility of the agent to the metal sites *in vivo*, nontoxic excretion, and no toxicity to the ligand–metal complex itself. Two final points must be made regarding the tenuous relationship between increased excretion of a toxic metal and the therapeutic efficacy of a given chelating agent. First, if the toxic metal produces a rapid and irreversible effect, then chelation and removal of the offending toxic agent may be of little, if any, benefit. Second, a chelating agent may bring about clinical improvement without any acceleration in metal excretion being detectable. This happens when the ligand–metal complex is an insoluble inert compound.

The remainder of this chapter will deal with the general properties of each of the major chelating agents (BAL, EDTA, penicillamine) including their solubility, structure, mechanism of action, excretion mechanism, and toxicity (Table 1).

BAL, or dimercaprol, was developed during World War II as a specific antidote for arsenic mustard gas. BAL represents one of the few logical approaches to the development of a useful therapeutic agent in pharmacology. The toxicity of mustard gas is related to its arsenic content, and the toxicity of arsenic results from its formation of stable compounds with the sulfhydral group of essential enzymes. These enzymes are thereby inhibited. A deliberate search for a ligand that had a stronger affinity for arsenic than endogenous ligands resulted in the discovery of the dithiol compound BAL (Fig. 1) as a specific antidote for arsenic. It should be

TABLE 1. *Clinically useful chelating agents*

Chelator	Dosage	Route of administration	Course
BAL	2.5–5.0 mg/kg	Deep i.m.	Repeat q 4 hr for 48 hr, then twice on day 3; once daily for next 5–10 days
EDTA	1.0 g in 500 cc 5% glucose in water or isotonic saline	i.v.	Administered over 1 hr twice a day for 3–5 days; then stop drug and evaluate whether further treatment is needed
Penicillamine	1.0–4.0 g/day	p.o.	250 mg tablet available; should be administered 30–45 min prior to meals

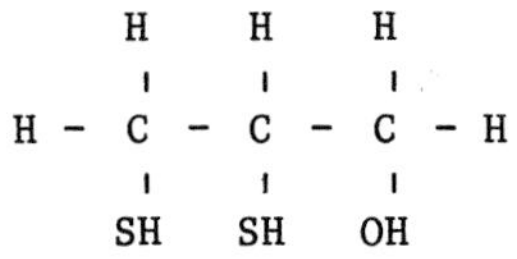

$$
\begin{array}{ccccccc}
& H & & H & & H & \\
& | & & | & & | & \\
H - & C & - & C & - & C & - H \\
& | & & | & & | & \\
& SH & & SH & & OH &
\end{array}
$$

DIMERCAPROL (BAL)

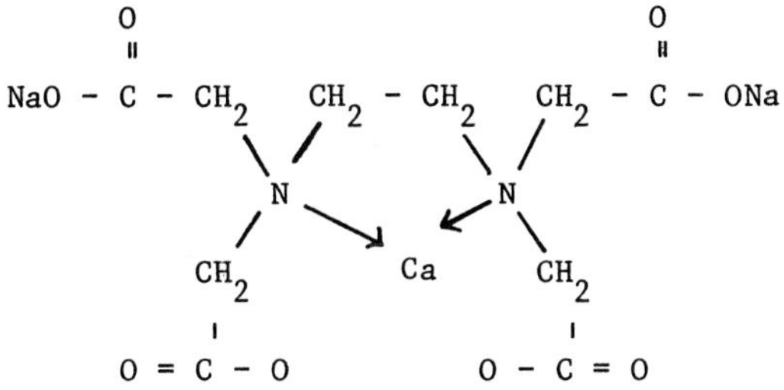

CALCIUM DISODIUM EDTA

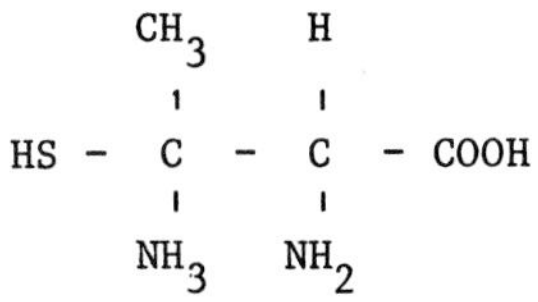

Penicillamine

FIG. 1. Structures of the three major chelating agents.

recalled that chelating agents are not specific for a single metallic ion, and BAL can also be employed to treat gold, silver, mercury, lead, and copper toxicity.

BAL is poorly soluble in water and therefore must be administered in a lipid solvent such as peanut oil. This limits its administration to intramuscular injection. The major portion of administered BAL is rapidly absorbed (within 30–60 min) and almost all of the drug is excreted in the urine within 4 hr. Numerous side effects accompany its administration and within 10 to 30 min of receiving the drug, up to 50% of patients will experience some of the following: anxiety, fatigue, dizziness, nausea and vomiting, headaches, paresthesia of the tongue and lips, rhinorrhea, and a rise in systolic and diastolic blood pressure. Antihistamines and epinephrine have both been reported to ameliorate some of these side effects. Although these reactions can be dramatic, they are usually transient and subside quickly. It is only in the occasional patient that the acute side effects are sufficient to either lower the dose administered or not administer it at all. Chronic treatment with BAL usually does not result in any toxic effects, although the injection sites may become quite painful, and an occasional sterile abscess will be produced.

EDTA is a polyaminopolycarboxylic acid (Fig. 1) that has been used as a markedly successful chelating agent since 1951 when it was first employed to treat lead toxicity. EDTA is available as either a calcium or sodium chelate. However, the sodium form is rather toxic because it can produce profound hypocalcemic problems, and therefore the calcium chelate is used in therapeutic settings. EDTA has a great affinity for zinc; however, this is rarely a toxic problem in humans. EDTA's affinity for other metals *in vivo* such as copper, iron, manganese, and even lead is not enough to increase any excretion of these metals very greatly. However, where lead is in excess in the body EDTA is an excellent chelator of lead. EDTA is not metabolically degraded and is excreted almost entirely in the urine. The excretion is dependent on glomerular filtration, not tubular excretion, since agents that block the tubular transport of organic acids do not interfere with EDTA excretion. EDTA is water soluble but is poorly absorbed from the gastrointestinal tract. Only 5% of an oral dose is absorbed because the calcium chelate of EDTA disassociates at the low pH of the stomach and the organic acid probably precipitates. EDTA is administered as an intravenous injection.

EDTA is associated with very few toxic reactions in humans, even after chronic use. However, in animal experiments, it is possible to produce proximal renal tubular lesions. These lesions can be reversed when EDTA administration is stopped. Whether the renal lesions are due to the ligand, the metal, or the ligand–metal complex is unsure. However, since EDTA alone can cause proximal renal tubular changes in the absence of excess metallic ions, it is reasonable to assume that EDTA alone may be responsible. An explanation for this effect may be that EDTA is forming stable ligand–metal chelates with endogenous trace elements and is suppressing and disrupting metal-controlled or metal-activated systems. EDTA is a drug with a high therapeutic index and is well tolerated by almost all patients.

D-penicillamine (Fig. 1) is obtained by the hydrolytic degradation of penicillin, and it was first identified in the urine of patients receiving penicillin. Penicillamine is valuable as a chelating agent because it is water soluble and the chelates it forms are also water soluble. Penicillamine is not metabolically degraded and is excreted almost entirely in the urine. In fact, approximately 80% of a given dose of penicillamine will be eliminated within 24 hr. Since up to 60% is absorbed after its oral administration, penicillamine has a therapeutic advantage over BAL and EDTA because it can be administered orally. Penicillamine has become the mainstay of chelation therapy in Wilson's disease, but it is also useful in the treatment of lead, mercury, and zinc intoxications. Penicillamine has also been used to promote excretion of cystine and thereby prevent urinary calculi in patients with cystinuria. Most recently there has been considerable enthusiasm about and use of penicillamine in the treatment of unresponsive rheumatoid arthritis.

Toxicity associated with the use of penicillamine can be divided into acute and chronic reactions. Acute reactions to penicillamine are similar to many acute allergic reactions to a drug. These include fever, malaise, urticaria, pleuritis, and eosinophilia. Although these reactions can be distressing, they should not be dose-limiting since, in the case of heavy metal intoxications and Wilson's disease, the chronic use of penicillamine may be life-saving. Some of the allergic responses can be suppressed by concomitant steroid administration. More chronic toxicity may be related to hematopoietic suppression, alteration in collagen formation, alteration in renal function, myasthenia gravis, and even hepatitis.

Considerable interest has focused on the ability of penicillamine to form stable thiozolidine complexes with pyridoxol-5-phosphate. This property makes penicillamine a pyridoxine antimetabolite. This has led to speculation that in the chronic use of penicillamine, as in Wilson's disease, the possibility of a pyridoxine-deficient polyneuritis exists. There have been no reports of clinical cases to support this hypothesis. In addition, the effect of pyridoxine deficiency on GABA synthesis may make chronic users of penicillamine more susceptible to seizures. Again this is not clearly discernible from clinical practice. As a result of the similarity in structure between penicillamine and penicillin, there have been reported occasional allergic cross-sensitive reactions. However, this is not at all a universal phenomenon, and many patients who are allergic to penicillin can tolerate penicillamine administration.

BIBLIOGRAPHY AND *SELECTED REVIEW

1. Cotsch, A., and Harmuth-Hoene, A. E. (1976): Pharmacology and therapeutic application of agents used in heavy metal poisoning. *Pharmacol. Ther.*, 1:1–118.
*2. Greenhouse, A. H. (1981): Heavy metals and the nervous system. In: *Clinical Neuropharmacology, Vol. 5*, edited by H. L. Klawans. Raven Press, New York (*in press*).
3. Levine, W. G. (1975): Heavy metals and heavy metal antagonists. In: *Pharmacological Basis of Therapeutics*, edited by L. S. Goodman and A. Gilman, pp. 912–923. Macmillan, New York.

Chapter 9

Essential Tremor

Essential tremor is a relatively benign monosymptomatic disorder of the nervous system. It is characterized clinically by a postural tremor that is most evident in the upper extremities, head, and neck, although the lower extremities may also be involved. It has also been described as a type of action tremor because the tremor is definitely exacerbated when the hands are used in maneuvers that require precision. In fact, the tremor can also be described as a type of intention tremor since the "finger to nose" and "heel to shin" test will exacerbate the movement although not as dramatically as seen in cerebellar disease. Although essential tremor has been described as a "constitutional monosymptomatic peculiarity" that can be scarcely regarded as a "disease" (2) its familial occurrence, progressive nature, and sometimes disabling movement problem certainly seem to rescue it from the category of "constitutional peculiarity" and raise it at least to the status of a disorder of the nervous system. When the symptoms occur in an isolated individual it is termed essential tremor; when in an individual over the age of 65, senile tremor; and with a family history, familial tremor.

Since essential tremor is neither life threatening nor life shortening the opportunity to examine the CNS post-mortem is not frequent. In those cases that have been examined pathologically, there is no distinctive CNS pathology. In fact, only five reported pathologic examinations in this disorder have been published, and the consensus is that there is no discernible pathology in the cerebello-olivary or extrapyramidal systems (6,13).

Essential tremor has occasionally been assumed to be a form *fruste* of the presenile cerebellar atrophies or to be linked to Parkinson's disease. Neither of these associations can be supported. It is interesting to note that essential tremor is often misdiagnosed as parkinsonism. Since essential tremor is not associated with bradykinesia, rigidity, postural reflex impairment, or with a resting tremor, it is often difficult to understand the source of confusion (7).

An interesting pathophysiologic postulate is that essential tremor represents an exaggeration of physiologic tremor. Physiologic tremor is the tremor that can be recorded in all people by the use of an accelerometer and that can be observed clinically in some normal individuals (8–12 Hz). This tremor is known to be exacerbated by anxiety and emotional stress. The mechanism that is responsible for the generation of physiologic tremor is not clearly defined. However, McAllister et al. (12) have presented evidence that physiologic tremor and essential tremor are different, because in their investigation the frequency of essential tremor was 6 to 8 Hz and that of physiologic tremor was 11 to 12 Hz.

Even though the basic organizational mechanisms underlying physiologic tremor are unknown, pharmacologic investigations have provided useful information. Marsden et al. (11) demonstrated that physiologic tremor can be increased by the administration of beta agonists and that this beta agonist-induced increase in tremor could be blocked by the prior administration of the beta antagonist propranolol. The increase in tremor was specifically related to beta receptors independent of vasodilatation. Although it is unclear exactly where these beta receptors are located, Young and Shahani (20) have suggested that they may be on the sensory region of small muscle fibers within the muscle spindle. The presence of a peripheral beta receptor, which when stimulated increases physiologic tremor to the degree that it becomes an action tremor, can in part explain the tremor seen in fright reactions, anxiety, pheochromocytoma, thyrotoxicosis, and in the therapy of asthma with beta agonists.

The usefulness of the beta receptor antagonist propranolol in essential tremor has been reported by several groups of investigators (3,17,18). Although there have been reports that propranolol is not effective in alleviating essential tremor (4,16), it has become increasingly clear that this beta blocker plays an important role in the treatment of this disorder. It is particularly useful in controlling intention tremor in the upper extremities and may make a significant difference to the patient in terms of being able to feed himself or to write legibly. This may be true even though propranolol may not abolish the tremor but may only markedly decrease its amplitude.

The efficacy of propranolol in essential tremor and the already described existence of a peripheral tremor mechanism that is dependent on beta adrenergic mechanisms raised the possibility that propranolol's effect on essential tremor was related to its peripheral pharmacologic activity. Young, Growdon, and Shahani (19) demonstrated that in patients with essential tremor the peripheral adrenergic tremor receptor mechanisms are intact. Intraarterial isoproterenol increased the amplitude of essential tremor in the injected limb with no effect on the contralateral limb, whereas intravenous or intraarterial propranolol prevented or acutely blocked the effect of isoproterenol. These investigators also demonstrated that intraarterial propranolol did not alter the amplitude or frequency of essential tremor. However, chronic oral propranolol in these same patients did have its expected efficacy in reducing tremor. Because the peripheral beta receptors were demonstrated to be blocked at a time when the essential tremor continued unchanged, it is suggested that propranolol's effect in essential tremor is mediated via central mechanisms. The role of central beta receptors in the CNS is very poorly defined at present.

Although propranolol is the treatment of choice in essential tremor, there are often markedly inconsistent therapeutic results. It has been suggested that these inconsistent results are related to individual variations in plasma levels after ingestion of the drug. Jefferson et al. (8) examined the dose–response relationship between tremor and plasma propranolol concentrations in 11 patients. Although there was a linear correlation between plasma propranolol concentration and ingested propranolol in a given patient, there was a very wide variation in plasma concentration among the patients for a given dose of propranolol. The study indicated that 7 of 11 patients improved at a plasma level of less than 20 ng/ml and that 9 of 11 patients improved at a plasma level of less than 40 ng/ml. The authors concluded that the effect of propranolol is not dose-dependent and that an effective plasma concentration can be achieved at low levels.

The critical difference between those patients who responded to propranolol and those who did not was not answered by this study.

The work of Sorensen and colleagues supports the observation that the plasma concentrations of propranolol are not correlated with suppression of essential tremor (15). In this study, 5 patients with essential tremor were given increasing doses of oral propranolol (up to 240 mg/day) and the percentage reduction of tremor was observed to be positively correlated with the daily dosage. The plasma propranolol levels varied widely and did not correlate with tremor reduction. In fact, all of the patients experienced measurable tremor reduction (20 to 68%) at a time when plasma propranolol could not be detected. These studies suggest that plasma drug levels are of little or no clinical use in the management of essential tremor patients. This is in contrast to the study of McAllister et al. (12), which demonstrated in an acute experiment that the intravenous administration of propranolol suppressed essential tremor and that the degree of suppression was directly correlated with the plasma propranolol concentration. However, the studies by Jefferson et al. (8) and Sorensen et al. (15) that examined the relationship between chronic oral propranolol and plasma concentration represent more accurate approximation of the clinical use of this drug than this acute intravenous study protocol.

There are certain groups of patients with essential tremor in whom the use of propranolol is contraindicated. This is particularly true for patients with chronic obstructive lung disease and asthma in whom the use of propranolol can precipitate dyspnea and wheezing. There have been two recent case reports illustrating this problem. In one case, a 65-year-old with chronic obstructive lung disease and essential tremor had marked amelioration of tremor with the administration of 160 mg/day of propranolol. However, this precipitated dyspnea on exertion and other respiratory symptoms. In the second case, a 37-year-old with asthma and essential tremor had the tremor ameliorated by propranolol at a dose of 150 to 200 mg/day. However, this precipitated markedly increased wheezing. In both these instances, the substitution of a different beta antagonist, metoprolol, resulted in amelioration of tremor and no return of bronchospastic symptoms (1,14).

Metoprolol is a beta receptor antagonist that is relatively selective in its action (predominant beta-1 blockade). Ljung (10) studied 22 patients with essential tremor and evaluated the usefulness of metoprolol and propranolol. This investigator reported that 19 of 22 patients had a favorable response to metoprolol (dose to 150 mg/day) and that this response occurred over a 4 to 12 month period. The 3 patients who did not respond to metoprolol also did not respond to propranolol.

Isoprenaline-induced exacerbation of tremor can be inhibited by premedication with propranolol; however, premedication with metoprolol will not inhibit this tremor exacerbation. This finding has been interpreted to suggest that the peripheral beta adrenergic mechanism in the forearm, discussed previously, is related to beta-2 receptor activity. The selective effect of beta antagonists on peripheral tremor as opposed to the consistent effect of beta antagonists on essential tremor is another piece of evidence that essential tremor is related to central mechanisms.

In further examinations of the effect of different beta antagonists on essential tremor, Jefferson et al. (9) investigated the effect of propranolol, sotalol, and atenolol in this disorder. Although the efficacy of propranolol has been strongly linked to beta-receptor antagonism, some investigators have suggested that its efficacy may be because of a less specific effect on membrane stabilization. In order to examine this, propranolol and sotalol were administered to patients. Sotalol is a nonselective beta antagonist that blocks both beta-1 and beta-2 receptors. Sotalol has no membrane stabilizing effects and, in addition, crosses the blood–brain barrier quite poorly. Sotalol and propranolol produced the same percent reduction in tremor in the 9 patients studied. In addition, atenolol (a selective beta-1 antagonist) in these same patients was demonstrated to be effective in reducing tremor but not as effective as either propranolol or sotalol. The authors concluded that since propranolol and sotalol induced equal tremor reduction, the membrane stabilizing effect of propranolol is not required to produce tremor reduction. Since a selective beta-1 antagonist produced less tremor reduction than nonselective beta antagonists, it was suggested that peripheral beta-2 receptors were involved in the mediation of essential tremor. Further studies of this nature with more selective beta antagonists will help to define the issue of beta-1 and beta-2 receptor involvement and the central or peripheral localization of these receptors.

It has been recognized that one of the features of the clinical history that an adult with essential tremor will often give is the salutary effect of alcohol on his tremor. In an attempt both to quantify the effect of alcohol on essential tremor and to delineate the possible site of ethanol action on the CNS in tremor amelioration, oral and intraarterial ethanol administration was examined in patients with essential tremor (5). These investigators again utilized the low dose intraarterial injection technique to attempt to study the isolated effect of a pharmacologic agent on peripheral tremor mechanisms. They demonstrated that local intraarterial injections of ethanol did not alter either the amplitude or the frequency of the oscillations seen in essential tremor. However, they also demonstrated that in these same patients oral ethanol (45 cc of 80-proof vodka in orange juice) produced an impressive decline in tremor within 10 to 15 min. It was concluded that, although the site of action within the CNS was not defined by their study, the study provided additional evidence that essential tremor originates from central mechanisms and not from peripheral ones.

There are, of course, action tremors that are much more influenced by peripheral tremor mechanisms. These have been alluded to previously in this chapter. In fact, essential tremor is undoubtedly also influenced to some degree by peripheral tremor mechanisms. This is demonstrated by the characteristic acute increase in symptomatology when these patients are anxious or are emotionally stressed. However, the pharmacologic evidence previously presented indicates that when peripheral tremor mechanisms are blocked, essential tremor continues, and this suggests a central origin for the tremor. The efficacy of chronic oral propranolol in essential tremor may, in fact, relate to its effect as a beta receptor blocker at both the central and peripheral beta receptors, the central effect being more responsible for overall suppression of tremor and the peripheral effect being responsible for preventing stress-induced exacerbation of the tremor.

BIBLIOGRAPHY AND *SELECTED REVIEW

1. Britt, C. W., and Peters, B. H. (1979): Metoprolol for essential tremor. *N. Engl. J. Med.*, 301:331.
2. Critchley, M. (1949): Observations on essential (heredofamilial) tremor. *Brain*, 72:113–139.
3. Dupont, E., Hansen, J. J., and Dalby, M. A. (1973): Treatment of benign essential tremor with propranolol. *Acta Neurol. Scand.*, 49:75–84.
4. Foster, J. B., Longley, B. P., and Stewart-Wynne, E. G. (1973): Propranolol in essential tremor. *Lancet*, 1:1455–1457.
5. Growdon, J. H., Shahani, B. T., and Young, R. R. (1975): The effect of alcohol on essential tremor. *Neurology (Minneap.)*, 25:259–262.
6. Herskovits, E., and Blackwood, W. (1960): Essential (familial, hereditary) tremor: A case report. *J. Neurol. Neurosurg. Psychiatry*, 32:504–511.
7. Hornabrook, R. W., and Nagurney, J. T. (1976): Essential tremor in Papua New Guinea. *Brain*, 99:659–667.
8. Jefferson, D., Jenner, P., and Marsden, C. D. (1979): Relationship between plasma propranolol levels and the clinical suppression of essential tremor. *Br. J. Clin. Pharmacol.*, 7:419–420.
9. Jefferson, D., Jenner, P., and Marsden, C. D. (1979): Beta adrenoreceptor antagonists in essential tremor. *J. Neurol. Psychiatr.*, 42:904–909.
10. Ljung, O. (1979): Treatment of essential tremor with metoprolol. *N. Engl. J. Med.*, 301:1005.
11. Marsden, C. D., Foley, T. H., Owen, D. A., and McAllister, R. G. (1966): Peripheral beta-adrenergic receptors concerned with tremor. *Clin. Sci.*, 33:53–65.
12. McAllister, R. G., Markesberg, W. R., Ware, R. W., and Howell, S. M. (1977): Suppression of essential tremor by propranolol: Correlation of effect with drug plasma levels and intensity of beta-adrenergic blockade. *Ann. Neurol.*, 1:160–166.
13. Mylle, G., and Von Bogaert, L. (1948): Dotreblement essential non familial. *Michr. Psychiat. Neurol.*, 115:80–90.
14. Riley, T., and Pleet, A. B. (1979): Metroprolol tartrate for essential tremor. *N. Engl. J. Med.*, 301:663.
15. Sorensen, P., Paulson, O. B., Steiness, E., and Jansen, E. C. (1981): Essential tremor treated with propanolol. *Ann. Neurol.*, 9:53–57.
16. Sweet, F. D., Blumberg, J., Lee, J. E., and McDowell, F. H. (1974): Propranolol treatment of essential tremor. *Neurology (Minneap.)*, 24:64–67.
17. Winkler, G. F., and Young, R. D. (1971): Propranolol: also for tremors. *Med. Wld. News*, 12:32.
18. Winkler, G. F., and Young, R. D. (1974): Efficacy of chronic propranolol therapy in action tremors of the familial, senile or essential varieties. *N. Engl. J. Med.*, 290:984–988.
19. Young, R. R., Growdon, J. H., and Shahani, B. T. (1975): Beta-adrenergic mechanisms in action tremor. *N. Engl. J. Med.*, 293:950–953.
*20. Young, R. R., and Shahani, B. T. (1979): Pharmacology of tremor. In: *Clinical Neuropharmacology, Vol. 4*, edited by H. L. Klawans, pp. 139–156. Raven Press, New York.

Chapter 10

Primary Writing Tremor

Over the last 10 years we have seen 6 patients, each with a chief complaint of difficulty in handwriting because of a tremor and each manifested a tremor related to the activation of specific muscles. The patients ranged in age from 16 to 42 years and the tremor was first noted at ages ranging from 8 to 54. In 2 patients the tremor was bilateral whereas in the other 4 it was exclusively right sided. None of the patients gave a history of similar involvement in other family members nor a history of encephalitis. Two had a history of perinatal hypoxia that could have been an etiologic factor. None of the 6 had any tremor at rest, 3 had a slight degree of postural tremor with the hand held in front of the body in the standard position and 3 had a very mild terminal intention tremor. All 6 had a gross sustained tremor that included a marked pronation/supination component that could be precipitated by either pronation of the wrist or forceful abduction of the fingers or both.

In all 6 patients the chief complaint was difficulty with handwriting. Patients with segmental dystonia (writer's cramp) present with difficulty in handwriting and can manifest myoclonic jerks on writing. However, none of these patients had any evidence of dystonia, and the abnormal movement was a rhythmic tremor in all. Rhythmic segmental myoclonus has been reported with a variety of lesions of the spinal cord, but the myoclonus in such patients occurs spontaneously and is not related to specific muscle activity. Several previous reports have described patients in whom specific muscle activity brought out a rhythmic tremor. Rothwell et al. described 1 patient with primary writing tremor in whom activity of the pronator teres caused a gross tremor but the patient's tremor lasted only a few seconds (2). Motor point anesthesia of the pronator teres abolished the tremor. Rondot, Korn, and Scherrer described a series of 25 patients with postural tremor of an entire limb, which was initiated by particular posture and could be relieved by selective anesthesia of the "inductor," a "pacemaker" muscle (1). In their study the most likely pacemaker muscles were the teres major (6 cases), infraspinatus (4 cases), biceps (5 cases), and triceps (2 cases). Unfortunately the clinical features of these patients were not described in any detail. The 6 patients, like the 1 patient of Rothwell et al., and the 25 patients of Rondot et al., were all characterized by the fact that specific muscle activity elicited the tremor that, in all but the 1 patient of Rothwell et al., persisted as long as the activity was sustained. This plus these authors' experience with motor point anesthesia suggests that proprioceptive muscle spindle input is necessary to elicit the tremor.

While having none of the characteristics of a parkinsonian tremor, these patients have some resemblance to benign essential tremor. A tremor that is present on action and maintains a posture is characteristic of this disorder and can certainly affect handwriting. The relationship of the tremor to specific activity as described here is not characteristic of benign essential tremor nor is the coarse nature of the tremor with prominent pronation/supination of the wrist.

The pharmacology of the tremor described here is also different than the pharmacology of benign essential tremor. The latter frequently improves with propanolol (See Chapter 9) and is unaffected by central cholinergic manipulation. The patients described here were not improved by propanolol but clearly were affected by cholinergic and anticholinergic agents. When given acutely, benztropine or scopolamine produce a markedly beneficial effect that was rapidly reversed by physostigmine. Long-term anticholinergic agents (usually benztropine) had a definitely beneficial effect.

BIBLIOGRAPHY

1. Rondot, M. D., Korn, H., Scherrer, J. (1968): Suppression of an entire limb tremor by anesthetizing a selective muscular group. *Arch. Neurol.*, 19:412–429.
2. Rothwell, J. C., Traub, M. M., Marsden, C. D. (1979): Primary writing tremor. *J. Neurol. Neurosurg. Psychiatry*, 42:1106–1114.

Chapter 11

Spasticity

Spasticity is defined as an abnormality in muscle tone which can be demonstrated as increasing muscular resistance to passive stretch. Classically this increasing resistance reaches a maximum, at which point it releases suddenly. This is the so-called clasp-knife response. Associated with the increased tone, there may also be paresis, increased deep tendon reflexes, and the presence of pathological reflexes. This simple description of spasticity belies the complexities of both its clinical meaning and its pathophysiology. A recent review article has stressed that the term "spasticity" may have up to six separate meanings depending on which clinical aspect of the abnormal muscle tone and related clinical findings are being described (7). Although the clinical definition can be belabored, it is important to recognize that spasticity is seen in a wide variety of neurologic conditions and, because of this, a uniform pathophysiologic or pharmacologic approach to the subject is hindered.

The anatomic substrate that is the final organizational level for the production of spasticity exists within the spinal cord. Suprasegmental lesions that involve descending pathways (most typically descending motor pathways) result in the pathophysiologic state that can produce spasticity by interaction with segmental spinal cord components. The segmental volitional motor organization that can become the substrate for the production of spasticity involves the interplay of the alpha and gamma motor neuron loops, the spinal cord interneurons, and the synaptic connections between these elements and the descending pathways. Many of these complex neurophysiologic relationships have recently been reviewed. The suprasegmental lesions that produce spasticity obviously involve altered function of these pathways, and this altered function in pharmacologic terms might involve alterations in transmitter uptake, release, synthesis, or storage. In addition, it is well described in the clinical literature that the development of spasticity may involve the passage of time, and this fact makes it reasonable that changes in neuronal receptor-site responses may also play a role in the evolution and production of spasticity. Since acetylcholine, serotonin, norepinephrine, and GABA have all been described as neurotransmitters in the spinal cord, and since these same pharmacologically active substances have also been described as neurotransmitters in the brain, and because there are additional putative neurotransmitters in the spinal cord (asparate, glutamate, glycine), a unifying approach to the pharmacology of spasticity is difficult.

Because there is no known specific neurotransmitter alteration that is responsible for spasticity, the pharmacologic agents that have been employed to treat spasticity will be discussed in relationship to their presumed sites of action. It should be recognized at the onset of this discussion that the segmental motor organization which is responsible for spasticity and which is the organization that pharmacologic therapy will attempt to interfere with is also the same motor organization that is responsible for normal volitional activity. Interference with spasticity may also interfere with normal motor activity. Overall, despite some decrease in elements of the spasticity syndrome produced by these agents, there is usually not an increase in motor strength.

Before discussing the three agents (diazepam, balclofen, and dantrolene) that are commonly used to treat spasticity, several general statements regarding neurotransmitter interaction at the segmental level are in order. These statements will provide background for understanding the proposed pharmacologic mechanism of these drugs. Afferent (Ia) nerve fiber from muscle spindle enters the spinal cord and can be involved in at least three, if not more, synaptic connections. These fibers can synape with alpha motor neurons (monosynaptic reflex) and provide an excitatory (depolarizing) stimulus. In this instance substance P is thought to be the responsible transmitter. The Ia afferents may excite interneurons that in turn form axo-axonic synapses on other Ia fibers to their evolving on the alpha motor neuron (presynaptic). This circuitry provides for presynaptic inhibition of the Ia fibers. The transmitter believed to be involved in the mediation of this event is GABA. A third possible synaptic connection for the terminating Ia fiber is with interneurons that in turn inhibit the corresponding antagonist muscle. There are undoubtedly other Ia circuits that are also involved in normal segmental physiology. The use of pharmacologic agents to alter segmental physiology will hopefully be expanded or improved as selective pharmacologic interference with these various transmitter-mediated events become possible.

BENZODIAZEPINES

These agents, particularly diazepam, are widely employed in the treatment of spasticity. Although they are acknowledged as having clinical efficacy, it is unclear exactly what their primary mechanism of action is and where its anatomic substrate is located. The benzodiazepines have been thought to have suprasegmental effects since they produce drowsiness, act as anticonvulsants, and have anxiolytic effects. It has been postulated that the efficacy of these agents in spasticity is related to suppression of descending pathways. On the other hand, there is evidence that diazepam increases primary afferent depolarization by enhancing presynaptic inhibition in the spinal cord. Since presynaptic inhibition in the spinal cord is related to the transmitter GABA, an interaction between diazepam and GABA is postulated. The molecular basis of the diazepam–GABA interaction is complex and this interaction is described more thoroughly in Chapter 23. However, this mechanism of action for benzodiazepines in spasticity relates it specifically to the segmental spinal cord organizational level. In addition, it has also been proposed that diazepam may have a direct effect on the contractile mechanism of muscle. It is, of course, possible that diazepam may affect spasticity both by suprasegmental suppression of descending pathways and interneuron pools and by segmental increases in presynaptic inhibition at the spinal cord level. This would explain some of the conflicting clinical evidence as to the effect of diazepam in complete and incomplete spinal cord lesions.

BACLOFEN

Interest in GABA-like compounds to treat spasticity developed because of the role of GABA in increasing presynaptic inhibition. If presynaptic inhibition is increased, then the excitatory influences on the alpha motor neuron pool are decreased. This results in reduced outflow from these neurons and subsequent reduction in muscle tone. Since GABA does not cross the blood-brain barrier, a lysophilic GABA derivative beta-(4-chlorophenyl)-GABA (baclofen) was developed (Fig. 1). This compound has been demonstrated to have clinical efficacy in the treatment of spasticity in patients with both complete and incomplete spinal cord lesions. This finding has led to the interpretation that at least some of the antispastic activity of baclofen is related to its action in the spinal cord, although there is no doubt that baclofen also has pharmacologic effects on suprasegmental regions of the CNS since it produces drowsiness and lethargy—subtle, sometimes uncomfortable mental changes—and has an effect on partial dystonias (spasmodic torticollis and levodopa-related dystonias).

Initially baclofen's mechanism of action on spasticity was related to suppression of alpha motor neurons, suppression of gamma motor neurons, reduction of post-tetanic potentiation, or facilitation of the Renshaw inhibitory loop. The success of baclofen in relieving spasticity seems to support its structure–activity relationship to GABA; however, it became apparent that whether GABA and baclofen share common mechanisms of action was open to doubt. The administration of baclofen does not alter endogenous levels of GABA. The iontophoretic application of GABA and baclofen to various spinal cord neurons depresses the spontaneous firing rate of these cells. However, the GABA antagonist bicuculline can abolish GABA-induced suppression of these neurons, whereas it does not abolish the baclofen-induced suppression. In addition, GABA and baclofen appear to have different physiologic effects when the primary afferent terminals in the spinal cord are

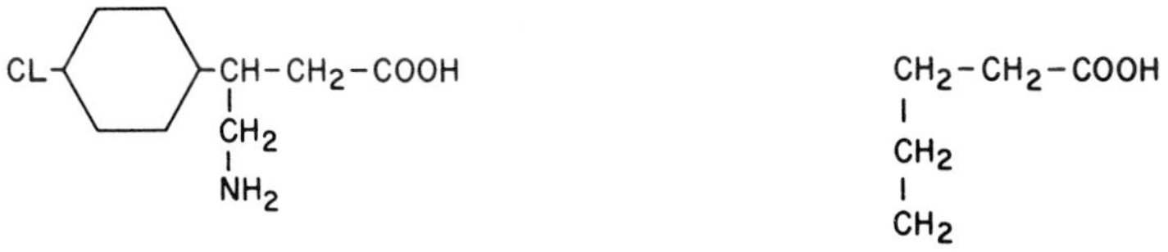

FIG. 1. Structure of baclofen (chlorophenyl GABA).

examined. GABA depolarizes these structures and baclofen hyperpolarizes them. These findings indicate that baclofen and GABA probably do not share the same mechanism of action.

There has been some discussion that baclofen's mechanism of action involves interaction with substance P. Substance P is an excitatory peptide that has been postulated to be the neurotransmitter released by the primary afferent fiber on the alpha motor neurons. If baclofen antagonized substance P by hyperpolarizing the primary afferent terminals, then this could explain its mechanism of action in spasticity. The interaction of substance P and baclofen remains speculative, and there is evidence that in fact no such direct antagonism exists.

Baclofen is clinically effective in relieving some of the components of the spasticity syndrome in patients. It has both suprasegmental and segmental pharmacologic effects, although it is currently believed that its effect in relief of spasticity is related to its effect on primary afferent terminals at the segmental level.

DANTROLENE

Dantrolene represents an entirely different pharmacologic approach to the treatment of spasticity. The drugs discussed previously had central effects that were thought to mediate their antispastic activities. Dantrolene's effectiveness in treating spasticity has been related to its effect on excitation–contraction coupling in muscle. Dantrolene is thought to interfere with the release of calcium from the sarcoplasmic reticulum. This action interferes with the contractile mechanism and thereby less tension develops in the muscle. This mechanism of action obviously has potential for interference with normal motor activity. Dantrolene has been reported to have several side effects including the induction of abnormal liver tests, and the question of drug-induced fatal hepatitis has been raised.

MISCELLANEOUS AGENTS OF THEORETICAL INTEREST

Glycine

Glycine is a pharmacologically active amino acid that passes the blood–brain barrier and that has been demonstrated to play an important role in segmental postsynaptic inhibition in the spinal cord. Glycine hyperpolarizes motor neurons and interneurons (3,11) and therefore depresses spasticity. Although the concentration of lumbar spinal cord glycine in patients with spasticity is unchanged (2), there is some evidence in animals that spasticity is associated with decreased glycine turnover (6). However, at the present time there have been only brief trials of glycine in spastic patients. These reports have claimed some success with glycine in the treatment of spasticity (1,10).

Thymoxamine

One of the descending bulbospinal pathways that terminates near the alpha motor neuron is thought to be noradrenergic. Since there is some evidence that noradrenergic spinal cord mechanisms are important to normal motor function, and since there is also evidence that there is increased fusimotor activity, which may in part be noradrenergically mediated in spasticity, a trial of thymoxamine, an alpha-adrenergic antagonist, was undertaken. Mai (8) studied 35 patients with spasticity and evaluated both clinical and electrical parameters of this syndrome before and after the acute intravenous administration of this agent. Since the acute effect of the drug was to ameliorate components of spasticity, the author concluded that alpha adrenergic mechanisms at both a suprasegmental and a segmental level were involved in the pathophysiology of spasticity.

Phenytoin

Although phenytoin is not useful clinically in the therapeutics of spasticity, a recent case report details an unusual toxic reaction to the administration of this drug. Stark (9) reported that a young patient with epilepsy who received an excessive dose of phenytoin developed, in addition to the usual signs of toxicity, increased muscular tone, clasp-knife response, increased deep tendon reflexes, and sustained clonus at both ankles. The original phenytoin level was approximately three times higher than the therapeutic level, and when the phenytoin level fell the signs of "spasticity" resolved. This unusual case report, although not helpful in understanding the pharmacology of spasticity, does serve as a reminder that the components of the spasticity syndrome can be organized on presumably normal anatomic substrates.

At the present time all agents used to treat spasticity share the problem that although they may alleviate some of the components of the syndrome, they all can potentially interfere with useful motor function. In addition, in all the clinical trials of these agents there has never been clear demonstration that the antispastic drugs improve functional motor activity, although it is clear that the alleviation of flexor spasms, painful spasms, and uncontrolled clonus can certainly benefit patients.

BIBLIOGRAPHY AND *SELECTED REVIEWS

1. Barbeau, A. (1974): Preliminary study of glycine administration in patients with spasticity. *Neurology (Minneap.)*, 24:392.
2. Boehme, D. H., Marks, N., and Fordice, M. W. (1976): Glycine levels in the degenerated human spinal cord. *J. Neurol. Sci.*, 27:347–352.
3. Bruggencate, G. T., and Engberg, I. (1968): Analysis of glycine actions on spinal interneurones by intracellular recording. *Brain Res.*, 11:446–450.
*4. Calne, D. B. (1975): Drug treatment of spasticity and rigidity. In: *Modern Trends in Neurology*, Vol. 6, edited by D. Williams, pp. 205–222. Butterworth, London.
*5. Davidoff, R. A. (1978): Pharmacology of spasticity. *Neurology (Minneap.)*, 28:246–251.
6. Hall, P. V., Smith, J. E., Lane, J., Mote, T., and Campbell, R. (1979): Glycine and experimental spinal spasticity. *Neurology (Minneap.)*, 29:262–266.
7. Landau, W. M. (1974): Spasticity: The fable of a neurological demon and the emperor's new therapy. *Arc. Neurol.*, 31:217–219.
8. Mai, J. (1978): Depression of spasticity by alpha-adrenergic blockade. *Acta Neurol. Scand.*, 57:65–76.
9. Stark, R. J. (1979): Spasticity due to phenytoin toxicity. *Med. J. Aust.*, 1:156–158.
10. Stern, P., and Bokonjic, R. (1974): Glycine therapy in 7 cases of spasticity. A pilot study. *Pharmacology*, 12:117–119.

11. Werman, R., Davidoff, R. A., and Aprison, M. H. (1968): Inhibitory action of glycine on spinal neurons in the cat. *J. Neurophysiol.*, 31:81–95.
12. Young, R. R., and Delwaide, P. J. (1981): Spasticity. *N. Engl. J. Med.*, 304:28–33.
13. Young, R. R., and Delwaide, P. J. (1981): Spasticity. *N. Engl. J. Med.*, 304:96–99.

Chapter 12

Myotonia

Myotonia is a delay in relaxation of a muscle or part of a muscle after voluntary forceful contraction or mechanical percussion. The prolonged muscle contraction is secondary to repetitive sarcolemmal depolarizations, which have a characteristic decrescendo pattern on electromyography. Myotonia as a symptom occurs in a large number of different disease states (see Table 1). Of these, myotonic muscular dystrophy (myotonia dystrophica, Steinert's disease, myotonia atrophica, MMD) is the most common and best studied.

The electrophysiologic basis of clinical myotonia is the repetitive discharge of single motor units. This repetitive firing often begins with a crescendo and characteristically ends in a decrescendo of both frequency and voltage amplitude. An EMG finding of myotonia is of considerable diagnostic value, but it is of limited value in following the course of the disease since the correlation between electrophysiologic myotonia and pharmacologic efficacy is very limited.

The diagnosis of myotonia requires both the occurrence of clinical manifestations and positive EMG evidence and excludes both prolonged muscle shortening without muscle action potentials, as seen in myxedema and McArdle's disease, and persistent muscle action potentials with significantly prolonged muscle contraction, as can be seen in denervation or polymyositis. Prolonged muscle contractions owing to neural stimulation such as tetanus, spasticity, and stiffman syndrome are also excluded.

The defect in myotonia appears to be sarcolemmal since the tendency toward repetitive sarcolemmal depolarization persists despite pharmacologic blockade of neural impulses with curare (4). The slow relaxation characteristic of myotonia is attributable primarily to the repetitive sarcolemmal depolarizations, which result

TABLE 1. *Forms of myotonia in man*

Myotonic muscular dystrophy
Myotonia congenita
Paramyotonia congenita with or without periodic paralysis
Chondrodystrophic myotonia (Schwartz-Jampel)
Drug-induced myotonia

in persistent muscle contraction. The resting membrane potential of muscle cells in patients with MMD has been shown to be low, although it is normal in patients with myotonia congenita (6). This change is probably not related to the myotonia since the critical depolarization (the amount of depolarization necessary to initiate an action potential) is normal (7). In myotonia congenita the chloride conductance of the muscle fibers is decreased and the potassium conductance is raised (1). It is generally believed that decreased chloride conductance is the basic defect that underlies the unstable myotonic membrane in this disorder and certain drug-induced myotonias (2).

Assuming that myotonia is caused by some alteration in muscle membrane physiology, which produces muscle fibers that are hypersensitive to mechanical, electrical, and chemical stimuli, any therapeutic agent that would restore the membrane toward normal should be an effective form of therapy. Such agents could act by altering ratios of intracellular to extracellular ions or by "stabilizing" the muscle membrane by some direct physiochemical means (13). It should be noted that the agents that are of value in the treatment of myotonia are a form of symptomatic therapy which acts only on the myotonia. The dystrophy of MMD is not relieved and continues to progress. The drugs used in the treatment of myotonia are listed in Table 2.

Quinine. The efficacy of quinine was originally thought to be due to a CNS effect of quinine but is now thought to be due to a direct membrane stabilizing effect on muscle membrane. The clinical efficacy of quinine is severely limited by a large number of side effects. Various minor side effects are common and result in low patient tolerance. These include nausea and vomiting, tinnitus, visual disturbances, confusion, and headache. These troublesome symptoms are all dose-dependent and result in a very low therapeutic index for quinine. As a result of these and other more serious but less common problems, quinine is now little used in myotonia. The major toxic side effects include vasculitis, bone marrow depression, retinal edema, nephropathy, and especially enhancement of the preexisting cardiac conduction defects that are frequent in MMD.

The effective dose of quinine in myotonia is highly variable. Symptomatic improvement is usually seen at a dosage level of 300 to 600 mg three to four times daily. After a single oral dose, peak plasma levels are reached in 1 to 3 hr.

TABLE 2. *Drugs that improve myotonia*

Myotonia-reducing drug	Mechanism of action
Quinine and quinidine	Increased refractory period
Procainamide	Decreased ionic permeability of sarcolemma
Phenytoin	Membrane stabilization, perhaps owing to increased sodium efflux

Procainamide. On the basis of the observation that procainamide reduces the repetitive firing of cardiac muscle, Geschwind and Simpson suggested that it might play a role in the treatment of myotonia (3). Given intravenously, procainamide was shown to ameliorate clinical myotonia. Since this original demonstration, numerous studies have confirmed the efficacy of procainamide in the treatment of myotonia.

Once again, minor but disturbing side effects are very common, dose-related, and severely limit patient acceptance. These include a characteristic, persistent bitter taste, anorexia, nausea, vomiting, flushing, hypotension, insomnia, emotional lability, and, rarely, hallucinations. Major but less common side effects include bone marrow depression, a lupus-like syndrome, and an intensification of preexisting cardiac conduction defects similar to that seen with quinine (12).

Following oral ingestion, peak plasma levels are reached in 1 hr. Procainamide is primarily excreted unchanged in the urine. In patients with normal renal function the biological half-life is approximately 3 to 4 hr. As with quinine, the dose necessary to produce clinical improvement shows a great deal of patient-to-patient variation. Most patients show significant clinical improvement on 3 to 4 g daily in divided doses. Current evidence suggests that procainamide must be given at least every 4 hr and preferably every 3 hr to maintain stable therapeutic plasma concentration (9).

Phenytoin. In 1967, Munsat suggested that phenytoin, a compound that has membrane-stabilizing activity, might be effective in myotonia (8). In a randomized double-blind crossover study of phenytoin, procainamide, and placebo, phenytoin was found to be as effective in relieving myotonia in MMD as procainamide. Phenytoin has the further advantage that it may in fact reduce the preexisting defects in cardiac conduction, which are often made worse by procainamide or quinine. Phenytoin is effective in myotonia at its usual anticonvulsant dosages and therapeutic blood levels. With such dosage, the efficacy of phenytoin in myotonia closely parallels that of procainamide, but phenytoin has a much more favorable therapeutic index. This results in a definite increase in ability of patients to take effective doses with many fewer and milder side effects. The efficacy of phenytoin has also been shown in myotonia congenita (15). In this form of myotonia the mechanism of action of phenytoin may be reversal of altered chloride conductance (2).

DRUG-INDUCED MYOTONIA

A number of pharmacologic agents are capable of inducing a syndrome in man that is similar if not identical to the myotonia that occurs in various disease states (Table 3). Most of these agents are either drugs used to reduce blood cholesterol such as 20-25 diazacholesterol (DAC) and triparanol, or monocarboxylic aromatic acids such as clofibrate (10,11,14,16).

DAC is an azosterol that was introduced in the 1960s for the treatment of hypercholesterolemia. It was soon discovered that DAC induced in some patients a myotonic syndrome characterized by features seen in clinical myotonia such as

TABLE 3. *Drugs that cause myotonia*

Hypocholestereschemic agents
   20-25 Diazacholesterol (DAC)
   Triparanol
Aromatic monocarboxylic acids
   Clofibrate
Miscellaneous agents
   Vincristine (1 case, relationship unclear)
   Propranolol (1 case, relationship unclear)

difficulty in relaxing the grip, percussion myotonia, EMG evidence of myotonia, and weakness, as well as other features reminiscent of MMD such as cataracts. Because of the high incidence of this syndrome, DAC is no longer used clinically. It is not of interest that a variety of DAC congeners are also able to elicit myotonia.

DAC-induced myotonia is of course not directly due to the ability of DAC to reduce elevated serum cholesterol to normal. DAC is believed to derive its anti-hypercholesteremic effect by inhibiting a specific enzyme that is necessary for the endogenous synthesis of Δ24-reductase. As a result of this blockade, the metabolic precursor to cholesterol, desmosterol (24-dehydrocholesterol), builds up in the plasma, erythrocytes, and more importantly muscle membrane. This accumulation of desmosterol replaces cholesterol in the sarcolemma and causes myotonia. Myotonia appears when approximately 50% of the cholesterol molecules in the sarcolemma are replaced by desmosterol. This can be brought about by either acute or chronic DAC treatment. This alteration of sarcolemma sterol content is associated with a marked decrease in membrane chloride conductance—the same physiological feature that occurs in myotonia congenita. This in turn causes the repetitive muscle action potentials that account for the delayed reaction of voluntary muscles similar to that observed in the myotonic diseases (11).

The reduction in chloride conductance is a direct result of demosterol replacement of cholesterol in the sarcolemmal membrane. The induced alteration in chloride conductance may be related to either decreased stability of the chloride channels or decreased solubility of chloride carriers. In either case, the decrease in chloride conductance results in repetitive action potentials that manifest themselves clinically as myotonia (10).

Triparanol was also used clinically for the treatment of hypercholesterolemia and, like DAC, is believed to act by selective inhibition of the reductase enzyme which, of course, results in the accumulation of desmosterol in plasma, erthrocyte, and muscle membrane. Unlike DAC, prolonged treatment with triparanol is required to induce myotonia. Triparanol is no longer used clinically because of the high incidence of cataracts and skin reactions.

Clomiphene, an antiestrogenic agent used clinically to induce ovulation, is chemically related to triparanol and causes the accumulation of desmosterol in various tissues, presumably by blocking the activity of Δ24-reductase. There is no evidence that it can induce myotonia, however.

A wide variety of aromatic monocarboxylic acids are capable of inducing myotonia in man or experimental animals. Clofibrate is the most clinically significant of these since it is used widely to reduce serum triglyceride levels despite its ability to induce myotonia. Other agents of this class capable of causing myotonia include indole acetic acid, indole ethanol (the precursor of indole acetic acid), and the herbicide 2,4 D (2,4-dichlorophenoxyacetic acid).

The mechanism by which these agents induce myotonia is not as well defined as the inhibition of Δ24-reductase by DAC and triparanol. These agents do, however, decrease chloride conductance in a manner which is qualitatively similar to that seen in both myotonia congenita and myotonia induced by Δ24-reductase inhibitors (2). The pathogenesis of this alteration is different, however. The agents may in some way bind to the sarcolemmal chloride carrier or to the outer rim of the chloride conductance channel. In either case, the resulting steric interference with the conductance of chloride results in myotonia. The observation that these agents can induce myotonia *in vitro* further supports the notion of a direct membrane effect. Phenytoin reverses both the myotonia and the alteration in chloride conductance caused by aromatic monocarboxylic acids (2).

Single cases of both vincristine- and propanolol-induced myotonia have been published. In both instances a definite causal relationship is unproven. It is quite possible that subclinical myotonia may have been present in both patients before treatment.

There are also a number of reports in the literature of either respiratory depression or abnormal muscular relaxation in myotonic patients given general anesthesia, and it has even been suggested that MMD patients are unusually sensitive to thiopentone. This abnormal sensitivity is not, however, clearly established and, like the reported anesthetic complications, may be primarily related not to the myotonia itself but to weakness of respiratory musculature or cardiopulmonary disease (5).

BIBLIOGRAPHY AND *SELECTED REVIEWS

1. Barchi, R. L. (1975): Myotonia. An evaluation of the chloride hypothesis. *Arch. Neurol.*, 32:175–180.
2. Furman, R. E., and Barchi, R. L. (1978): The pathophysiology of myotonia produced by aromatic carboxylic acids. *Ann. Neurol.*, 4:357–364.
3. Geschwind, N., and Simpson, J. A. (1955): Procainamide in the treatment of myotonia. *Brain*, 78:81–91.
4. Hoffman, W. W., Alston, W., and Rowe, G. (1966): A study of individual neuromuscular junctions in myotonia. *Electroencephalogr. Clin. Neurophysiol.*, 21:521–537.
5. Kaufman, L. (1960): Anesthesia in dystrophia myotonia: a review of the hazards of anesthesia. *Proc. Soc. Med.*, 53:183–188.
6. Lipicky, R. J. (1977): Studies in human myotonic dystrophy. In: *Pathogenesis of Human Muscular Dystrophies*, edited by L. P. Rowland, pp. 729–738. Excerpta Medica, Amsterdam.
7. McComas, A. J., and Mrozek, K. (1968): The electrical properties of muscle fiber membranes in dystrophia mytonica and montonia congenita. *J. Neurol. Neurosurg. Psychiatry*, 31:441–447.
8. Munsat, T. L. (1967): Therapy of myotonia. *Neurology*, 17:359–367.
*9. Munsat, T. L., and Scherfe, R. T. (1979): Myotonia. In: *Clinical Neuropharmacology, Vol. 4*, edited by H. L. Klawans. pp. 83–108. Raven Press, New York.

10. Peter, J. B., Campion, D. S., Dromgoole, S. H., Nagatoma, T., and Andiman, R. M. (1975): Similarities and differences between human myotonia and drug-induced myotonia in rats. In: *Recent Advances in Myology*, edited by W. G. Bradley, D. Gardner-Medwin, and J. N. Walton, pp. 434–440. Excerpta Medica, Amsterdam.

11. Peter, J. B., and Fiehn, W. (1973): Diazacholesterol myotonia: accumulation of desmosteral and increased adenosine triphosphate activity of sarcolemma. *Science*, 179:910–912.

12. Prockop, L. D. (1966): Myotonia, procaine amide, and lupus-like syndrome. *Arch. Neurol.*, 14:326–330.

13. Roses, A. D., Butterfield, A., Appel, S. H., and Chestnut, O. B. (1975): Phenytoin and membrane fluidity in myotonic dystrophy. *Arch. Neurol.*, 32:535–538.

14. Rudel, R. (1976): The mechanism of pharmacologically induced myotonia. In: *Membranes and Disease*, edited by L. Bolis, J. F. Hoffman, and A. Leaf, pp. 207–213. Raven Press, New York.

15. Thompsen, C. E. (1972): Diphenylhydantoin for myotonia congenita. *N. Engl. J. Med.*, 289:893.

16. Winer, N., Klachko, D. M., Baer, R. D., Langley, P. L., and Burns, T. W. (1966): Myotonic response induced by inhibitors of cholesterol biosynthesis. *Science*, 153:312–313.

Chapter 13

Stiff Person Syndrome

Stiff person syndrome (SPS) is a rare clinical disorder characterized by increased muscular stiffness and involuntary spasms that was first described by Moersch and Woltman (7). In a truly remarkable display of restraint, the initial patient in their original series was seen in 1924, and it was not until 1956 and 13 patients later that the full clinical syndrome was reported by them. The disorder initially presents with symptoms of stiffness, tightness, and rigidity as well as with intermittent spasms of the involved muscles. In almost all cases reported, there was a gradual onset with slow progression of signs and symptoms. Neurologic examination is normal except for the finding of persistent, marked increase in muscle tone. The muscle tone is most unusual and has been described as "feeling like stone." Superimposed on this increased tone are intermittent, painful muscular spasms. These spasms may occur spontaneously or may be induced by sudden noises, passive or active movement of the involved muscles, emotional upsets, or tactile stimuli. The spasms themselves are associated with increased tone, pain, tachycardia, and profuse sweating. The pattern of muscle involvement is symmetric, proximal, and usually begins in the legs and back with subsequent spread. The most severely affected muscles are those of the back and abdomen. Functional difficulties related to the increased muscle tone are reflected in severe problems of motor mobility. The face is usually spared, although dysphagias may be a problem. There is no known familial incidence, and the syndrome usually presents between ages 30 and 60. In the rare case that has come to neuropathologic examination, there have been no obvious CNS lesions (1).

The etiology of the syndrome remains entirely unknown. Laboratory investigations have tried to establish a link between the increased muscle tone and impaired carbohydrate metabolism or thyroid dysfunction. Neither of these two metabolic problems is clearly related to this syndrome. Although CSF abnormalities have not been previously reported, a recent case report of CSF studies in a single patient with SPS indicates that although total protein is normal, the IgG is increased. Although there was no CSF pleocytosis, the authors suggested that this elevation of IgG might indicate a subacute inflammatory process (5). Replication of the finding reported and extensive further investigation are required. The most valuable clinical laboratory examinations in this syndrome have been muscle biopsy, nerve conduction velocities, and electromyographic studies. In all instances, nerve conduction velocities have been reported to be normal. Routine biopsy has never revealed any changes distinctive of a primary muscle disorder. EMG evidence and histochemical studies have also not revealed any primary muscle involvement. The EMG reveals a characteristic electrical abnormality. There is constant activity of motor unit potentials in involved muscles similar to the firing pattern seen in normal muscle during volitional activity or postural contraction. This firing persists despite conscious effort to relax the involved muscles. There is no evidence from the EMG of fibrillations or fasciculations, and the motor unit potentials are of normal configuration. Neurophysiologic investigations have resulted in the finding that general anesthesia, spinal anesthesia, peripheral nerve block, and the use of depolarizing or hyperpolarizing neuromuscular blockers will all decrease tone prior to interference with and paralysis of volitional muscle activity.

Hypotheses related to the etiology of SPS have centered on suprasegmental and spinal cord segmental organizational levels. The wide range of theories available reflect the current lack of understanding of the basic pathophysiology and the apparent absence of CNS pathological lesions. As a starting point, it is apparent that the increased muscle tone has a final organizational pathway in the anterior horn cell and its motor unit. This is recognized because selective peripheral motor nerve blockade and myoneural blocking agents will reduce the increased tone. However, there is no clinical, histochemical, or electrical evidence that an abnormality of the anterior horn cell exists. In addition, the volitional or passive movement of an affected muscle will often result in activation and increased tone in uninvolved muscles. This latter phenomenon supports the concept that segmental or suprasegmental organizational components are involved in the pathophysiology of this syndrome. A pharmacologic analysis of this syndrome must attempt to synthesize the organizational components apparently implicated with the therapeutic knowledge that diazepam is a truly remarkable treatment (3).

Diazepam, although effective as a therapeutic agent, lacks a precisely defined pharmacologic mechanism of action. There is no question that diazepam has both suprasegmental and segmental influence. If SPS is related to descending suprasegmental influences, then it is possible that diazepam's ability to suppress suprasegmental neuronal pools may be its mechanism of action in this syndrome. Although there are no data with regard to any specific central neurotransmitter deficiency, excess, or imbalance, there are some data with regard to urinary metabolites of norepinephrine. 3-Methoxy-4-hydroxyphenylglycol (MHPG) in the urine is thought to be derived from central norepinephrine catabolism. Schmidt et al. (10) reported in a single patient that urinary MHPG excretion rates were elevated in SPS and that the degree of elevation correlated with severity of symptoms. In addition, diazepam's therapeutic efficacy in this instance was correlated with decreased MHPG excretion. This preliminary evidence could support the concept that SPS is related to increased activity of descending noradrenergic systems. Nutt et al. (8) have provided an additional piece of evidence regarding altered nonadrenergic function in this syndrome. They reported that the plasma and CSF of a patient with SPS who was off medication had abnormally high concentrations of norepinephrine. It is of note that in this same patient other centrally active substances and catabolic products including HVA, 5-HIAA, GABA, glycine, and substance P were all normal in the CSF. However, diazepam is also known to have segmental pharmacologic influences. Diazepam increases primary afferent depolarization by its effect on presynaptic inhibition. Spinal cord presynaptic inhibition is believed to be mediated by GABA, and therefore diazepam is believed to interact with GABA systems (see Chapter 10 for further discussion of this issue). This, of course, could explain diazepam's efficacy in SPS. However, it does not aid in understanding the basic pathophysiology since it does not absolutely delimit the pathophysiologic process to the segmental level insofar as whatever phenomenon is disturbing the anterior horn cell pool could be beneficially affected by this proposed action on primary afferent depolarization.

At the segmental level, other transmitter abnormalities have been proposed to account for the apparent increase in activity of the anterior horn cells. These include loss of recurrent inhibition (acetylcholine) and loss of inhibitory interneuron (glycine) activity. Schmidt et al. (10) administered physostigmine to a patient with SPS in an attempt to enhance central cholinergic influences. They reported no effect and concluded that cholinergic synapses were not involved in SPS. Since glycine is believed to be a postsynaptic inhibitory transmitter utilized by spinal interneurons, a decrease in glycinergic activity might relate to increased anterior horn cell activity. The administration of glycine to patients with SPS did not have clinical efficacy, and the glycine hypothesis is not believed to be pivotal (4,10).

Attempts at manipulating other neurotransmitter systems have also not been particularly helpful. Increasing serotonergic influence was examined in a single patient without result (4). Manipulation of the nonadrenergic systems has also been evaluated in a single patient (8). Thymoxamine, an alpha-adrenergic antagonist, ameliorated muscle rigidity and spasms but produced sedation as well. The use of propanolol for low-dose, beta-adrenergic antagonism produced no clinical effect. Levodopa administration, on the other hand, has been reported to increase muscular tone and spasms (2,4,10). Although this last finding is not useful therapeutically, it may be theoretically useful in formulating a hypothesis concerning which neurotransmitters are involved in SPS. The finding that levodopa increased symptomatology in SPS was used by Guilleminault et al. (2) to propose SPS to be related to an imbalance between catecholaminergic and GABA systems. Actually this proposal has received additional support from the studies already discussed, since there is evidence that excessive norepinephrine activity is related to increasing symptoms. Diazepam's segmental effect may be to increase primary afferent depolarization that is mediated by GABA, and therefore diazepam may be acting by increasing GABAergic influences. It has been reported that baclofen, a GABA derivative, may also decrease symptoms (6). However, baclofen's relationship to the GABA system, despite its being a GABA derivative, is doubtful. Increased catecholaminergic influence increases symptoms, and increased GABA influence decreases symptoms, so that an imbalance between catecholamines and GABA may be the most reasonable explanation at this time for SPS. This, of course, is based on preliminary pharmacologic evidence and a lack of anatomic correlations.

Therapeutically, SPS can be managed fairly well with diazepam. The problem often is with diagnosis, but once this is accomplished truly remarkable efficacy can be achieved with diazepam (20–300 mg/day). Clonazepam has also been reported to be beneficial in doses approximately one-tenth that of diazepam (9,11). This may be of benefit in patients in whom diazepam causes excessive drowsiness. In our own experience, diazepam and related agents and baclofen have proven to be the most useful drugs. Whereas the literature is replete with reports of excellent therapeutic responses, not all patients respond that dramatically in the long run, and some may require large doses of more than one agent and still have significant disabilities.

BIBLIOGRAPHY

1. Gordon, E. E., Januszko, D. M., and Kaufman, L. (1967): A critical survey of stiff-man syndrome. *Am. J. Med.*, 42:582–599.
2. Guilleminault, C., Sigwald, J., and Castaigne, P. (1973): Sleep studies and therapeutic trial with levodopa in a case of stiffman syndrome. *Eur. Neurol.*, 10:89–96.
3. Howard, F. M. (1963): A new and effective drug in the treatment of the stiff-man syndrome: Preliminary report. *Mayo Clin. Proc.*, 38:203–212.
4. Mamoli, B., Heiss, W.-D., Maida, E., and Podreka, I. (1977): Electrophysiological studies on the "stiff-man" syndrome. *J. Neurol.*, 217:111–121.
5. Marda, E., Reisner, T., Summer, K., and Sandoz-Eggesth, H. (1980): Stiff-man syndrome with abnormalities in CSF and computerized tomography findings. *Arch. Neurol.*, 37:189–193.
6. Mertens, H. G., and Ricker, K. (1968): Ubererregbarkeit der gamma-motoneurone beim "stiff-man" syndrom. *Klin Wochenschr.*, 46:33–42.
7. Moersch, F. P., and Woltman, H. W. (1956): Progressive fluctuating muscular rigidity and spasm ("stiff-man" syndrome): Report of a case and some observations in 13 other cases. *Mayo Clin. Proc.*, 31:421–427.
8. Nutt, H. G., William, A. C., Lolse, C. R., and Chase, T. N. (1979): Cerebrospinal fluid neurotransmitters in the stiff man syndrome. *Neurology*, 29:536.
9. Nyland, H., Mellgren, S. I., and Frovig, A. G. (1979): Stiff man syndrome with central and peripheral neuron manifestations. *J. Neurol.*, 219:171–176.
10. Schmidt, R. T., Stahl, S. M., and Spehlman, R. (1975): A pharmacologic study of the stiff-man syndrome. Correlation of clinical symptoms with urinary 3-methoxy-4-phenyl glycol excretion. *Neurology*, 25:622–626.
11. Westblom, U. (1977): Stiff man syndrome and clonazepam. *J.A.M.A.*, 237:1930.

Chapter 14

Muscle Relaxants

A separate chapter dealing with "centrally" acting muscle relaxants is more in keeping with tradition and clinical practice than with a rational approach to the pathophysiologic problem seen with increased muscle tone or with the suspected action of these drugs. In 1910 Antodyne (3-phenoxy-1,2-propanediol) was introduced as an analgesic and antipyretic. Shortly after, it was noted that in laboratory animals this compound could produce flaccid paralysis. It was this agent's effect on muscle that led to multiple structure–activity experiments attempting to produce better and more efficient central muscle relaxants. All muscle relaxants have sedative effects in addition to any specific muscle relaxant activity, and these combined clinical actions in part are the explanation for the clouded understanding of the pharmacologic properties of this class of drugs (1–3).

Muscles in spasms are in a state of involuntary sustained contracton and not only exhibit increased tone but are also frequently both hard and tender.

The clinical situations in which muscle relaxants are most commonly used are those settings in which muscles spasms are secondary to inflammation or trauma. These obviously include fractures, sprains, arthritis, nerve root compression, and inflammation of the muscle itself. In many instances the muscle spasm may contribute to both pain and disability. It is presumed, although certainly not proved, that local inflammation and trauma produce increased muscle tone through afferent pathways which then activate segmental polysynaptic neuronal pathways. Since the centrally acting muscle relaxants do not affect neuromuscular transmission, nerve conduction velocity, or muscle excitability, their activity has been related to their effect on interneuron pools. The pharmacologic action of muscle relaxants is related to suppression of spinal cord polysynaptic reflexes. Brainstem polysynaptic reflexes are also inhibited, and there is no question that with the clinically used muscle relaxants a central sedative effect also occurs. Although it is possible to differentiate between muscle relaxants with strong sedative effects (e.g., meprobamate, diazepam) and those with fewer sedative effects (methocarbamol) and more presumed selective action on spinal cord polysynaptic pathways, it is of interest that the latter group has never been demonstrated in controlled clinical trials to be effective. The widespread clinical use of muscle relaxants and their apparent anecdotal usefulness is probably related to their antianxiety and sedative activity. There is also evidence that in order to obtain muscle relaxation in animals with the centrally active muscle relaxants, dosages 5 to 10 times higher than the suggested intravenous dose in man must be employed. The oral administration of muscle relaxants in man at the dosages clinically employed could not reasonably be expected to produce muscle relaxation by a specific relaxant effect.

It seems relatively simplistic to state that muscle relaxants act by suppressing polysynaptic neuronal pools. Since the segmental organization of increased muscle tone has been discussed elsewhere in this text (Chapters 10 and 12) in different contexts, there is no value in discussing it again. However, it will be recalled that several drugs are employed in the treatment of both spasticity and SPS because of their ability to affect specific components of motor organization. Diazepam, baclofen, glycine, and dantrolene should be considered in the treatment of muscle spasm. Of course, diazepam is extensively and successfully used in this setting, but the others have not been. Surely pharmacologic agents that affect the final motor organization at the segmental level should be effective in the treatment of muscle spasms.

Extensive structure–activity investigations which began with Antodyne eventually led to the development of mephenesin, an alpha-substituted glycerol ether (Fig. 1). Mephenesin is the most extensively studied muscle relaxant and usually serves as the prototype for a discussion of these drugs, but it was never demonstrated to be clinically effective and, in fact, is not clinically available for use. In further attempts to prolong the action and increase the activity of mephenesin, carbamates of the glycerol monoethers were investigated. This led to the development of methocarbamol (Robaxin) and chlorphenesin carbamate (Maolate). These drugs were used clinically with some reported success, although the reservations previously mentioned must be considered. In further structure–activity investigations, synthetic chemists have developed, among others, orphenadrine citrate (Norflex), carisoprodal (Soma), and chlorzoxazone (Paraflex), which are also used clinically as muscle relaxants. The difficulties in interpretation of their pharmacologic site of action remain their widespread effects on both suprasegmental and segmental neuronal systems. All structures of these muscle relaxants are illustrated in Fig. 1.

MUSCLE CRAMPS

Muscle cramps are painful spasmodic involuntary contractions of a single muscle. The contracted muscle often moves the adjacent joint, but it does not result in an abnormal posture as is seen in dystonia. To be a cramp, the spasm must last at least several seconds. Muscle cramps are often painful. Table 1 lists the more common causes of muscle cramps. These diseases should always be kept in mind in any patient presenting with cramps. On the other hand, almost everyone at one time or another has muscle cramps. These occur most commonly after unusual exercise and are self-limited. In occasional patients they can be so frequent and severe as to be incapacitating. Usually an isolated muscle cramp is alleviated by actively stretching the involved muscle. In those instances where the cramps are recurrent or are symptomatic of some other etiology, pharmacologic treatment may be required.

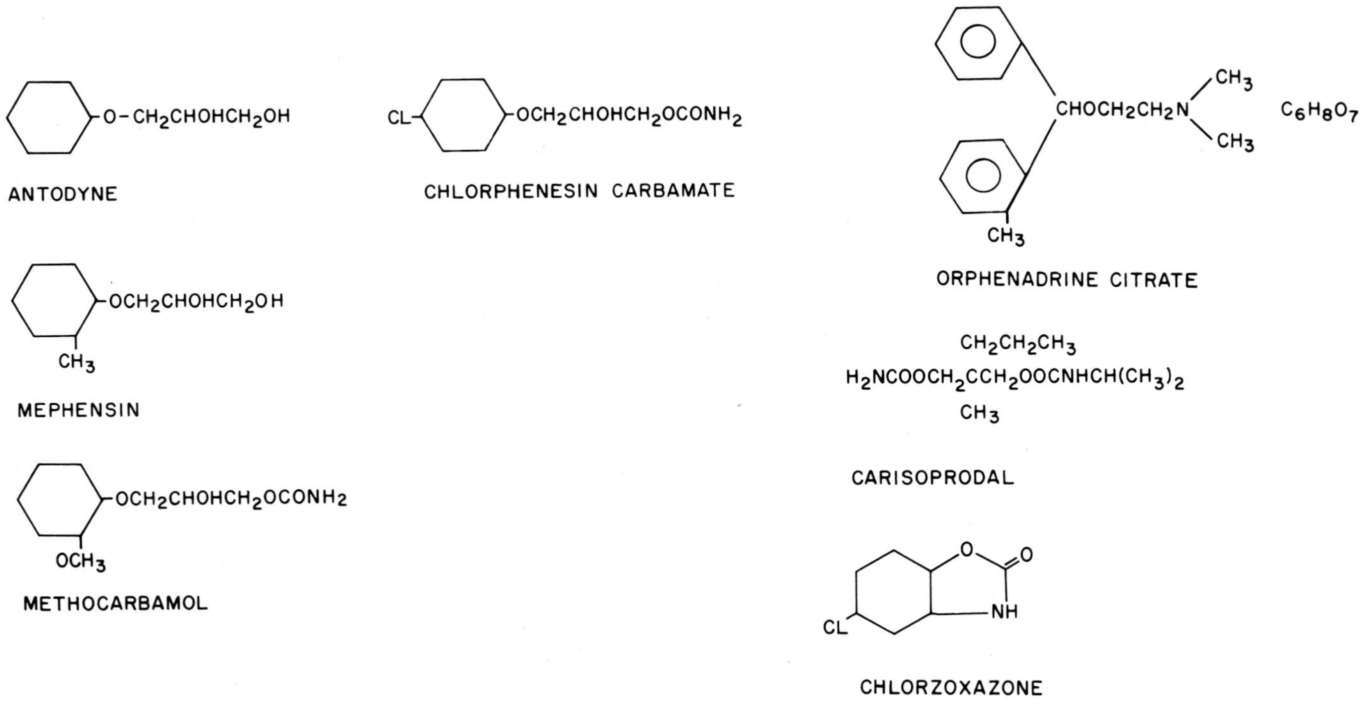

FIG. 1. Structures of various muscle relaxants.

TABLE 1. *Etiologies of muscle cramps*

Marked muscle activity
Dehydration
Salt depletion
Pregnancy
Hyperthyroidism
Partially denervated muscle

Drug induced
    Diuretics
    Clofibrate
    Anticholinesterase drugs

Muscle relaxants, quinine sulfate, and the other pharmacologic agents that affect segmental motor physiology (e.g., dantrolene, baclofen) have often been reported to be helpful in these circumstances.

BIBLIOGRAPHY

1. Donahue, H. B., and Kimura, K. K. (1968): Synthetic centrally acting skeletal muscle relaxants. In: *Drugs Affecting the Central Nervous System*, edited by A. Burger, pp. 265–326. Arnold Publ., London.
2. Franz, D. N. (1975): Drugs for Parkinson's disease: centrally acting muscle relaxants. In: *The Pharmacological Basis of Therapeutics*, edited by L. S. Goodman and A. Gilman, pp. 227–244. Macmillan, New York.
3. Smith, C. M. (1965): Relaxants of skeletal muscle. In: *Physiological Pharmacology, Vol. 2: The Nervous System, Part B. Central Nervous System Drugs*, edited by W. S. Root and F. G. Hofmann, pp. 2–96. Academic Press, New York.

Chapter 15

Myoclonus

Myoclonus, a term originally used by Friedreich, describes a brief shocklike contraction of a voluntary muscle or group of muscles which can involve virtually any part of the body. Myoclonic movements originate in the CNS and require intact lower motor neuron innervation, a feature that distinguishes myoclonus from fasciculation. Involuntary muscle contractions resulting from incomplete injury of a motor nerve (facial hemispasm, for example) are differentiated from myoclonus on a similar physiologic basis and are clinically identified by the presence of muscle atrophy in association with the spontaneous movement disorder. Myoclonus and dystonia are differentiated by the brevity of the former, whereas differentiation from chorea is based on the lack of complex movements and posturing in myoclonus. Involuntary tics and habit spasm may be indistinguishable from myoclonus on examination, but differentiation is usually made on the basis of additional clinical features such as coprolalia, or typical choreatic movements, not seen with myoclonus.

In clinical practice, myoclonic movements are frequently described by using a number of different terms that relate to specific anatomic areas of involvement or hypothetical pathophysiologic models. Asterixis identifies a metabolic myoclonic disorder evident in the outstretched hands, opsoclonus refers to a myoclonic movement disorder involving conjugate gaze. Other terms such as segmental myoclonus, palatal myoclonus, or polymyoclonia imply a specific anatomic distribution. Still others, like reflex myoclonus, intention myoclonus, or reticular reflex myoclonus, relate to proposed pathophysiologic mechanisms involved in production of the movements.

This terminology has been applied in a haphazard fashion, and different terminology describing identical movements has been employed. Similar ambiguity exists in the myoclonic epilepsies, in which convulsive phenomena and myoclonic movements are rarely viewed as separable entities. This is best illustrated by the frequent inclusion of epilepsy partialis continua (which appears to be a focal convulsive disorder) in most reviews of myoclonus.

In the present discussion, we have used a system of classification that has been derived from physiologic studies and empirical clinical observation. The basic premise of this system is that myoclonus is a distinct movement disorder that occurs in the context of a wide variety of disorders as well as in the normal individual. Regardless of the setting in which myoclonus occurs, the basic neuronal substrate responsible for the movements is probably the same and should be amenable to similar therapeutic measures.

The second premise is that myoclonus may arise at different levels of the CNS and that different mechanisms may be involved in the production of myoclonic movements at each level. Over a number of years we have attempted to correlate the clinical features of various myoclonic movements with what is known about the proposed "myoclonus-producing regions" of the CNS and to organize therapy on this basis.

Myoclonus is seen in a large number of settings, summarized in Table 1. Physiological studies suggest that most myoclonic movements can be subdivided into one of three general categories: segmental or focal, brainstem or "reticular," and cortical. Detailed discussions of the experimental data supporting this subdivision are extensively reviewed in other publications and will not be reviewed in detail here (2).

Segmental myoclonus refers to the presence of typical myoclonic movements in a restricted segmental motor distribution. The movements are usually rhythmic and frequently persist during sleep. Muscle atrophy is absent, although radicular sensory and segmental reflex loss is frequently evident. Sensory stimulation does not modify the movements (5,10,11).

This disorder is believed to represent autonomous activation of the alpha motor neuron pool resulting from irritation at the level of the afferent sensory system or from destruction of inhibitory interneuronal elements at the segmental level. The primary process leading to this pattern of dysfunction may be traumatic, infectious, neoplastic, or vascular. Segmental myoclonus may involve the spinal cord or the bulbar musculature (palatal myoclonus) and may spread to contiguous segments over time. Intoxication with agents known or believed to block inhibitory spinal cord transmitters (tetanus, strychnine, systemic penicillin) may lead to segmental myoclonic activity at multiple levels. In these situations, the lack of pathologic damage in the afferent sensory system may produce a picture of stimulus-sensitive myoclonus, a feature rarely encountered in segmental myoclonus of other etiologies.

Brainstem-mediated myoclonus appears to arise from the caudal region of the reticular system, possibly from the nucleus gigantocellularis (10). Activation of this region follows urea infusion in experimental animals and leads to multifocal myoclonic movements that progress to generalized myoclonic jerks. Various sensory stimuli appear capable of eliciting generalized myoclonic movements, and the overall picture resembles an enhanced form of the normal startle response. The characteristics of this system imply that it lacks any somatotopic organization in its output and receives convergent sensory input from the lemniscal and reticular systems. Movements originating from this region continue after decortication and are distally blocked by spinal transsection. The cerebellum and cerebral cortex appear to exert an inhibitory influence on output from the brainstem myoclonic center. In a clinical setting, myoclonic movements arising at this level are usually symmetric and resemble the startle response. Axial and proximal limb muscles are

TABLE 1. *Conditions in which myoclonus is prominent*

Focal lesions of the CNS (includes vascular, infectious and neoplastic etiologies)	
Spinal	Segmental myoclonus
Brainstem	Palatal myoclonus
Inborn errors of metabolism	Hexosaminidase A deficiency
	Hexosaminidase A and B deficiency
	Beta-galactosidase deficiency
	Wilson's disease
	Phenylpyruvic oligophrenia
Metabolic and drug-induced	Uremia
	Hepatic failure
	Postanoxic
	Bromides
	Tetanus
	Strychnine
	Penicillin
	L-5-HTP (in Down's syndrome)
	Levodopa
	Imipramine
	Amitriptylline
	Chloralose
	Piperazine
Infectious	Viral encephalitis
	Jacob Creutzfeld disease
	SSPE
Associated with epilepsy	Nonspecifically with various convulsive disorders
	Myoclonic epilepsy
	Some cases of dyssynergia cerebellaris Myoclonica
In association with cerebellar dysfunction	Dyssynergia cerebellaris myoclonica (syndrome of Ramsay Hunt)
	Ataxia, myoclonus, and opsoclonus in association with carcinoma
	Dancing eyes, dancing feet syndrome (with or without neuroblastoma)
	Some cases of paramyoclonus multiplex
Primary sleep disorder	Pathologic nocturnal myoclonus Cataplexy
Primary myoclonic disorders	Hereditary essential myoclonus
	Paramyoclonus multiplex
	Infantile spasms (cryptogenic)
Normal	Startle response
	Nocturnal myoclonus
	REM-sleep-related

preferentially involved, and the movements often persist during sleep. In some cases myoclonic activity may be present only during sleep (13).

Myoclonic movements may occur spontaneously, or they may be induced by a variety of sensory stimuli. The sensory modality inducing myoclonus does not appear to be as critical in identifying this form of myoclonus as the generalized pattern of the ensuing myoclonic movement.

In many cases, the EEG remains unchanged during periods of myoclonic jerking, whereas in others paroxysmal activity is simultaneously apparent. It has been suggested that spontaneous activity of the brainstem myoclonic region may be projected rostrally as well as caudally, and data from experimental studies appear to support this theory (10). The critical point is that an abnormal EEG in association with myoclonic movements does not necessarily imply a cortical origin for the disorder.

The third form of myoclonus encountered clinically is thought to originate in the cortex. In this form of myoclonus, the EEG is usually abnormal, and frequently an enhanced somatosensory evoked response can be demonstrated (10). Sensory stimulation results in a myoclonic movement in the general area of the site of stimulation and is best elicited with activation of the muscle stretch receptors. The clinical movement observed is "action or intention myoclonus." In such patients, attempts at moving a limb are interrupted by myoclonic movements, which disappear when the limb is at rest. The phenomenon is usually encountered after diffuse anoxic brain damage and in the context of some lipidoses.

Frequently such patients will also have episodes of generalized myoclonic activity identical to those seen in patients with presumed brainstem-mediated myoclonus. This suggests that a close interaction exists between the cortex and the brainstem in the mediation of myoclonic movements, and separation of two distinct movement disorders in such patients is often difficult. In our own experience, therapy directed at suppressing action myoclonus sometimes worsens coexistent generalized myoclonic activity and suggests that the two movement patterns may arise at different levels and be differentially sensitive to therapy.

Table 2 summarizes the clinical features we have utilized to differentiate myoclonic movements. Table 3 groups recognized myoclonic disorders into the three categories (insofar as this is currently possible).

ANIMAL MODELS OF MYOCLONUS

In the same way that there are numerous human forms of myoclonus, there are also different patterns of animal myoclonus, occurring after various toxic exposures and anatomic lesions. Infusions of phenol, sodium santonin, chloralose, strychnine, and organochlorides produce myoclonic jerks in animals (22a). The level of organization of the myoclonus is not identical for these various toxins, since chloralose-induced myoclonus is abolished by spinal cord transection, in contrast to that induced with phenol or strychnine where the jerks continue even after the cord is severed from supraspinal connections. Klawans et al. reported the production of myoclonus in young guinea pigs given 5-HTP, the immediate amino acid precursor of serotinin (14a). The myoclonus intensity correlated directly with elevated whole brain serotonin levels. Furthermore, it was specifically blocked by methysergide, a serotonin antagonist, while adrenergic, cholinergic, and dopaminergic antagonists did not inhibit the behavior. Working with the same model, Chadwick and colleagues lesioned 5-HTP-treated animals at the spinal or midbrain level (1a). Decerebrate animals continued to show myoclonus, suggesting the behavior is orga-

TABLE 2. *Subdivision of myoclonic disorders*

Segmental myoclonic disorders	Spinal segmental myoclonus (includes brachial, lumbar, etc.)
	Palatal myoclonus
	Other cranial myoclonic disorders
	Multisegmental myoclonus with strychnine, penicillin, tetanus intoxication
Brainstem myoclonic disorders	Nocturnal myoclonus
	Levodopa-induced myoclonus
	Hereditary essential myoclonus
	Paramyoclonus multiplex
	Dyssynergia cerebellaris myoclonus
	Dancing eyes, dancing feet syndrome
	Paraneoplastic opsoclonus, myoclonus, and ataxia
	Uremia
	Intoxications with imipramine, amitriptylline, L-5-HTP, chloralose
	? Infantile spasms
	? some cases of GM_1, GM_2, gangliosidosis
	? some cases of myoclonic epilepsy
	? myoclonus in association with epilepsy
	? in slow virus infections (Jacob Creutzfeld disease, SSPE)
	? generalized myoclonus in postanoxic action myoclonus
Cortical myoclonus	Postanoxic action myoclonus
	GM_1 and GM_2 gangliosidosis
	Some cases of myoclonic epilepsy

nized caudal to the midbrain. After spinal cord transection, the myoclonus was inhibited below the lesion, indicating that descending spinal paths are important to the behavior. Further segmental lesions have not been performed.

THERAPY

Myoclonic movements frequently arise in the context of more widespread disease processes. The first object of therapy is to rule out treatable etiologies, before embarking on a course of pharmacological therapy. When this point in evaluation has been reached, it is useful to categorize the movement disorder on the basis of clinical and laboratory studies, as we have previously outlined.

As mentioned above, the therapy of these disorders is largely empirical, and the following discussion should not be taken as a dogmatic outline of therapy. Therapeutic agents are offered in each category in the order that we usually follow in clinical practice. This sequence is based on the efficacy of the agent relative to other forms of treatment and, to a degree, on the relative toxicity of the agents under discussion. Dosages have been omitted in view of the wide variability in individual response. We usually employ one agent at a time and slowly increase

TABLE 3. *Characteristics of various myoclonic movements*

	Clinical features	Associated features	EEG	Sensory dependence
Segmental	Rythmic, segmental usually assymetric	Segmental reflex loss, frequent sensory loss	Normal	Usually absent (except in various intoxications)
Brainstem	Generalized, irregular, or multifocal, usually symmetric	Variable, may be seen in isolation, frequently associated with cerebellar dysfunction	Frequently normal; sensory evoked potentials normal	Frequently present
Cortical	Absent at rest; induced by movement; frequently restricted to region being moved	Evidence of widespread cortical dysfunction often evident	EEG dysrhythmia with myoclonus often observed; enhanced sensory evoked potentials	Present

TABLE 4. *Therapy of myoclonic movements*

Segmental	Clonazepam
	Tetrabenazine
Brainstem	Methysergide
	Cyproheptadine
	Corticosteroids
	ACTH
	Clonazepam
	Nitrazepam
	Diazepam
	Valproic acid
Cortical	L-5-HTP (with decarboxylase
	inhibitor)
	L-tryptophan
	Valproic acid
	Clonazepam
	Diazepam
	? Levodopa

dosage until a maximal clinical effect is observed or until signs of toxicity develop. If some improvement is observed, a second agent is usually added in an attempt to improve control. In the case of serotonin blocking agents and indirect serotonin agonists, an adverse response to one group (in the form of increased myoclonic activity) is usually followed by a trial of an agent with opposing activity.

Segmental Myoclonus

In all forms of this disorder (including those involving the cranial musculature), clonazepam appears to be the most successful form of therapy (7,11). Favorable results have also been reported following the administration of tetrabenazine (11). The precise mechanism of action is unknown but is thought to be related to inhibition of polysynaptic activation at the site of myoclonic activation. Diazepam would also be expected to be effective but has not been extensively employed. In our own experience, the sedative effects of diazepam appear to limit its usefulness in segmental myoclonus. Serotonergically active agents do not appear to have any efficacy in segmental myoclonus, and phenobarbital and reserpine have been reported to be ineffective as well (11).

Brainstem Myoclonus

This group encompasses the majority of myoclonic movement disorders encountered in clinical practice. All forms of therapy reported in this group have not been employed in all of the conditions grouped under this heading, and some agents have been applied only to specific disorders. Where applicable, these specific settings are indicated.

Cases of isolated myoclonus (lacking associated abnormalities in the EEG) have been successfully treated with central serotonergic blocking agents. Methysergide and cyproheptadine inhibit myoclonic movements observed following chronic levodopa therapy (14) and appear to be effective in some cases of dyssynergia cerebellaris myoclonica and paramyoclonus mutliplex (6). Pathologic nocturnal myoclonus also appears to respond to cyproheptadine in the few cases in which it has been used (*personal observation*). The efficacy of serotonin-blocking agents in other forms of presumed brainstem myoclonus has not been investigated.

Corticosteroids and adrenocorticotrophic hormone have been used in the therapy of infantile spasms and infantile polymyoclonia (dancing eyes, dancing feet syndrome; myoclonic encephalopathy of Kinsbourne) (12,18,21). The mechanism of action is unclear and the pathophysiology of either disorder is not completely understood. We have grouped these disorders under the heading of "brainstem myoclonus" with some reservation because the role of cortical mechanisms in these disorders is unclear. The induction of myoclonus with associated EEG alterations has been reported in patients with Down's syndrome who have received L-5-HTP (3). This suggests that some forms of infantile spasms may rely on central serotonergic mechanisms and bear some similarity to the myoclonic movements observed in other "brainstem" myoclonic movement disorders.

Corticosteroids are known to accelerate the peripheral metabolism of serotonin precursors (15) and markedly inhibit L-5-HTP-induced myoclonus in experimental animals (*personal observation*). Corticosteroids are also known to inhibit GABA-T and to raise central levels of GABA (1). Either mechanism might explain the therapeutic effect observed following corticosteroid therapy in infantile polymyoclonia or infantile spasms. Unfortunately, the effect of specific serotonin blocking agents has not been studied in either of these disorders, nor have steroids been utilized in the therapy of myoclonic disorders reported to respond to methysergide or cyproheptadine. Although current data suggest that all these disorders may share similar pathophysiologic mechanisms, further studies are necessary to clarify this possibility.

Other agents advocated in the treatment of infantile spasms include diazepam, nitrazepam, and clonazepam, but these agents are usually employed after a trial of corticosteroid therapy (17,18,23). An isolated report of successful treatment with L-5-HTP has appeared, but similar results have not been reported subsequently.

The myoclonic epilepsies appear to respond to the same agents that are effective in infantile spasms, although in this disorder corticosteroids appear to have little long-term efficacy (18). Generalized seizures in these disorders are usually treated with conventional anticonvulsants and may not predictably respond to treatment directed at suppression of myoclonic movements.

Valproic acid has recently been reported to be useful in the treatment of myoclonic epilepsy (22). This agent is effective in suppressing L-5-HTP-induced myoclonus in the guinea pig, which may suggest application in myoclonic disorders that respond to corticosteroid therapy. Extensive clinical experience with this agent has not yet been reported in myoclonic conditions other than myoclonic epilepsy.

Cortical Myoclonus

Action myoclonus appears to respond to L-5-HTP and may also be reduced after administration of L-tryptophan (4,8,9). The therapeutic response may be dramatic, although the mechanism of action involved is still unclear. Other agents that have been successfully utilized in action myoclonus include clonazepam (7,9), diazepam (20), and valproic acid (19).

In our own experience, treatment with serotonin precursors appears to be most beneficial in action myoclonus, whereas coexistent generalized myoclonic movements appear to respond following the addition of diazepam, clonazepam, or valproic acid. In some patients generalized myoclonic movements and action myoclonus respond differentially to various forms of therapy, which may suggest that pathologic conditions giving rise to action myoclonus may also alter the response of other (probably brainstem) sites capable of initiating myoclonic discharges.

Haloperidol and methysergide have been utilized in the treatment of action myoclonus, and both have been reported to worsen the disorder (16). In some cases, levodopa alone and in combination with a decarboxylase inhibitor is reported to improve action myoclonus (16). The role of dopaminergic systems in action myoclonus is still very unclear but does not appear as important as alteration in serotonergic activity.

A summary of therapeutic agents and the myoclonic disorders in which they are employed is presented in Table 4.

BIBLIOGRAPHY AND *SELECTED REVIEWS

1. Banay-Schwartz, M., DeGuzman, T., and Lajtha, A. (1979): The effect of corticosteroids on amino acid content of brain tissue preparations. *Psychoneuroendocrinology*, 4:207–217.
1a. Chadwick, D., Hallett, M., Jenner, P., and Marsden, C. D. (1978): 5-hydroxytryptophan induced myoclonus in guinea pigs. *J. Neurol. Sci.*, 35:157–165.
*2. Charlton, M. H. (Ed.) (1975): *Myoclonic Seizures*. Roche Medical Monograph Series, Excerpta Medica, Amsterdam.
3. Coleman, M., Boullin, D., and Davis, M. (1971): Serotonin abnormalities in the infantile spasm syndrome. *Neurology*, 21:421–424.
4. De Lean, J., Richardson, J., and Hornykiewicz, O. (1976): Beneficial effects of serotonin precursors in postanoxic action myoclonus. *Neurology*, 26:863–868.
5. Glatt, S., Klawans, H. L., Weiner, W. J., and Nausieda, P. (1979): Myoclonic disorders responsive to serotonergic blockade. Presented at the 31st Annual Meeting of the American Academy of Neurology, Chicago, April 24–28.
6. Garcin, R., Rondot, P., and Guiot, G. (1968): Rhythmic myoclonus of the right arm as the presenting symptom of a cervical cord tumor. *Brain*, 91:75–84.
7. Goldberg, M., and Dorman, J. (1976): Intention myoclonus: Successful treatment with clonazepam. *Neurology*, 26:24–26.
8. Growdon, J. H., Young, R. R., and Shahani, B. T. (1976): L-5-hydrotryptophan in treatment of several different syndromes in which myoclonus is prominent. *Neurology (Minneap.)*, 26:1135–1140.
9. Hallett, M., Chadwick, D., Adam, J., and Marsden, C. (1977): Reticular reflex myoclonus: A physiologic type of human posthypoxic myoclonus. *J. Neurol. Neurosurg. Psychiatry*, 40:253–264.

10. Halliday, A. (1975): The neurophysiology of myoclonic jerking: A reappraisal. In: *Myoclonic Seizures*, edited by M. H. Charlton, pp. 1–29. Roche Medical Monograph Series, Excerpta Medica, Amsterdam.

11. Hoehn, M., and Cherington, M. (1977): Spinal myoclonus. *Neurology*, 27:942–946.

12. Kinsbourne, M. (1962): Myoclonic encephalopathy of infants. *J. Neurol. Neurosurg. Psychiatry*, 5:271–276.

13. Kisbourne, M., and Rosenfeld, D. (1975): Nonprogressive myoclonus. In: *Myoclonic Seizures*, edited by M. H. Charlton, pp. 30–59. Roche Medical Monograph Series, Excerpta Medica, Amsterdam.

14. Klawan, H. L., Goetz, C. G., and Bergen, D. (1975): Levodopa induced myoclonus. *Neurology*, 32:331–334.

14a. Klawans, H. L., Goetz, C. G., and Weiner, W. J. (1973): *Neurology*, 23:1234–1237.

15. Knox, W., Piras, M., and Tokuyama, K. (1966): Induction of tryptophan pyrrolase in rat liver by physiologic amounts of hydrocortisone and secreted glucocorticoids. *Enzym. Biol. Clin.*, 7:1–10.

16. Lhermitte, F., Peterfalvi, M., Marteau, R., Gazengel, J. V., and Serdaru, M. (1971): Pharmacological analysis of a case of postanoxic intention and action myoclonus. *Rev. Neurol. (Paris)*, 124:21–34.

17. Millichap, J. G., and Ortiz, W. R. (1966): Nitrazepam in myoclonic epilepsies. *Am. J. Dis. Child.*, 112:242–248.

18. Myers, G. (1975): The therapy of myoclonus. In: *Myoclonic Seizures*, edited by M. H. Charlton, pp. 121–160. Roche Medical Monograph Series, Excerpta Medica, Amsterdam.

19. Rollinson, R. D., and Gilligan, B. (1979): Postanoxic action myoclonus (Lance–Adams syndrome) responding to valproate. *Arch. Neurol.*, 36:44–45.

20. Sherwin, I., and Redmon, W. (1969): Successful treatment in action myoclonus. *Neurology*, 19:846–850.

21. Sorel, L., and Dusaucy-Bouloye, A. (1958): A propos de 21 das d'hypsarhythmie de Gibbs: Son traitment spectaculaire par l'ACTH. *Acta Neurol. Belg.*, 58:130–136.

22. Tomlinson, E. B. (1974): Progressive myoclonic epilepsy: The response to sodium Di-n-propyl-acetate. *Proc. Aust. Assoc. Neurol.*, 11:203–208.

22a. Van Woert, M. H. and Hwang, E. C. (1978): Biochemistry and pharmacology of myoclonus. In: *Clinical Neuropharmacology, Vol. 3*, edited by H. L. Klawans. Raven Press, New York.

23. Weinberg, W. A., and Harwell, J. L. (1965): Diazepam in myoclonic seizures. *Am. J. Dis. Child.*, 109:123–127.

Chapter 16

Anticonvulsants: Mechanism of Action and Drug Selection

From a clinical standpoint, a seizure can be defined as the overt behavioral manifestation of sudden excessive hypersynchronous gray matter (usually cortical) discharges. It is probably best to assume that every epileptic seizure begins as a focal neuronal discharge which can either be cortical or subcortical. This local paroxysmal discharge induces either focal or more generalized dysfunction by spreading either locally or diffusely along neuronal pathways. Differences in the site of the initial focus and its method of spread result in the myriad clinical varieties of seizures. The symptoms of any particular attack are the result of the function of that part of the brain which is involved, e.g., consciousness is characteristically lost when the upper brainstem and thalamus are involved, whereas motor movements result from involvement of the motor cortex.

One of three things can happen when a group of neurons develops a hypersynchronous abnormal discharge:

(a) The discharge may remain localized solely to that original group of neurons.

(b) The discharge may spread locally without becoming generalized.

(c) The discharge may spread throughout the entire brain.

In the first two instances, the seizures are called partial, whereas in the third instance the seizure is called generalized. Table 1 shows the 1974 revised clinical classification of seizures of the International League Against Epilepsy. This classification is based on presumed site and spread.

Most of the agents in common use as anticonvulsants are listed in Table 2. It is obvious that a wide variety of chemical structures show anticonvulsant activity. Traditionally it has been taught that there is a close relationship between the structure of these agents and their anticonvulsant properties. This concept was derived from analysis of many of the older anticonvulsants. It is true that nearly all of the barbiturates, hydantoins, acetylureas, succinimides, and oxazolidinediones share certain structural characteristics (see Fig. 1). A ring structure containing carbon, oxygen, and nitrogen is common to most of these agents. Drugs that are effective against tonic–clonic seizure activity have one or more phenyl groups substituted at the fifth carbon atom of the ring. Alkyl groups at the same location protect against absence attacks, whereas straight carbon chains at either the nitrogen or carbon atom are related to sedation.

TABLE 1. International classification of seizure disorders

Partial seizures beginning locally
    Partial seizures with elementary symptoms generally without impairment of consciousness
        With motor symptoms (includes Jacksonian)
s324With special or somatosensory symptoms
        With autonomic symptoms
        Compound (or mixed) forms
    Partial seizures with complex symptomatology generally with impairment of conscious awareness (includes psychomotor)
        With impaired consciousness only
        With cognitive symptoms
        With mood (affective) symptoms
        With psychosensory symptoms
        With psychomotor automatisms
        With compound (mixed) symptoms of the above
    Partial seizures which generalize secondarily
Generalized seizures (i.e., bilateral, symmetrical, and without clinical evidence of focal or lateralized onset)
        Absences (so-called petit mal)
        Bilateral massive epileptic myclonus
        Infantile spasms
        Tonic seizures
        Clonic seizures
        Mixed tonic-clonic seizures
        Atonic seizures
        Akinetic seizures
Unilateral seizures (predominantly)
Unclassified epileptic seizures (usually so classified because of incomplete historical data)

TABLE 2. *Commonly used anticonvulsants*

Hydantoins	Succinimides
Phenytoin	Ethosuximide
Mephenytoin	Methsuximide
Ethotin	Phensuximide
Barbiturates	Benzodiazepines
Phenobarbitol	Diazepam
Mephobarbitol	Clonazepam
Primidone	Acetylureas—phenylacetylurea
Carbamazepine	Miscellaneous, less commonly used
Branched chain amino acid—valproic acid	anticonvulsants
Oxyazolidinediones	Acetazolamide
Trimethadione	Dextroamphetamine
Paramethadione	ACTH
	Paraldehyde
	Bromide
	Imipramine

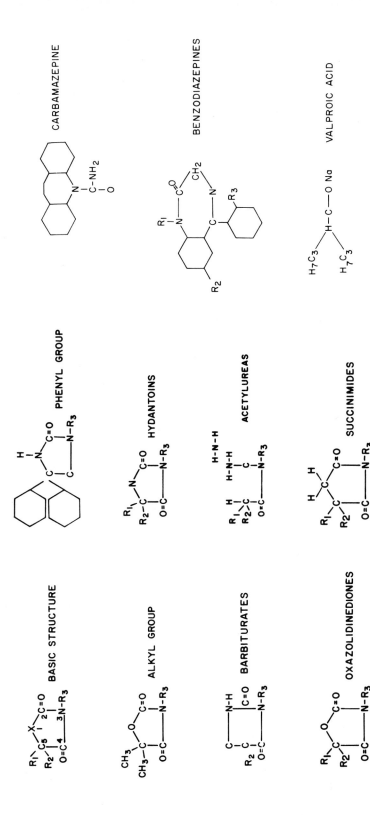

FIG. 1. Structures of major anticonvulsants.

Recent discoveries cast some doubt on the validity of classic structure–activity theory. Valproic acid (sodium dipropylacetate; see Fig. 1) is a simple branch chained organic acid which is very effective against absence and myoclonic seizures but has a broad range of efficacy. This drug was actually found to have anticonvulsant activity serendipitously when it was used as a vehicle to help dissolve agents related to those shown in Fig. 1 in an attempt to find a new classically structured anticonvulsant. When used as a vehicle, valproic acid proved to have greater anticonvulsant activity than the test drugs.

As pointed out by Schmidt and Wilder (24), an ideal antiepileptic drug should be able to suppress seizures completely at a dose level that produces no other signs or symptoms of drug effect. It should be taken orally at a low cost and be free of toxic effects and occasional idiosyncratic reactions in sensitized patients. The margin of safety between the therapeutic dose andone causing serious side effects should be high. Laboratory determinations of serum levels of the anticonvulsant should be simple and inexpensive to perform. Withdrawal of the ideal anticonvulsant should not produce symptoms or incite seizures, and tolerance to continued use should not develop. Unfortunately, such an agent has yet to be discovered.

It is a fair statement that the exact mechanisms of action of the various anticonvulsants are not completely known. The various experimental models that are used for evaluation and screening of anticonvulsant agents are far from perfect, and the results obtained with such models do not parallel the effects in epileptic patients. Despite these problems, enough is known about many of these agents to help in understanding their activities and uses in patients.

HYDANTOINS—PHENYTOIN

Virtually all the basic experimental work on hydantoins has been done with phenytoin, which may be the best studied of all anticonvulsants. It is usually believed that the remaining hydantoins have properties similar to phenytoin.

In various animal models phenytoin has been shown to: (a) suppress the local spread of epileptiform activity from a cortical focus without suppressing the interictal activity of the focus (19), and (b) suppress propagation of epileptiform activity to the contralateral cortex, subcortical centers, and other areas without suppressing simple projection of the discharge (28,30). Many of these properties have been demonstrated in the hippocampus, amygdala, and anterior nucleus of the thalamus as well as in the cortex and diencephalon. Although phenytoin does not increase the seizure threshold for such convulsant agents as strychnine, picrotoxin, or pentylenetetrazol, it does block the tonic phase of tonic–clonic seizures induced by the last two agents. The failure of phenytoin to block strychnine-induced seizures is interpreted as evidence that phenytoin does not facilitate inhibition, because strychnine-induced seizures are usually attributed to loss of inhibition.

Phenytoin inhibition of posttetanic potentiation (PTP) is usually thought to account for its various anticonvulsant activities such as local spread of a focal discharge and propagation of the discharge to distant areas of the brain.

PTP is a marked increase in the amplitude of a monosynaptic response to a single electrical stimulus that is observed immediately after a series of repetitive (tetanic) stimuli. This type of effect could play a role in both the local spread of a focal discharge and the distant propagation of seizure activity. The inhibition of PTP may also account for the ability of phenytoin to block the tonic phase of various experimentally induced seizures and generalized tonic or tonic–clonic convulsions in man, since PTP is probably involved in the pathophysiology of tonic seizures.

Phenytoin inhibition of PTP is attributed to its ability to stabilize neuronal membranes. It must be remembered that this property has been demonstrated primarily in peripheral nerves. The mechanism by which phenytoin stabilizes membranes is not entirely clear, and several possible mechanisms have been suggested including: (a) stimulation of the sodium pump (18), (b) inhibition of passive loss of sodium (7), (c) inhibition of calcium-dependent processes such as neurotransmitter release (20), and (d) competitive inhibition of calcium uptake into the neuron (13). Which, if any, of these is responsible for the physiologic effects of phenytoin is unclear.

A second, entirely different physiologic mechanism has also been proposed. Phenytoin has been shown to facilitate Purkinje cell discharges, a phenomenon which might suppress seizure activity (16).

In general, the ability of phenytoin to inhibit PTP is thought to be related to the clinical efficacy of this agent against generalized tonic–clonic seizures and partial seizures.

BARBITURATES—PHENOBARBITAL

As in the case of the hydantoins, most of the preclinical investigations of barbiturates have been restricted to a single agent, phenobarbital. Primidone has also been studied but to a lesser degree. With some exceptions for primidone, all other barbiturates are believed to have properties similar to phenobarbital.

It is generally believed that barbiturates act primarily at synapses, as opposed to the general neuronal membrane effect of the hydantoins. The ability of barbiturates to inhibit synaptic transmission occurs in both monosynaptic and polysynaptic pathways with a slight selectivity for the latter. This cannot really account for the anticonvulsant activity of the barbiturates. The effect of these agents on repetitive activity in polysynaptic pathways is much more likely to be a factor in their anticonvulsant activity. The initial stimulus is unaffected but the response to subsequent stimuli is greatly suppressed. At times, the response to the first stimulus is even enhanced, a phenomenon which might explain the fact that phenobarbital can exacerbate spike-and-wave absence attacks (petit mal discharges), which consist of single excitatory bursts followed by prolonged inhibitory phases.

Barbiturates affect synaptic function at all levels of the CNS. Although the midbrain seems to be more sensitive to the effect of barbiturates, this selectivity is more likely to be related to the sedative activity of these drugs than to their anticonvulsant activity.

The barbiturates have been shown to inhibit seizures induced by strychnine, pentylenetetrazol, and picrotoxin and to inhibit focal epileptiform discharges and spread of seizure activity. All of these properties have been attributed to their ability to inhibit synaptic transmission of repetitive stimuli (24).

The barbiturates with anticonvulsant properties include phenobarbital; metharbital, which is metabolized to phenobarbital; mephobarbital, which is metabolized to barbituric acid; and primidone, which is metabolized to phenobarbital (see below). It is clear that the sedative effects of the barbiturates are not related to their anticonvulsant activity. Barbiturates are of value in generalized (especially tonic–clonic) seizures and partial seizures.

PRIMIDONE

Primidone is converted to two metabolites: phenobarbital and phenylethyl malonic acid (PEMA). It is not entirely clear how much each of these compounds contributes to the anticonvulsant activity of primidone (11,24). PEMA probably plays a major role (but not the only one) since it is more effective than phenobarbital against electroshock-induced seizures. Clinically, primidone is also different from phenobarbital, having greater efficacy against partial complex seizures. Its major use is in the treatment of partial complex seizures and generalized tonic–clonic seizures.

CARBAMAZEPINE

This agent has been shown to inhibit selectively transmission in the anterior ventral nucleus of the thalamus, a structure that is thought to have a function in the generalization and spread of seizures (14). It has also been claimed to inhibit synaptic transmission in the spinal trigeminal nucleus (9) and to have some ability to inhibit PTP (17). Which, if any, of these properties contribute to the efficacy of carbamazepine against generalized and partial complex seizures is unclear.

BRANCHED CHAIN AMINO ACIDS—VALPROIC ACID

It has been proposed that the primary effect of valproic acid is biochemical rather than physiologic. This drug is a competitive inhibitor of GABA-transaminase, the major enzyme involved in the catabolism of GABA. By inhibiting GABA-transaminase it produces increased brain GABA levels (25). This may only occur, however, with levels that are significantly greater than those which have therapeutic efficacy. GABA is primarily an inhibitory neurotransmitter, so that increasing GABA activity might well have anticonvulsant effects. Interestingly, valproic acid blocks seizures induced by both picrotoxin and bicuculine, which are due to competitive inhibition of GABA at GABA receptors (8). It has been suggested that valproic acid blocks the neuronal and glial uptake of GABA, which would increase GABA activity without much effect on its concentration. The exact mechanism remains unclear. It has a wide spectrum of clinical activity including generalized (especially myoclonic) and partial seizures.

OXYAZOLIDINEDIONES

Of these, only trimethadione has been studied thoroughly. These agents preferentially block pentylenetetrazol-induced seizures. Because the mechanism whereby pentylenetetrazol induces seizures is unclear, this sheds limited light on the mechanism of action of these agents. The main effect of trimethadione appears to be to raise seizure threshold by inhibiting the response to repetitive stimuli within the thalamus (23). It also blocks the spread of a cortical epileptogenic activity to the thalamus (19). Its ability to block abnormal activity, both inhibitory and excitatory, in the corticothalamic system may account for its clinical efficacy in absence attacks, since a corticothalamic-cortical system is thought to be involved in such seizures.

SUCCINIMIDES

The exact mechanism of action of ethosuximide is unclear but may be similar to that of trimethadione (22). Little is known about the mechanism of action of the other members of this group except that they tend to protect against pentylenetetrazol and electroshock convulsions.

BENZODIAZEPINES

Diazepam inhibits a variety of experimentally induced seizures (including strychnine-, picrotoxin-, and tetanus-induced) but its efficacy is most marked in inhibiting pentylenetetrazol-induced seizures. The mechanism of its anticonvulsant activity is unclear. The following mechanisms have been proposed: (a) increased Purkinje cell activity (15), (b) increased presynaptic inhibition (12), and (c) increased postsynaptic inhibition (21).

Its major use as an anticonvulsant is in the treatment of status epilepticus.

The preclinical profile of clonazepam is similar to that of diazepam. In man it suppresses generalized seizure activity better than focal seizure activity (2).

ACETYLUREAS

Phenylaceturea has a broad clinical spectrum including generalized tonic–clonic seizures, absence seizures, and partial complex seizures. It possesses both hydantoin-like properties, e.g., prevention of the tonic phase of various experimentally induced seizures, and barbiturate-like properties, e.g., increasing a variety of seizure thresholds (24). Its toxicity precludes its clinical use.

MISCELLANEOUS ANTICONVULSANTS

Acetazolamide. Acetazolamide is a carbonic anhydrase inhibitor. Its anticonvulsant activity is thought to be related to inhibition of cerebral carbonic anhydrase activity with the subsequent accumulation of H_2CO_3. This results in decreased intracellular sodium and increased intracellular potassium, which together reduce neuronal excitability. It has some efficacy in absence seizures.

Amphetamines. Amphetamines, including both dextroamphetamine and methamphetamine, have been used as adjuncts to other anticonvulsants. They are usually used in an attempt to decrease the sedation caused by various anticonvulsants but also have some minor anticonvulsant effect on generalized seizures, both tonic–clonic and absence. The mechanism is unclear, although the ability of these agents to cause desynchronization of electrical activity may play a role (24).

ACTH. ACTH has striking efficacy against infantile spasms but little other clinical indication in the treatment of seizures. The mechanism of this effect is unclear. Rarely, a young patient with absence attacks will also improve on ACTH.

Paraldehyde. Paraldehyde is a polymer of acetaldehyde and is still occasionally used in the treatment of status epilepticus. Its mechanism of action is unknown.

Bromides. Bromides are rarely used today, and their anticonvulsant activity is believed to be due to their generalized depressant effect on neuronal excitability.

Imipramine. Imipramine is occasionally of value in absence and myoclonic–astatic seizures. The mechanism of action is unproven (10).

Chloroquine and quinacrine. Chloroquine and quinacrine have been said to possess anticonvulsant activity in absence attacks but this is not the general experience.

Pyridoxine. is only of value in seizures owing either to pyridoxine deficiency (which can be iatrogenic; see Chapter 7) or to pyridoxine dependency.

SELECTION OF ANTICONVULSANTS

It is obvious from the large number of agents available and the wide variety of clinical epileptic conditions that there is no one agent for all situations. In fact, there is not any universal acceptance of any one agent in most individual clinical situations. In this section we shall present a brief summary of the major clinical problems and the drugs that have shown efficacy for each.

Status Epilepticus

There is no one way to treat status epilepticus (SE). A variety of pharmacologic approaches have been and continue to be advocated. The general management of a patient with SE is beyond the scope of pure pharmacology and will not be included here. The interested reader is referred to the review by Duffy and Lombroso (6). The following regimes are in use today.

Intravenous Phenytoin

Intravenous phenytoin is the approach we tend to favor and has the advantage of not only treating SE but at the same time, instituting effective long-term anticonvulsant therapy. It is usually effective without suppressing respiratory function (29). Intravenous phenytoin should be given at no more than 100 mg/min and is usually given at 50 mg/min (especially in elderly patients or patients with cardiorespiratory disease). It rapidly enters the brain and can be effective within 30 min. The usual dose is approximately 15 mg/kg. Since i.m. phenytoin is poorly and irregularly absorbed, this method of administration should not be used (4).

Intravenous Barbiturates

The classic approach in treating SE involves the intravenous use of sodium amobarbital along with intramuscular phenobarbital. The former is used to halt the SE, whereas the latter is used to produce longer-term anticonvulsant activity so that the rapid disappearance of the amobarbital will not be followed by recurrence of SE. Amobarbital is usually given at 50 to 100 mg/min in an adult with a total dose per injection of 500 mg or less. The recommended dose of i.m. phenobarbital varies from 2 to 4 mg/kg. If necessary, a second dose of amobarbital can be given 1 hr later. We personally do not use amobarbital because of its tendency for respiratory suppression and its short duration of activity, which necessitates both repeated injections (with increased risk of respiratory depression) and simultaneous use of i.m. phenobarbital. If we use an intravenous barbiturate, we tend to use phenobarbital and usually only as a secondary drug if intravenous phenytoin has not proven to be sufficient. We then give 2 mg/kg, which can be repeated q 6 to 8 hr.

Intravenous Diazepam

Intravenous diazepam may be the most widely used treatment for SE because it frequently has efficacy within minutes (1). Its disadvantages are: (a) It tends to cause respiratory depression. (b) There is a failure to build up any long-term anticonvulsant activity, so that SE may recur. This would require repeated injections with increased risk of respiratory depression. (c) Interaction with barbiturates may cause severe respiratory depression.

We tend to use this only after phenytoin has proved insufficient. In this situation, the phenytoin supplies the long-term anticonvulsant effect. Diazepam should be given slowly ($<$ 1 mg/min) with a total dose/injection of up to 10 mg in adults and 5 mg or less in children.

Parenteral Paraldehyde

Parenteral paraldehyde is rapidly absorbed after oral, rectal, or intramuscular administration. Intramuscular administration is not recommended because of the risk of sterile abscesses. Intravenous administration is not recommended because of the risk of pulmonary edema and in the treatment of SE, it is usually given rectally and is probably most widely used in children. The recommended dosage in children is 1 mg/year not to exceed 5 mg. This can be repeated in 1 hr and then in 2 to 4 hr. Normally paraldehyde is metabolized primarily by the liver with acetaldehyde as the major metabolite. The agent is therefore not useful in patients on disulfiram (Antabuse), which elevates the levels of paraldehyde and acetaldehyde. In patients with liver disease, the rate of excretion of paraldehyde is slowed with a greater percentage of the drug excreted through the lungs. This has led to a belief in many areas that paraldehyde is an agent of choice in the treatment of ethanol withdrawal seizures in chronic alcoholics with liver dysfunction. In view of the hepatotoxicity of the drug, we prefer to use a barbiturate in this setting and see little reason to initiate therapy with paraldehyde.

Combined Approach

The combined approach is what we often advocate. It involves starting with phenytoin and then adding either phenobarbital or diazepam as required.

A number of variations of SE require different pharmacologic approaches. These include:

(a) Petit mal or absence status. Diazepam is often remarkably effective for this (6).

(b) Partial complex ("temporal lobe") status. We favor i.v. phenytoin followed by diazepam, if necessary.

(c) Epilepsia partialis continua ("focal status"). Although often difficult to control, this is not life threatening and should not be overtreated. Diazepam rarely, if ever, has a permanent effect although it may temporarily stop the seizure. We do not recommend it here. Instead, we use phenytoin followed by phenobarbital, and we supplement this as necessary with carbamazepine p.o. Two special conditions for all practical purposes are entirely refractory to anticonvulsants and so that the use of anticonvulsants should therefore be avoided. These are (i) seizures associated with paroxysmal lateralized epileptiform discharges (PLEDs) and (ii) seizures associated with nonketotic hyperglycemic coma.

(d) Phenytoin-induced myoclonic status. This rare condition usually responds well to paralydehyde.

Before embarking on the treatment of status epilepticus, one should be confident of the diagnosis. The occurrence of a single seizure in a hospital setting does not require the administration of massive doses of anticonvulsants.

Partial Seizures

Partial seizures with elementary symptoms respond to the following recommended regimes:

(a) phenobarbital alone especially in children;

(b) phenytoin alone;

(c) phenobarbital and phenytoin especially in adults;

(d) carbamazepine either alone or in combination with phenobarbital, but especially the former (27);

(e) primidone alone or in combination;

(f) valproic acid alone or in combination (3).

Because of experimental evidence suggesting that phenobarbital is effective at suppressing an active seizure focus and preventing the development of "mirror foci," we believe that all patients with such a focus should receive phenobarbital. If the patient cannot be managed on phenobarbital alone, we add a second drug (phenytoin or carbamazepine) in addition to the phenobarbital. Obviously, primidone could be substituted for phenobarbital.

Partial seizures with complex symptomatology tend to be more difficult to manage, but recommended regimes include the following:

(a) phenobarbital and phenytoin;

(b) carbamazepine either alone or in combination with phenobarbital or phenytoin, but especially the former (27);

(c) primidone alone or in combination;

(d) valproic acid alone or in combination (3).

Partial seizures with secondary generalization respond to the following:

(a) phenobarbital alone especially in children;

(b) phenytoin alone;

(c) phenobarbital and phenytoin especially in adults;

(d) carbamazepine either alone or in combination with phenobarbital or phenytoin, but especially the former (27);

(e) primidone alone or in combination;

(f) valproic acid alone or in combination (3).

Patients with partial seizures with complex symptomatology and those with partial seizures with secondary generalization both have active focal discharges and in our opinion require phenobarbital for the reasons cited above. Children are more likely to be managed on phenobarbital alone than adults. Virtually all adults, in our experience, eventually require combined therapy. For combined therapy we add either phenytoin or carbamazepine to phenobarbital. We reserve the use of primidone or valproic acid for those situations where control cannot be established with adequate levels of the above agents.

Generalized Seizures

Absences often respond initially to a wide variety of agents, but tolerance can develop rapidly. Recommended drugs include:

(a) ethosuximide,

(b) valproic acid,

(c) trimethadione or paramethadione,

(d) acetazolamide,

(e) clonazepam.

Trimethadione was the first agent to show specific efficacy in the treatment of absence attacks and was at one time the drug of choice. Following its introduction, ethosuximide, because of its greater safety, quickly replaced trimethadione as the drug of choice. Today ethosuximide and valproic acid are the most widely used drugs in patients with absence attacks. We tend to start patients on ethosuximide, but this may be based more on our experience with this drug than any evidence that it is more effective than valproic acid. We also tend to use acetazolamide and clonazepam before resorting to trimethadione. A drug to which a patient has become refractory often proves useful after a few months of withdrawal. This is especially true of acetazolamide.

Phenobarbital may make absences worse. Phenytoin may cause myoclonic status. Myoclonic seizures may respond best to:

(a) valproic acid,

(b) clonazepam.

In treating patients with absences or myoclonic seizures, one should keep in mind that the concomitant use of valproic acid and clonazepam is hazardous (see Chapter 18) and multidrug regimens should not combine these agents. For details on the treatment of myoclonus, see Chapter 15.

Infantile spasms may respond to ACTH, and at times benzodiazepines are of some but limited value.

Mixed tonic–clonic, tonic, clonic, and atonic seizures are treated with the following:

(a) phenobarbital alone especially in children;

(b) phenytoin alone;

(c) phenobarbital and phenytoin especially in adults;

(d) carbamazepine either alone or in combination with phenobarbital or phenytoin, but especially the former (27);

(e) primidone alone or in combination;

(f) valproic acid alone or in combination (3).

Most adults with generalized seizures, including those with partial seizures with secondary generalization, unfortunately cannot be adequately controlled on phenobarbital or phenytoin alone and require more than one anticonvulsant. It is always best to start a patient on only one drug. Theoretically, of course, it would be difficult to be sure that any particular patient might not respond to a single drug therapy. Furthermore, the exact cause of an idiosyncratic reaction (e.g., skin rash) would be difficult to interpret in a patient placed simultaneously on two new drugs. In most adults, especially those with a defined focus on EEG, we tend to add a second drug within a few weeks without waiting for another seizure. As a result our initial therapy in such patients consists of phenytoin and phenobarbital in combination.

Febrile Seizures

If pharmacologic intervention is necessary in acute febrile seizures, either diazepam or phenobarbital is usually sufficient (6). The question of long-term anticonvulsant therapy in these patients remains controversial. Like Wolf, we recommend chronic phenobarbital in all patients who have had two seizures as well as in those with one seizure and two or more of the risk factors for epilepsy, such as family history of epilepsy, age under 1 year at the time of the initial febrile seizure, neurologic damage prior to the febrile seizure, or severe (i.e., multiple) seizures during initial episode (31). The phenobarbital should probably be continued until age 4. The practice of advising that phenobarbital be administered when fever develops in a patient with a history of febrile seizures (on a p.r.n. basis) is not uncommon. The major benefit of such therapy would appear to be to the physician, who is reluctant to treat a patient chronically but unwilling to withhold treatment altogether. Since febrile seizures usually follow early rapid elevations in body temperature, an oral dose of phenobarbital is ineffective at inhibiting the convulsion and serves to prolong postictal sedation. The treatment of febrile seizures should be viewed as an "all or none" decision.

Neonatal Seizures

These are frequently metabolic and respond to therapy aimed at the metabolic defect rather than standard pharmacotherapy. This therapy includes correction of hypoglycemia, hypocalcemia, and hypomagnesemia as well as giving pyridoxine for possible deficiency or dependency. If anticonvulsants are needed we tend to recommend phenobarbital (20 mg i.v. in two divided doses and maintenance of 3–5 mg/kg) and/or phenytoin (20 mg i.v. in two divided doses and maintenance of 4–6 mg/kg) (5).

Eclampsia

Usually control of hypertension is the recommended therapy in this condition. If seizures persist after blood pressure has been brought under control, they usually signal the presence of an additional cerebral lesion. In these cases phenytoin and barbiturates are the preferred therapeutic agents. The use of magnesium sulfate in eclamptic seizures is a practice that persists in spite of little data to support its efficacy in this setting. We do not recommend its use.

Ethanol-Related Seizures ("Rum Fits")

Generalized convulsions occurring in the first 48 hr of ethanol abstinence rarely require chronic anticonvulsant therapy. In most cases a few convulsions occur in a short time but rarely progress to status epilepticus. By the time orally administered agents have reached therapeutic levels, the period of seizures may have passed and obviated the need for intervention. The prophylactic administration of phenobarbital or parenteral phenytoin early in withdrawal might offer a degree of protection from convulsions on a theoretical basis, but the opportunity for such treatment is limited (since most patients present acutely following an initial seizure). The only pitfall in treatment is ascribing all convulsions in such patients to ethanol and missing the occasional case of hypomagnesemia, hypoglycemia, or central nervous system infection. The presence of focal seizures or a persistently abnormal EEG in an abstinent state are the only settings in which chronic anticonvulsant treatment is employed. In the remainder of cases abstinence is curative and remains the sole form of therapy.

BIBLIOGRAPHY AND *SELECTED REVIEWS

1. Bell, D. S. (1969): Dangers of treatment of status epilepticus with diazepam. *Br. Med. J.*, 1:159–161.
2. Browne, T. R. (1976): Clonazepam: A review of a new anticonvulsant drug. *Arch. Neurol.*, 33:326–332.
*3. Calne, D. (1979): Valproic acid in epilepsy. In: *Clinical Neuropharmacology, Vol. 4*, edited by H. L. Klawans, pp. 31–38. Raven Press, New York.
4. Dam, M., and Olsen, V. (1966): Intramuscular administration of phenytoin. *Neurology*, 16:288–292.
5. Dodson, W. E. (1979): Pharmacology and treatment of epilepsy in childhood. In: *Clinical Neuropharmacology, Vol. 4*, edited by H. L. Klawans, pp. 1–30. Raven Press, New York.
*6. Duffy, F. H., and Lombroso, C. T. (1978): Treatment of status epilepticus. In: *Clinical Neuropharmacology, Vol. 3*, edited by H. L. Klawans, pp. 41–56. Raven Press, New York.
7. Escueta, A. V., and Appel, S. H. (1971): Diphenylhydantoin and potassium transport in isolated nerve terminals. *J. Clin. Invest.*, 50:1977–1984.

8. Frey, H. H., and Loscher, W. (1976): Di-propylacetate profile of anticonvulsant activity in mice. *Arzneim. Forsch. Drug Res.*, 26:299–301.

9. Fromm, G. H., and Killian, J. M. (1967): Effect of some anticonvulsant drugs on the spinal trigeminal nucleus. *Neurology*, 17:275–280.

10. Fromm, G. H., Wessel, H. B., Glass, J. D., Alvin, J. D., and Van Horn, G. (1978): Imipramine in absence and myoclonic-astatic seizures. *Neurology*, 28:953–957.

11. Gallagher, B. B., Smith, D. B., and Mattson, R. H. (1970): The relationship of the anticonvulsant properties of primidone to phenobarbital. *Epilepsia*, 11:293–301.

12. Haefely, W., Kulesar, A., Moehler, H., Pieri, L., Polc, P., and Schaffner, R. (1975): Possible involvement of GABA in the central actions of benzo-diazepines. In: *Mechanism of Action of Benzo-diazepines*, edited by E. Costa and P. Greengard, pp. 131–151. Raven Press, New York.

13. Hasbain, M., Pincus, J. H., and Lee, S. (1974): Diphenylhydantoin and calcium movement in lobster nerves. *Arch. Neurol.*, 31:250–254.

14. Holm, E., Kelleter, R., Hinemann, H., and Homann, K. F. (1970): Elektrophysiologiche analyse der wirkungen von (behun) carbamazepine auf das (behun) der katze. *Pharmakopsychiatr. Neuropsychopharmalkol.*, 3:187–200.

15. Julien, R. M. (1972): Cerebellar involvement in the antiepileptic action of diazepam. *Neuropharmacology*, 11:683–691.

16. Julien, R. M., and Halpren, L. M. (1972): Effects of diphenylhydantoin and other antiepileptic drugs on epileptiform activity and Purkinje cell discharge rates. *Epilepsia*, 13:387–400.

17. Krupp, P. (1969): The effects of tegretol on some elementary neuronal mechanisms. *Headache*, 9:46–53.

18. Lewin, J., and Bleck, V. (1968): The effect of diphenylhydantoin on cortex sodium potassium activated ATPase. *Neurology*, 20:419.

19. Morrell, F., Bradley, W., and Ptashne, M. (1959): Effect of drugs on discharge characteristics of chronic epileptogenic lesions. *Neurology*, 9:492–498.

20. Pincus, J. H., and Lee, S. H. (1973): Diphenylhydantoin and calcium: Relation to norepinephrine release from brain slices. *Arch. Neurol.*, 29:239–244.

21. Raabe, W., and Gumnit, R. J. (1977): Anticonvulsant action of diazepam: Increase of cortical postsynaptic inhibition. *Epilepsia*, 18:117–120.

22. Radan, C., and Esplin, B. (1977): Effects of ethosuximide on transmission of repetitive impulses and apparent rates of transmitter turnover in the spinal monosynaptic pathway. *J. Pharmacol. Exp. Ther.*, 201:320–325.

23. Schallek, W., and Kuehn, A. (1963): Effects of trimethadione, diphenylhydantoin and chlordiazepoxide on after-discharges in the brain of cat. *Proc. Soc. Exp. Biol. Med.*, 112:813–817.

*24. Schmidt, R., and Wilder, B. J. (   ): *Epilepsy*. F. A. Davis, New York.

25. Simler, S., Ciesielski, L., Maitre, M., Randrianarisoa, H., and Mandel, P. (1973): Effect of sodium n-dipropylacetate on audiogenic seizures and brain gamma-aminobutyric acid level. *Biochem. Pharmacol.*, 22:1701–1708.

*26. Tower, D. M. (1960): *Neurochemistry of Epilepsy*. Charles Thomas, Springfield, Ill.

*27. Troupin, A. S. (1978): Carbamazepine in epilepsy. In: *Clinical Neuropharmacology, Vol. 3*, edited by H. L. Klawans, pp. 15–40, Raven Press, New York.

28. Wilder, B. J. (1969): Laboratory evaluation of antiepileptic drugs. *Epilepsia*, 10:237;260–261;380.

29. Wilder, B. J., Ramsay, R. E., Willmore, L. J., Fuessner, G. F., Perchalski, R. J., and Shumate, J. B. (1977): Efficacy of intravenous phenytoin in the treatment of status epilepticus. *Ann. Neurol.*, 1:511–518.

30. Wilder, B. J., and Schmidt, R. P. (1965): Propagation of epileptic discharge from chronic neocortical foci in monkey. *Epilepsia*, 6:297–309.

31. Wolf, S. M. (1979): Controversies in the treatment of febrile convulsions. *Neurology*, 29:287–289.

*32. Woodbury, D. M. (1969): Mechanisms of action of anticonvulsants. In: *Basic Mechanisms of the Epilepsies*, edited by H. H. Jasper, A. A. Ward, Jr., and A. Pope, pp. 647–681. Little Brown and Company, Boston.

Chapter 17

Anticonvulsants: Blood Levels

Anticonvulsants, like most drugs, demonstrate a definite relationship between clinical efficacy and plasma concentration. There is also a direct relationship between intoxication and plasma concentration. Fortunately, the therapeutic index is such that for most patients, at least some degree of efficacy is usually achieved with concentrations below those which cause intoxication. The level necessary to suppress seizures does, however, vary significantly among patients, perhaps in part being related to the characteristics of each patient's epileptic process. There is also individual variability in susceptibility to intoxication. Despite these problems, empirical therapeutic ranges of plasma levels of antiepileptic drugs can be defined. Ranges of plasma levels that will induce toxicity in most patients can also be defined. The development of tolerance to toxic but not anticonvulsant effects will alter this during chronic therapy. Despite these problems, the use of "therapeutic" and toxic dose ranges is often very valuable. In all situations, the physician must pay attention to both the laboratory value and the patient.

Plasma levels are, of course, usually related to daily dose levels: Lower doses produce lower levels, and higher doses produce higher levels. A number of factors influence the relationship between dose taken and blood level obtained. These include: (a) absorption, (b) biotransformation, (c) plasma binding capacity, and (d) rate of elimination. These factors vary from individual to individual and may change in any one individual over time. Despite these problems, it is still possible and worthwhile to define ranges of blood levels observed in most patients with the usual doses of a particular drug (see Table 1). The concept of an expected blood-level range with a given dose gives the treating physician useful information, because the discovery of levels too low or too high for a particular dose may help him diagnose possible noncompliance, drug–drug interactions, or unusual rates of drug absorption, biotransformation, and elimination.

In order to understand the pharmacokinetics of the various drugs, certain properties must be defined.

First-order kinetics. This describes the biotransformation or elimination of a drug in which there is a direct relationship between the concentration of the drug and the rate of biotransformation or elimination.

Saturation, or zero-order kinetics. This describes the situation in which the biotransformation system is acting at its maximal rate (saturated) so that the amount of drug transformed is constant over time and no longer related to concentration.

TABLE 1. *Relationship between dosage and blood level for selected anticonvulsants*

Anticonvulsant	Daily dosage (mg)	Steady-state level (μg/ml)
Phenytoin	300–400	5–20
Mephenytoin		
Ethylphenylhydantoin	300–500	20–40
Phenobarbital	90–150	10–30
Primidone	750–1,250	5–15
PEMA		10–25
Phenobarbital		10–30
Ethosuximide	750–1,500	30–80
Carbamazepine	800–1,200	4–8
Trimethadione	900–1,500	
Dimethadione		300–900
Valproic acid	750–1,500	30–80

Biological half-life. The time required to eliminate one half of a drug from a particular compartment, e.g., plasma half-life.

Steady state. A state in which intake of a drug and its elimination and/or biotransformation are equal, so that its concentration remains stable or steady. There is obviously a direct relationship between half-life and time required to reach a steady state. This is usually believed to be 4 to 6 times the half-life.

The exact indication for when and how often to order blood level estimations is still unsettled. Kutt believes that blood level estimations are practical in the following situations (15):

(a) after onset of treatment to ascertain the individual's effective level in response to a specific dose

(b) after a change of the dose

(c) after addition of new medication, antiepileptic or other, that is known to be associated with interactions with drugs the patient is receiving

(d) poor seizure control

(e) evidence of intoxication, especially in a patient on multiple drugs

(f) periodically, to reinforce compliance.

Like other clinical procedures, these must be individualized for each patient. Since most anticonvulsants have relatively long plasma half-lives and reach the steady-state ith a given dose only after an appropriate time of continuous administration, blood levels examined too soon after initiation or alteration in dosage will not indicate the maximum steady-state level.

Many anticonvulsant drugs are bound to plasma proteins to some degree. A variety of conditions including uremia, hepatic disease, intake of other protein-bound drugs, and the normal newborn period will decrease the protein binding (11). As a result, the total plasma level will be lower but the percent unbound will be increased with several effects:

(a) Biotransformation and elimination are increased, i.e., decreased half-life.

(b) More drug will reach the brain than would with comparable total plasma levels under normal binding conditions, so that usually effective and toxic ranges are both shifted downward.

It might seem that under such circumstances unbound levels should be measured. Because of technical problems, this is not yet possible.

The major anticonvulsants, their active metabolites, as well as the usually therapeutic plasma concentrations and biologic half-life are listed in Table 2.

PHENYTOIN

The most common ranges of efficacy and toxicity are listed in Table 3. Most patients begin to show efficacy at levels of 10 μg/ml or more, although occasional patients, especially children, may respond to lower levels. The relationship of increasing levels to degree of intoxication is shown also in Table 3 (3). This is subject to individual variation and adaptation. Tolerance is not uncommon, so that patients on chronic therapy may be symptom-free despite moderately toxic levels. Rarely, intoxication may be associated with an increase in seizure frequency (27). Levels of 10 to 20 μg/ml are the best therapeutic range for most patients since such levels are usually associated with significant efficacy without any significant toxicity.

Some patients will require higher levels for significant efficacy. The half-life of phenytoin is usually estimated as 18 to 24 hr, and it usually takes 5 to 10 days with

TABLE 2. *Half-lives and therapeutic plasma levels*

Anticonvulsant	Usual serum half-life (hr)	Time needed to reach steady state (days)	Usual therapeutic range (μg/ml)
Phenytoin	18–24	5–10	10–20
Mephenytoin	24–48	7–14	25–40[a]
Ethylphenylhydantoin	72–96	14–21	25–40[a]
Phenobarbital	72–120	14–21	20–40
Primidone	6–12	2–4	5–15
PEMA	10–15	3–6	5–25
Phenobarbital	72–120	14–21	20–40
Ethosuximide			
(Adults)	60	8–12	
(Children)	30 ± 6	4–6	40–100
Methsuximide	1–2		
N-desmethylmeth-suximide	35–45	10–14	20–50
Carbamazepine	12–18	2–4	5–10
Trimethadione	10–20	4–8	
Dimethadione	4 or more days	several wks	600–1,200
Diazepam	2–10	7–10	
	20–60		
Clonazepam	20–40	6–12	0.02–0.100
Valproic acid	5–12	2–4	50–100

[a]Combined mephenytoin and ethylphenylphenytoin level.

TABLE 3. *Effects of phenytoin levels*

Level (µg/ml)	Effect
0–10	Subtherapeutic Suspect noncompliance or rapid metabolism; may be therapeutic if decreased plasma binding (e.g., uremia)
10–20	Therapeutic; could be toxic if decreased plasma binding
20–30	Mild toxicity; nystagmus and at times mild ataxia; if decreased plasma binding, toxicity may be more severe; may be tolerated without toxicity during chronic therapy
30–40	Moderate toxicity Ataxia prominent; during chronic therapy some patients may be symptom-free (tolerance)
> 40	Severe toxicity; ataxia, depressed level of consciousness, and at times, encephalopathy; such levels can rarely be tolerated without evidence of toxicity

a given dose of phenytoin to reach a steady-state (Table 2). It has recently been shown that oral phenytoin loading in adults with 0.20 mg/kg given in two to four divided doses in 3 to 24 hr or less can achieve and maintain therapeutic levels for 18 to 24 hr after initiation of loading (6,20). Adult doses of 300 to 400 mg daily (4–6 mg/kg) usually produce blood levels of 5 to 20 µg/ml (Table 1). Children usually require higher doses (in milligrams per kilogram) to maintain comparable levels. After puberty this difference diminishes. The steady state depends largely on the individual specific rate of phenytoin biotransformation. This is determined by genetic makeup and environmental factors such as liver function and the state of enzyme induction (13). An initial increase of dosage may result in a fairly linear increase in blood level, but further increases of dosage will become nonlinear with rapid increases in the resulting blood level. This is due to a shift from first-order to zero-order kinetics and depends on the individual saturation point of the phenytoin-metabolizing enzyme system. In most patients this saturates at somewhere near 20 µg/ml. In patients with levels in the high therapeutic range (15–20 µg/ml) any increase in dosage should be done in small increments such as 30 to 50 mg/day with monitoring of actual blood levels before any further increase. In patients with high phenytoin levels (e.g., 50 µg/ml), half-lives of 40 to 60 hr have been observed. In such a situation any decrease resulting from discontinuation of therapy would be slow. Such patients are best managed by frequent monitoring of the blood levels, with phenytoin being withheld until the patient is at or near therapeutic levels.

Normally 90% or more of phenytoin is bound to plasma proteins, especially albumin. There is an inverse relationship between the side effects of phenytoin and serum albumin levels. The lower the albumin level, the higher is the incidence of side effects (22). Newborns have lower levels of serum proteins, which bind less drug. As a result, the percentage of unbound phenytoin in the plasma of newborns may be considerably higher than the usual 7 to 8%. Similarly, uremics bind only approximately 70 to 80% so that the free phenytoin level is relatively high and our concepts of toxic and therapeutic levels must be shifted downward considerably (see Table 3) (11).

Phenytoin and Drug Interactions

A whole host of drugs can interfere with the life cycle of phenytoin and thus affect its plasma concentration and at times its half-life. Drug interaction can involve induction of enzymes involved in phenytoin metabolism. Phenobarbital and phenytoin itself are prototypes of enzyme inducers. In clinical situations involving multiple anticonvulsants such as phenytoin, phenobarbital, and primidone, this is rarely a problem. While Cucinell (7) showed that phenobarbital added to phenytoin decreased plasma phenytoin levels, others (4) could not duplicate these results, perhaps because phenytoin itself is an enzyme inducer so that the addition of a second inducer has little effect. There are reports, however, that ethanol may at times reduce phenytoin levels perhaps by enzyme induction. Both carbamazepine and valproic acid may also decrease phenytoin levels. This may, in part, involve enzyme induction, but the major factor appears to be decreasing the binding of phenytoin resulting in lower levels but increased unbound effective fractions (28).

A variety of drugs can interfere with phenytoin metabolism and cause unexpectedly high levels. These are listed in Table 4 in decreasing order of probability. Disulfiram may be considered as the prototype of these agents. It interferes with phenytoin hydroxylation and prolongs the half-life, resulting in elevated levels. Bishydroxycoumarin-increased phenytoin levels occur only rarely. More important are the diminished bishydroxycoumarin values induced by phenytoin or phenobarbital in patients being anticoagulated. In such patients, increasing the dose of bishydroxycoumarin overcomes this effect, but, if phenytoin or phenobarbital is then withdrawn, excessive anticoagulation can result in hemorrhaging.

As mentioned above, both carbamazepine and valproic acid can decrease phenytoin binding. Salicylate and phenylbutazone displacement of phenytoin has also been reported. Phenytoin may also affect the levels of other nonanticonvulsant

TABLE 4. *Drugs that increase phenytoin concentrations and prolong half-life[a]*

Disulfiram	Diazepam
Sulthiame	Sulfamethiozole
Isoniazid	Phenylbutazone
Bishydroxycoumarin	Sulfhaphenazone
Phenyramidol	Ethosuximide
Phenobarbital	Chlorpromazine
Primidone	Prochlorperazine
Chloramphenicol	Chloridiazepoxide
Methylphenidate	Propoxyphene

[a]Listed in decreasing order of probability.
Adapted from Kutt (13).

drugs. Some of these are listed in Table 5. These changes usually result from enzyme induction or decreased plasma protein binding as in the case of thyroxine.

MEPHENYTOIN

Mephenytoin is metabolized to ethylphenylhydantoin (Table 1). Both agents have antiepileptic action. In the steady-state, ethylphenylhydantoin blood levels are four to 10 times higher than those of mephenytoin (26). It appears that the half-life of mephenytoin is 1 to 2 days and that of ethylphenylhydantoin is 3 to 4 days (Table 2). More recent data suggest that the half-life of mephenytoin may be as short as 7 hr, so that most of the anticonvulsant activity may be provided by ethylphenyl-hydantoin (24). Protein binding of mephenytoin and ethylphenylhydantoin is probably in the range of 50 to 70% (15). Combined blood levels may be more easily obtained and sufficient for clinical purposes (26). The usual combined therapeutic levels are probably between 24 and 40 μg/ml with levels of 25 μg or more required for efficacy and levels above 40 μg/ml being frequently associated with toxicity (Table 2). The common clinical dose of 300 to 500 mg daily produces total me-phenytoin blood levels ranging from 20 to 40 μg/ml (Table 1).

ETHOTOIN

This hydantoin is not often used because of limited efficacy and has been little studied. It has a short half-life of approximately 5 hr, which may be the major factor in limiting its clinical usefulness (24).

PHENOBARBITAL

The usual therapeutic dose range of phenobarbital is 20 to 40 μg/ml (Table 2). It usually requires levels of at least 15 to 20 μg/ml for anticonvulsant efficacy, although when used in combination with other agents lower levels may have some efficacy. Sedation is common if not ubiquitous when phenobarbital therapy is initiated, but in many patients tolerance does develop over time. Continuous sedation is not infrequent with levels over 40 or 50 μg/ml, although some patients on long-

TABLE 5. *Drugs whose plasma concentrations are decreased by phenytoin*

Digitoxin
Bishydroxycoumarin
Metyrapone
Dexamethasone
Cortisol
25-Hydroxycholecalciferol
Thyroxine

term therapy have developed sufficient tolerance to levels even in this range. Occasionally children develop hyperkinetic behavior when placed on phenobarbital.

The half-life of phenobarbital is quite long, and 2 to 3 weeks is often required to reach steady state (Table 2). In adults, 90 to 150 mg per day will result in steady state levels of 10 to 30 μg/ml (Table 1). In children, higher mg/kg doses are often needed. Unlike phenytoin, saturation kinetics does not occur even with excessive serum levels. Approximately 15 to 30% of phenobarbital is excreted metabolically unchanged; therefore excessive accumulation may occur with decreased urinary function. Alkalinization of the urine will increase phenobarbital excretion and decrease serum levels. Acidification will do the opposite. Valproic acid has been shown to decrease phenobarbital excretion because of urine acidification and result in elevated phenobarbital levels (28).

PRIMIDONE

Primidone is metabolized into two metabolites: PEMA and phenobarbital. As mentioned in Chapter 15, primidone itself and both phenobarbital and PEMA may contribute to the anticonvulsant activity, although the role of PEMA has not been definitely proven. Furthermore, there are few blood level data on PEMA. The plasma half-life of primidone is short, and it reaches steady state within a few days (Table 2). The half-life of PEMA is thought to be somewhat longer and it therefore takes correspondingly longer to reach steady state, whereas the characteristics of phenobarbital are as stated above (Table 2). Little, if any, protein binding occurs with primidone.

Patients with significant efficacy from primidone usually have blood levels of over 5 μg/ml. Signs of intoxication, especially excessive sedation, are common early in the course of therapy even with low levels, but tolerance does develop so that most patients on chronic therapy can tolerate levels of 15 μg/ml. Patients on chronic primidone therapy who do not develop tolerance to sedation usually have primidone levels over 15 μg/ml and phenobarbital levels over 40 μg/ml. Because of this 5 to 15 μg/ml is taken to be the usual therapeutic level of primidone itself.

The usual adult dosage of primidone of 750 to 1,250 mg/kg results in the following steady state levels (Table 1):

    (a) primidone, 5 to 15 μg/ml
    (b) PEMA, 10 to 25 μg/ml
    (c) phenobarbital, 10 to 30 μg/ml.

Patients on phenytoin may have higher phenobarbital:primidone ratios (approximately two) (12). The ratio of phenobarbital to primidone can also be used to estimate compliance. This is because a phenobarbital level of less than or near to that of primidone is usually seen during the first week of therapy, while during chronic therapy the phenobarbital level is often three times the level of primidone. Patients who have stopped or reduced their primidone and then restarted it just before seeing their physician will have a low ratio. Like phenytoin, carbamazepine will enhance that conversion and produce higher phenobarbital:primidone blood level ratios. Isoniazid can inhibit primidone conversion to phenobarbital and produce low phenobarbital:primidone blood level ratios (21). Decreased renal function can result in the accumulation of both primidone and phenobarbital. No reliable data are available on the other barbiturates.

CARBAMAZEPINE

Carbamazepine is metabolized into one active metabolite, carbamazepine 10-11 epoxide, which contributes to the overall anticonvulsant effect. However, this contribution is limited since its concentration is usually three to four times lower than that of carbamazepine itself. Furthermore, data on blood levels of this compound are still scanty. The half-life of carbamazepine is fairly short (12–18 hr) and it usually takes 2 to 4 days to reach a steady state (Table 2). The half-life of the epoxide is less. Approximately 75% of circulating carbamazepine is bound to plasma protein, whereas only 50% of the epoxide is protein-bound. Even if the plasma concentration of this metabolite is low compared to that of the parent compound, the percent that is unbound and therefore active is higher. In the long run it may be that the total of the two will be the best guide (15).

The usual therapeutic range is said to be 5 to 10 μg/ml (see Table 2) (23). This estimation is not as clear as in the case of phenobarbital or phenytoin since carbamazepine is frequently given to patients on other anticonvulsants. Levels over 4 or 6 μg/ml have been observed to result in efficacy both when carbamazepine is used by itself and when it is used with other anticonvulsants. Levels over 10 or 12 μg/ml have been found to result in intoxication that is similar to that induced by phenytoin. The relationship between blood level and degree of toxicity is not as direct for carbamazepine as it is for phenytoin. Additive, if not synergistic effects on signs of intoxication have been observed between carbamazepine at levels of 2 to 4 μg/ml and phenytoin at levels of over 20 μg/ml. On rare occasions excessive levels of carbamazepine are associated with increased seizures (25).

In adults, 800 to 1,200 mg carbamazepine daily produces steady state blood levels of 4 to 8 μg/ml (Table 1). The epoxide metabolite levels are usually 20 to 40% of this. Higher milligram-per-kilogram doses are needed in children to maintain comparable levels. Self-induction of carbamazepine metabolism may occur since blood levels tend to decline with chronic administration. Barbiturates and/or hydantoins lower the blood level of the parent compound by enzyme induction and at the same time increase the level of metabolite.

ETHOSUXIMIDE

In children, the plasma half-life of ethosuximide is approximately 30 hr and it takes 4 to 6 days to reach steady state. In adults, these figures are 60 hr and 8 to 10 days (Table 2). As with primidone, plasma protein binding is negligible. In both children and adults the usual therapeutic blood level is between 40 and 100 μg/ml since 40 μg/ml or more are usually required for definite efficacy, and sedation as well as nausea and vomiting tend to occur with levels over 100 μg/ml (17). In adults, 750 to 1,500 mg usually produces levels of 30 to 80 μg/ml (Table 1). Again, higher mg/kg doses are needed in children to produce the same steady state levels. Saturation kinetics do not occur.

METHSUXIMIDE AND PHENSUXIMIDE

Methsuximide itself has an extremely short half-life and most of its anticonvulsant activity is probably due to a metabolite, desmethylmethsuximide, which has a much longer half-life and usually requires 10 to 14 days to reach steady state (Table 2). The concentrations of the parent compound in the plasma are extremely low, whereas those of the metabolite are 20 to 50 μg/ml with the common clinical doses (18).

Porter et al. have recently published a study of the clinical efficacy of phensuximide and methsuximide in relationship to plasma concentrations of each agent and its desmethyl metabolites in 5 patients with intractable seizures. Phensuximide and desmethylphensuximide both had half-lives of approximately 8 hr and because of this accumulated only to low levels. Methsuximide itself had a very short half-life (less than 2 hr) but its active desmethyl metabolite had a long half-life (almost 40 hr) and built up to reasonable levels (> 40 μg/ml). These differences in half-lives and resultant circulating levels were thought to account for the fact that methsuximide had a greater anticonvulsant effect than phensuximide (19).

TRIMETHADIONE

Trimethadione (TMO) is rapidly metabolized to dimethadione (DMO). Both of these are active anticonvulsants and can be measured in plasma. The parent compound has a short half-life (10–20 hr) and can take 4 to 8 days to reach a steady state (Table 2). DMO has a much longer half-life and does not reach steady state for several weeks. During chronic therapy the levels of DMO are much higher than those of TMO so that DMO probably accounts for most of the anticonvulsant activity. DMO levels of 600 to 1,200 μg/ml are generally thought to be therapeutic. The usual clinical doses of 900 to 1,500 mg daily result in steady state DMO levels ranging from 300 to 900 μg/ml (Table 1). The TMO levels are approximately one-twentieth of this and quite variable (1).

DIAZEPAM

Diazepam is rapidly metabolized to desmethyldiazepam, which, like the parent compound, is an active anticonvulsant. The initial half-life of diazepam is short (2–10 hr), but it is highly lipid soluble and exhibits redistribution kinetics so that its overall half-life is variously estimated as up to 20 to 60 hr (22). Because of this prolonged half-life and redistribution kinetics, excessive diazepam in the treatment of SE can result in prolonged coma. It can easily take 7 to 10 days to reach steady state (see Table 2). The therapeutic range is not clearly defined but may be between 0.2 and 1.2 μg/ml for diazepam and a bit higher for desmethyldiazepam (2).

CLONAZEPAM

Clonazepam has a half-life of 20 to 40 hr and would reach steady state in 6 to 12 days. The known metabolites are probably inactive. Usual therapeutic range is said to be 0.020 to 0.1 µg/ml (see Table 2) (9).

VALPROIC ACID

Valproic acid has a half-life of 5 to 12 hr so that plasma levels tend to fluctuate greatly. Fifty to 100 µg/ml is considered a reasonable therapeutic range (see Table 2) (5).

BIBLIOGRAPHY AND *SELECTED REVIEWS

1. Booker, H. E. (1972): Trimethadione and other oxazolikinediones: Relation of plasma levels to clinical control. In: *Antiepileptic Drugs*, edited by D. M. Woodbury, J. K. Penry, and R. P. Schmidt, pp. 403–407. Raven Press, New York.
2. Booker, H. E., and Celesia, G. G. (1973): Serum concentrations of diazepam in subjects with epilepsy. *Arch. Neurol.*, 29:191–194.
3. Booker, H. E., and Darcey, B. (1973): Serum concentrations of free diphenylhydantoin and their relationships to clinical intoxication. *Epilepsia*, 14:171–184.
4. Buchanan, R. A., and Sholiton, L. J. (1972): Diphenylhydantoin: Interaction with other drugs. In: *Antiepileptic Drugs*, edited by D. M. Woodbury, J. K. Penry, and R. P. Schmidt, pp. 181–192. Raven Press, New York.
5. Calne, D. B. (1979): Valproic acid in epilepsy. In: *Clinical Neuropharmacology, Vol. 4*, edited by H. L. Klawans, pp. 31–38. Raven Press, New York.
6. Cranford, R. E., Leppik, I. E., Patrick, B., Anderson, C. B., and Kostick, B. (1978): Intravenous phenytoin: Clinical and pharmacokinetic aspects. *Neurology*, 28:874–880.
7. Cucinell, S. A. (1972): Phenobarbital: Interactions with other drugs. In: *Antiepileptic Drugs*, edited by D. M. Woodbury, J. K. Penry, and R. P. Schmidt, pp. 319–328. Raven Press, New York.
*8. Dodson, W. E. (1979): Pharmacology and treatment of epilepsy in childhood. In: *Clinical Neuropharmacology, Vol. 4*, edited by H. L. Klawans, pp. 1–30. Raven Press, New York.
9. Dreifuss, F. E., Penry, J. K., Rose, S. W., Kupferberg, H. J., Dyken, P., and Sato, S. (1975): Serum clonazepam concentrations in children with absence seizures. *Neurology*, 25:255–258.
*10. Eadie, M. J. (1976): Plasma level monitoring of anticonvulsants. *Clin. Pharmacokinet.*, 1:52–66.
11. Ebadi, M. (1975): The pharmacokinetic basis of therapeutics with special reference to drugs used in neurology. In: *Advances in Neurology, Vol. 13*, edited by W. J. Friedlander, pp. 333–380. Raven Press, New York.
12. Fincham, R. W., Schottelius, D. D., and Sahs, A. L. (1974): The influence of diphenylhydantoin on primidone metabolism. *Arch. Neurol.*, 30:259–262.
13. Kutt, H. (1971): Biochemical and genetic factors regulating dilantin metabolism in man. *Ann. N.Y. Acad. Sci.*, 179:704–722.
*14. Kutt, H. (1975): Interactions of antiepileptic drugs. *Epilepsia*, 16:393–402.
*15. Kutt, H. (1978): Anticonvulsant blood levels in the management of epileptic patients. In: *Clinical Neuropharmacology, Vol. 3*, edited by H. L. Klawans, pp. 1–14. Raven Press, New York.
*16. Kutt, H., and Penry, J. K. (1974): Usefulness of blood levels of antiepileptic drugs. *Arch. Neurol.*, 31:283–288.
17. Penry, J. K., Porter, R. J., and Dreifuss, F. E. (1972): Ethosuximide: Relation of plasma levels to clinical control. In: *Antiepileptic Drugs*, edited by D. M. Woodbury, J. K. Penry, and R. P. Schmidt, pp. 431–441. Raven Press, New York.
18. Porter, R. J., Penry, J. K. Lacy, J. R., Newmark, M. E., and Kupferberg, H. J. (1977): The clinical efficacy and pharmacokinetics of phensuximide and methsuximide. *Neurology*, 27:375–376.
19. Porter, R. J., Penry, J. K., Lacy, J. R., Newmark, M. E., and Kupferberg, H. J. (1979): Plasma concentrations of phensuximide, methsuximide and their metabolites in relation to clinical efficacy. *Neurology*, 29:1509–1513.
20. Record, K. E., Rapp, R. P., Young, A. B., and Kostenbouder, H. B. (1979): Oral phenytoin loading in adults: Rapid achievement of therapeutic plasma levels. *Ann. Neurol.*, 5:268–270.

21. Sutton, G., and Kupferberg, H. J. (1975): Isoniazid as an inhibitor of primidone metabolism. *Neurology*, 25:1179–1181.
22. Swett, C., Jr. (1973): Diphenylhydantoin side effects and serum albumin levels. *Clin. Pharmacol. Ther.*, 14:529–532.
23. Troupin, A. S. (1978): Carbamazepine in epilepsy. In: *Clinical Neuropharmacology, Vol. 3*, edited by H. L. Klawans, pp. 15–40. Raven Press, New York.
24. Troupin, A. S., Friel, P., Lovely, M. P., and Wilensky, A. J. (1979): Clinical pharmacology of mephenytoin and ethotoin. *Ann. Neurol.*, 6:410–414.
25. Troupin, A. S., and Ojeman, L. M. (1975): Paradoxical intoxication: A complication of anticonvulsant administration. *Epilepsia*, 16:753–758.
26. Troupin, A. S., Ojeman, L. M., and Dodrill, C. B. (1976): Mephenytoin: A reappraisal. *Epilepsia*, 17:403–414.
*27. Wilder, B. J. (1978): Anticonvulsant drug toxicity. In: *Clinical Neuropharmacology, Vol. 3*, edited by H. L. Klawans, pp. 57–84. Raven Press, New York.
28. Wilder, B. J., Willmore, L. J., Brune, J., and Villarreal, H. J. (1978): Valproic acid: Interaction with other anticonvulsant drugs. *Neurology*, 28:892–896.

Chapter 18

Anticonvulsants: Toxicity

The various anticonvulsants can produce a wide variety of toxic side effects which can be divided into two major groups:

(a) Toxicity related to the CNS effects. These are somewhat predictable and often reflect the limited therapeutic indices of these agents.

(b) Toxicity unrelated to the CNS effects. These are in general not predictable, bear no relationship to the therapeutic index of the individual agent, and are often idiosyncratic in nature.

NEUROLOGIC TOXICITY

Acute CNS toxicity results from iatrogenic, accidental, or intentional overdosage. When therapeutic levels are exceeded, the anticonvulsant agents have an increasing effect on normal neuronal function. As pointed out by Wilder, four separate systems are usually involved (28):

(a) cerebellovestibular, producing signs ranging from nystagmus to ataxia and severe dysnergia;

(b) higher cortical function, varying from mild difficulty with concentration or recent memory to severe disorientation;

(c) reticulocortical activating system, ranging from lethargy to frank coma with respiratory suppression;

(d) motor, including chorea, asterixis, and at times myoclonus and even seizures.

In theory, the different anticonvulsants affect specific CNS systems differentially. This should result in accurate clinical diagnosis of the specific offending agent in a patient on more than one anticonvulsant. In practice, this theory does not hold up. In patients receiving more than one anticonvulsant who have neurologic toxicity, the offending agent usually cannot be definitely identified on clinical grounds alone. Only plasma drug levels make an accurate diagnosis possible. With this information, the dosage can be selectively reduced with less of a chance of increasing the frequency of seizures or even precipitating status epilepticus by reducing the dosage of the wrong drug.

In general, agents with strong hypnosedative properties such as barbiturates, primidone, and diazepam produce a syndrome of cortical dysfunction with progressive depression of level of consciousness at times associated with loss of higher cortical functions. Severe toxicity produces frank coma with a marked tendency for respiratory depression but without marked ataxia or motor involvement. Benzodiazepines may depress cardiorespiratory function at low levels of toxicity in patients with reduced respiratory reserve and in young children.

Phenytoin and other hydantoins initially cause cerebellovestibular dysfunction followed by progressive alteration in higher cortical function, motor signs including chorea, dystonic postures, myoclonic jerks and even generalized seizures and finally stupor and coma (9). The pattern seen with carbamazepine is less well defined but probably similar (21). Ethosuximide and methsuximide probably produce a syndrome somewhat reminiscent of hypnosedatives in which loss of higher cortical function and reticulocortical involvement are most prominent. Oxazolidinediones act similarly. Valproic acid seems to resemble the hydantoins but with less motor involvement.

Clinical cerebellar dysfunction, lethargy, and altered mentation are frequently encountered during chronic therapy with anticonvulsants. These symptoms are usually directly related to elevated levels of one or more antiepileptic drugs and usually disappear rapidly when the appropriate drug or drugs are reduced or withdrawn. Whether these agents, as a result of subclinical chronic low-grade or even recurrent severe toxicity, can produce permanent pathological changes in the CNS remains controversial. Numerous reports of pathological changes in the CNS, resulting from long-term anticonvulsant therapy, have been published, but identical pathologic changes can also be caused by hypoxia owing to repeated generalized seizures. Many, if not most, pathological specimens are from patients who have had severe and usually poorly controlled seizure disorders. Another problem hindering the interpretation of these studies is the fact that these patients have usually received multiple anticonvulsants. Animal studies unfortunately have not clearly settled this issue.

A number of neuropathologic studies have attributed degeneration of the cerebellum to either excessive or prolonged phenytoin therapy (10,11). Dam found similar if not identical changes in patients on long-term phenytoin therapy but attributed these changes to repeated convulsions and resultant hypoxia (7).

Studying the acute effects of high doses of phenytoin in animals, Snider and Del Cerro have described a variety of electron-microscopic alterations including proliferating spiral membranes arising from Purkinje cells, abnormal mossy and basket cell terminals, and altered Bermann astrocytes (23). These investigators attributed these changes to direct phenytoin toxicity, whereas Dam (7) has interpreted identical changes as the effect of either technical artifact or hypoxia. In general, most clinicians believe that phenytoin can result in permanent cerebellar degeneration and ataxia but seem to be much more willing to accept this relationship in patients with a definite history of clinically significant phenytoin toxicity.

The term "phenytoin encephalopathy" is used to describe a syndrome consisting of increasing frequency of seizures, EEG changes, and clinical evidence of diffuse encephalopathy (9). Many of these patients manifest changes in seizure patterns with an increase in tonic or opisthotonic components, whereas some patients demonstrate increased CSF protein and mild pleocytosis. This syndrome is usually attributed to chronic toxicity and usually responds well to withdrawal of phenytoin. The syndrome is fortunately rare.

Folate deficiency has been suggested as a possible cause for this syndrome, but this conjecture is unproven (20). Folate deficiency as measured by serum and red cell folate levels is quite common in patients chronically receiving anticonvulsants, especially phenytoin. Any significance of this deficiency is unknown except for drug-induced megaloblastic anemia.

The mechanism by which the anticonvulsant drugs alter folate metabolism is not completely clear. Folate absorption, the metabolism of folate coenzymes, and tissue utilization of folate have been reported to be influenced by anticonvulsants. Folate administration has been shown to reduce the hematologic and perhaps some other side effects resulting from anticonvulsant drug administration. Although it has been reported that folate administration increases seizure frequency, this has not been the clinical experience of most physicians treating patients with epilepsy. Because of folate's central role in nucleoprotein synthesis, prolonged severe folate deficiency might theoretically produce widespread CNS injury. However, such changes have not been reported in patients with anticonvulsant-induced megaloblastic anemia (28).

Peripheral neuropathy has also been attributed to chronic anticonvulsant treatment. Lovelace and Horwitz reported absent ankle and knee reflexes in 18% of their patients (16). Sensory signs were also present in some. In more than half of the patients tested, nerve conduction velocities were decreased. In another study, patients on phenytoin for 10 or more years were found to have both neurologenic changes on electromyography and slowed nerve conduction velocities (8). In general, evidence of neuropathy correlated well with higher plasma phenytoin levels. There are apparently two forms of phenytoin-induced neuropathy. Some patients develop a transient neuropathic syndrome owing to acute toxicity and associated with clearly toxic phenytoin levels. The second and more common syndrome is one of chronic, usually subclinical, neuropathy, which is found in patients on chronic phenytoin for many years but without "toxic" phenytoin levels. Low folate values have been reported in some patients with neuropathy, but folate therapy has not been shown to reverse the neuropathy.

The combined use of clonazepan and valproic acid has been reported to induce status epilepticus in a number of cases. The basis of this response is not currently understood. Concomitant use of these agents is not recommended.

TOXICITY UNRELATED TO THE CNS

Anticonvulsants also produce numerous side effects which are not related to their effect on the CNS, are usually not dose-related, and are essentially nonpredictable.

Three such reactions involve genetic predisposition (5):

(a) anticonvulsant drug-induced acute crisis in acute intermittent porphyria (autosomal recessive),

(b) phenytoin intoxication caused by hydroxylation deficiency (autosomal dominant), and

(c) phenytoin intoxication associated with concurrent isoniazid therapy in patients with deficient acetyltransferase (autosomal recessive).

These acute "idiosyncratic" reactions, which are all uncommon, are listed in Table 1. The skin reactions are often explosive and require immediate drug withdrawal and, if severe, steroid treatment.

Hemopoietic System

Megaloblastic anemia occurs in fewer than 1% of epileptics on chronic anticonvulsant therapy and is usually seen in patients on phenytoin either alone or in combination with phenobarbital. This has also been occasionally reported in patients on only phenobarbital or primidone and uniquely in one patient on mephenytoin. Anemia can occur at any time during chronic therapy, and pregnancy or poor diet may increase the risk. The anemia is due to folic acid deficiency as reflected by subnormal serum and red cell folate levels and always responds to treatment with folic acid, even in doses as low as 25 to 500 μg daily. Improvement following withdrawal of the offending drugs has also been noted. There is a 10% relapse rate following cessation of vitamin therapy. Although the incidence of frank megaloblastic anemia is low, macrocytosis as a reflection of folic acid deficiency is much more common, as are megaloblastic changes in the bone marrow (20).

Coagulation defects and resultant bleeding have been reported in infants born to mothers on phenobarbital and/or phenytoin (18,24). The bleeding is directly related to deficiency of vitamin K-dependent coagulation factors (II, VII, IX, and X) in the infant, even in the presence of normal maternal clotting factors. Both phenytoin and phenobarbital readily cross the placenta and accumulate in the liver of the unborn infant where they act competitively with vitamin K and prevent production of vitamin K-dependent clotting factors. Vitamin K has been shown both to prevent and to treat this coagulation defect, and it has been recommended that pregnant women receiving these drugs be given small doses of vitamin K before delivery, and that the neonate be given 1 mg at birth although the efficacy of the latter is unclear. Postpartum vitamin K is clearly not sufficient since hemorrhages have occurred both in utero and during delivery.

As with almost any drug, agranulocytosis, pancytopenic, neutropenia, leukopenic, thrombocytopenia, and aplastic anemia can occur with the commonly used anticonvulsants phenytoin, phenobarbital, primidone, and ethosuximide. These reactions are all, fortunately, uncommon. There are numerous reports of bone marrow depression due to carbamazepine therapy. These reports usually involve elderly patients receiving carbamazepine for trigeminal neuralgia. Bone marrow depression is apparently less frequent in younger patients receiving carbamazepine as an anticonvulsant. A transient decrease in WBC count and occasionally in RBC count occurs in many patients early in the course of carbamazepine therapy. This common phenomenon is transient and not a harbinger of aplastic anemia. When carbamazepine is to be used, a CBC should be done prior to initiating therapy and the

TABLE 1. *More common nonneurologic toxic effects of anticonvulsants*

Effect	Drug	Mechanism
Skin		
Erythemia multiforme	All anticonvulsants	Allergy
Exfoliative dermatitis		
Stevens-Johnson syndrome		
Epidermal necrosis		
Morbilliform rash		
Urticaria		
Hematopoiesis		
Leukopenia	Carbamazepine	Allergy or direct toxicity
Granulopenia	Mephenytoin	
Aplastic anemia	Phenacemide	
Agranulocytosis	Trimethadione	
Thrombocytopenia	Succinimides	
Pancytopenia[a]		
Megaloblastic anemia	Phenytoin	Folic acid deficiency
	Phenobarbital	
	Primidone	
Liver		
Hepatocellular damage	Phenacemide	Allergy or direct toxicity
	Mephenytoin	
	Phenytoin	
	Valproic acid	
Kidney		
Nephrotic syndrome	Trimethadione	Unknown
Lymphoid tissue		
Lymphomatous change	Phenytoin	Unknown
Pseudo-Hodgkin's disease	Primidone	
Lymphadenopathy	Mephenytoin	
	Trimethadione	
Immune system		
Lupus erythematosus reaction	Phenytoin	Possibly tissue-mediated with drug haptene immune reaction
Periarteritis nodosa reaction	Trimethadione	
Thyroiditis	Primidone	
Myasthenic syndrome	Carbamazepine	
	Succinimides	
	Mephenytoin	
Gastrointestinal system		
Nausea, vomiting, diarrhea, anorexia	Succinimides	Direct irritation; effect on chemoceptor trigger zones
	Primidone	
	Carbamazepine	
	Phenytoin	
	Valproic acid	

[a]Phenytoin, phenobarbital, and primidone rarely cause significant bone marrow depression. However, if the white blood count is serially measured after institution of therapy, mild-to-moderate depression of the white blood cells transiently occurs.

Adapted from Wilder (28). This table lists only the more common or significant toxicities and only those agents which have been more frequently reported to cause such problems.

patient should be followed closely for the first 2 years with serial WBC counts and hematocrits. After 2 years, evaluation every 3 to 6 months is probably adequate.

Possibly Immune-Related Disorders

Lymphadenopathy, which can resemble Hodgkin's disease and malignant lymphoma, is a rare complication of hydantoin therapy that usually occurs within a few months of institution of phenytoin and often, but not always, is associated with other drug-related problems such as rash or fever (22).

IgA production is reduced in some patients during long-term hydantoin administration, but a cause and effect relationship remains unproven (25).

A reversible clinical picture identical to systemic lupus erythematosus (SLE) is rarely seen in patients on long-term anticonvulsants, especially phenytoin, although it can also occur in patients on phenobarbital, primidone, and ethosuximide (1). Positive SLE preps and, more frequently, antinuclear antibodies are often seen in asymptomatic patients (20). The prevalence of antinuclear antibodies increases with the administration of multiple drugs, and it has been suggested that the drugs may alter nuclear components in many patients, but this only precipitates SLE in otherwise predisposed individuals.

Approximately two dozen cases of phenytoin-induced hepatitis, occasionally fatal, have been reported (19). This usually consists of mixed hepatocellular damage with cholestatis and necrosis, and it appears as part of a multisystem involvement including rash, fever, lymphadenopathy, and leukocytoses. Delayed hypersensitivity may be involved. Valproic acid can produce dose-related alteration in hepatic function, and several cases of fatal hepatitis have occurred in patients receiving valproic acid in addition to other anticonvulsants (29).

Paraldehyde has been reported to induce fatty changes and toxic hepatitis. This complication may occur with acute poisoning or may be seen after chronic administration.

Connective Tissue and Skin

Gingival hyperplasia occurs in up to 40% of patients on phenytoin and much less frequently in patients receiving other anticonvulsants (15). The prevalence is higher in children and adolescents than in adults. In adults the occurrence is inversely related to the degree of oral hygiene. Most patients with gingival hyperplasia have phenytoin levels in the usual therapeutic range. It has been suggested that the phenytoin-induced depression of serum and salivary IgA is the major predisposing factor to gingivitis and gum hypertrophy induced by phenytoin. Management consists of withdrawal of phenytoin, if possible; meticulous oral hygiene; and often gingivectomy.

Coarsening of the facial features owing to generalized thickening of the subcutaneous tissues of the face and scalp occurs in some patients on prolonged high-dosage antiepileptic therapy, especially those in chronic institutions (14). Severe involvement is sometimes referred to as "hydantoin facies" and is usually restricted to patients on multiple drugs for poorly controlled seizure disorders who frequently have levels of phenytoin and phenobarbital above the therapeutic range. At times, such patients have a combination of drug-induced features including acne, cholasma, hypertrichosis, coarsening of features, and gum hypertrophy so that they markedly resemble each other.

Dupuytren's contractures seem to be more common in epileptic patients on anticonvulsants, but the mechanism is unclear. Hirsutism is a well recognized side effect of chronic anticonvulsant therapy and includes both generalized and facial hirsutism. This is most commonly seen with phenytoin and is frequently irreversible, although it may regress slightly after withdrawal of the drug. It is unrelated to drug dose, drug level, or endocrine dysfunction. In both adolescents and adults, acne may be exacerbated, and occasionally hydantoins may cause a cholasma-like rash.

Skeletal System

Although frank osteomalacia or rickets are uncommon problems of chronic antiepileptic therapy, radiological or biochemical evidence of metabolic bone disease is much more common. There appears to be a relatively higher prevalence of metabolic bone disease and vitamin D deficiency in Great Britain than in the U.S., probably owing to a relatively lower dietary intake of vitamin D and less exposure to sunlight (12). Osteomalacia-related myopathy has even been attributed to anticonvulsants (17). Many drug effects may contribute to this problem including decreased calcium uptake from intestinal mucosa (phenytoin and to a lesser extent phenobarbital), enhanced metabolism of vitamin E (phenytoin and phenobarbital), and alterations in parahormone activity (phenytoin). The precise mechanism is unproven (3).

In a significant number of patients receiving phenytoin, both serum calcium and 25-hydroxycholecalciferol (the major active metabolite of cholecalciferol) concentrations are decreased, whereas alkaline phosphatase values are increased (27). Oral hydroxycholecalciferol can reverse laboratory findings and treat the osteomalacia or rickets (6). It has been suggested that patients should be maintained on supplemental vitamin D to prevent the development of metabolic bone disease.

A variety of endocrine effects have been attributed to anticonvulsants, especially phenytoin, but these are rarely if ever a clinical problem (20,28).

Miscellaneous Problems

Trimethadione often induces hemeralopia, or day blindness, at low dosage levels. This effect is secondary to direct drug action on the ganglion cell layer of the retina and often is reported in the absence of other signs of toxicity. Of the anticonvulsants, trimethadione is the one most frequently indicated as a cause of nephrotic syndromes.

Two of the less commonly used anticonvulsants have marked toxicity. The first is phenacemide (phenylacetylurea). Although this is an effective anticonvulsant with a broad range of efficacy, adverse effects are unfortunately frequent and severe. These include (a) behavioral effects such as personality changes, aggression, paranoia, and even depressive psychotic reactions; (b) toxic hepatitis; and (c) aplastic anemia. The other is the hydantoin, mephenytoin. This is metabolized by N-demethylation to Nirvanol, which was withdrawn from the market because of its severe toxicity. Skin rash, fever, lymphadenopathy, leukopenia, pancytopenia, agranulocytosis, hepatotoxicity, periarteritis, and lupus erythematosus have occurred with greater frequency with this agent than other anticonvulsants.

Teratogenic Effects

Congenital anomalies are more common in infants of epileptic mothers, whether the mother received anticonvulsants during pregnancy or not. The highest incidence, however, occurs in children born to mothers who received treatment during pregnancy. Although this difference could be due to either the severity of maternal disease or the drugs, most of the data suggest that the latter is the major factor. The relative incidence of congenital malformation is shown in Table 2, based on studies of Janz (13) and Speidel and Meadow (26). The overall risk of congenital anomalies is definitely increased in the children of treated epileptics. Some increase is also found in children of untreated epileptics. It must be mentioned that it is not known

TABLE 2. *Incidence of congenital malformations*

Status of mother	Malformations
Drug-treated epileptic mothers	88 of 1,461 live births (6%)
Untreated epileptic mothers	19 of 455 live births (4.2%)
Nonepileptic mothers	2,940 of 117,176 live births (2.5%)

TABLE 3. *Frequency of congenital malformations in 1,726 children of epileptic mothers treated during pregnancy*

Malformation	Incidence
Orofacial clefts	1.8%
Congenital heart disease	1.5%
Skeletal abnormalities	1.0%
Anencephaly	0.3%
Microcephaly	0.3%
Hydrocephaly	0.1%
Neural tube defects	0.3%
Hypospadias	0.5%
Intestinal atresia	0.3%

Adapted from Janz (13).

TABLE 4. *Drug regimen in pregnancy followed by birth of children with selected malformations*

Regimen	Orofacial clefts[a]		Heart lesion[a]	
	A	B	A	B
Barbiturates	24	5	15	6
Hydantoins	18	4	13	1
Oxazolidinediones	5	2	4	2
Carbamazepine			0	1
Ethosuximide	2	0		
Benzodiazepines	1	0	1	

[a]A, as part of regimen including two or more anticonvulsants; B, as sole anticonvulsant. Adapted from Janz (13).

whether children of mothers who convulse during pregnancy are at greater risk of malformation than those whose mothers are free of seizures. Fetal hypoxia in the first trimester could easily cause malformations. The types of congenital malformations seen and the incidence of occurrence are shown in Table 3. The overall increased incidence is mostly due to the large increase in incidence of orofacial cleft defects and less significant increase of heart lesions. While all anticonvulsants are probably potential causes of teratogenic effects, phenytoin and phenobarbital are the best studied in this regard. Table 4 shows the relative frequency with which different agents have been implicated. This gives no data as to relative incidence with these agents.

Epileptic women also have an increased incidence of complications during pregnancy and labor (4).

BIBLIOGRAPHY AND *SELECTED REVIEWS

1. Alarcon-Segovia, D. (1969): Drug induced lupus syndromes. *Mayo Clin. Proc.*, 44:664–681.
2. Alarcon-Segovia, D., Fishbein, E., Reyes, P. A., Dies, H., and Shwadsky, S. (1972): Antinuclear antibodies in patients on anticonvulsant therapy. *Clin. Exp. Immunol.*, 12:39–47.
3. Bell, R. D., Pak, C. Y. C., Zerwekh, J., Barilla, D. B., and Vasko, M. (1979): Effect of phenytoin on bone and vitamin D metabolism. *Ann. Neurol.*, 5:374–378.
4. Bjerkedal, T., and Bahna, L. (1973): The course and outcome of pregnancy in women with epilepsy. *Acta Obstet. Gynecol. Scand.*, 52:245–248.
*5. Booker, H. E. (1979): Idiosyncratic reactions to the antiepileptic drugs. *Epilepsia*, 16:171–181.
6. Christiansen, C., Rodbro, P., and Lund, M. (1973): Incidence of anticonvulsant osteomalacia and effect of vitamin D: Controlled therapeutic trial. *Br. Med. J.*, 4:695–701.
7. Dam, M. (1972): Diphenylhydantoin: Neurological aspects of toxicity. In: *Antiepileptic Drugs*, edited by D. M. Woodbury, J. K. Penry, and R. P. Schmidt, pp. 227–235. Raven Press, New York.
8. Eisen, A. A., Woods, J. F., and Sherwin, A. L. (1974): Peripheral nerve function in long-term therapy with diphenylhydantoin. *Neurology*, 24:411–417.
*9. Glaser, G. H. (1972): Diphenylhydantoin toxicity. In: *Antiepileptic Drugs*, edited by D. M. Woodbury, J. K. Penry, and R. P. Schmidt, pp. 219–226. Raven Press, New York.
10. Gratak, N. R., Santoso, R. A., and McKinney, W. M. (1976): Cerebellar degeneration following long-term phenytoin therapy. *Neurology*, 26:818–820.
11. Haberland, C. (1962): Cerebellar degeneration with clinical manifestation in chronic epileptic patients. *Psychiatr. Neurol. (Basel)*, 143:29–44.
12. Hunter, J., Maxwell, J. D., Stewart, D. A., Parsons, V., and Williams, R. (1971): Altered calcium metabolism in epileptic children on anticonvulsants. *Br. Med. J.*, 4:202–204.

*13. Janz, D. (1975): Teratogenic risks of antiepileptic drugs. *Epilepsia*, 16:159–169.

 14. Lefebvre, E. B., Haining, R. G., and Labbe, R. F. (1972): Coarse facies, calvarial thickening and hyperphosphatasia associated with long-term anticonvulsant therapy. *N. Engl. J. Med.*, 286:1301–1302.

 15. Livingston, S., and Livington, H. L. (1969): Diphenylhydantoin gingival hyperplasia. *Am. J. Dis. Child.*, 117:265–270.

 16. Lovelace, R. E., and Horwitz, S. J. (1968): Peripheral neuropathy in long-term diphenylhydantoin therapy. *Arch. Neurol.*, 18:69–77.

 17. Marsden, C. D., Reynolds, E. H., Parsons, V., Harris, R., and Ducehn, L. (1973): Myopathy associated with anticonvulsant osteomalacia. *Br. Med. J.*, 4:526–527.

 18. Mountain, K. R., Hirsch, J., and Gallus, A. S. (1970): Neonatal coagulation defect due to anticonvulsant drug treatment in pregnancy. *Lancet*, 1:265–268.

 19. Parker, W. A., and Shearer, C. A. (1979): Phenytoin hepatotoxicity: A case report and review. *Neurology*, 29:175–178.

*20. Reynolds, E. H. (1975): Chronic antiepileptic toxicity: A review. *Epilepsia*, 16:319–352.

 21. Reynolds, E. H. (1975): Neurotoxicity of carbamazepine. In: *Advances in Neurology, Vol. 2, Complex Partial Seizures and Their Treatment*, edited by D. D. Daly and J. K. Penry, pp. 345–354. Raven Press, New York.

 22. Saltzstein, S. L., and Ackerman, L. V. (1959): Lymphadenopathy induced by anticonvulsant drugs and mimicking clinically and pathogenically malignant lymphomas. *Cancer*, 12:164–182.

 23. Snider, R. S., and Del Cerro, M. (1972): Diphenylhydantoin: Proliferating membranes in cerebellum resulting from intoxication. In: *Antiepileptic Drugs*, edited by D. M. Woodbury, J. K. Penry, and R. P. Schmidt, pp. 237–245. Raven Press, New York.

 24. Solomon, G. E., Hilgartner, M. W., and Kutt, H. (1972): Coagulation defects caused by diphenylhydantoin. *Neurology*, 22:1165–1171.

 25. Sorrell, T. C., Forbes, I. J., Burness, F. R., and Rischbieth, R. H. C. (1971): Depression of immunological function in patients treated with phenytoin sodium (sodium diphenylhydantoin). *Lancet*, 2:1233–1235.

 26. Speidel, B. D., and Meadow, S. R. (1972): Maternal epilepsy and abnormalities of the fetus and newborn. *Lancet*, 2:839–843.

 27. Stamp, T. C. B., Round, J. M., Rowe, D. J. F., and Haddad, J. G. (1972): Plasma levels and therapeutic effect of 25-hydroxycholecalciferol in epileptic patients taking anticonvulsant drugs. *Br. Med. J.*, 4:9–12.

*28. Wilder, B. J. (1978): Anticonvulsant drug toxicity. In: *Clinical Neuropharmacology, Vol. 3*, edited by H. L. Klawans, pp. 57–84. Raven Press, New York.

 29. Willmore, L. J., Wilder, B. J., Bruni, J., and Villarreal, H. J. (1978): Effect of valproic acid on hepatic function. *Neurology*, 28:961–964.

Chapter 19

Anticonvulsants in Trigeminal Neuralgia and Other Related Syndromes

Patients with a variety of chronic pain syndromes often respond to treatment with anticonvulsants. The use of anticonvulsants in these diverse disorders began with the observation that phenytoin was frequently of value in ameliorating trigeminal neuralgia (tic douloureux). To this day, the use of anticonvulsants in the treatment of pain is best documented and perhaps best understood in this disorder. In most of the other disorders, the trials with anticonvulsants have usually been uncontrolled. Despite this, the efficacy observed in disorders for which there is often no reasonable alternative form of treatment has resulted in increasing acceptance of this therapeutic approach.

TRIGEMINAL NEURALGIA

The general acceptance of the concept that anticonvulsants could be of use in the treatment of trigeminal neuralgia followed the work of Iannone et al. (11). If anticonvulsants are given intravenously in doses of 100 to 250 mg, pain relief can sometimes occur within minutes. The oral doses required for sustained relief (400–600 mg/day) are often above that which can be tolerated because of ataxia and lethargy. Since most of the data on phenytoin in trigeminal neuralgia was obtained before the widespread use of blood level determination, it is not clear what the therapeutic phenytoin level is for the treatment of this disorder. It appears, however, that many if not all patients require levels that are above the usually accepted anticonvulsant range. Only approximately one-half of all patients can be managed chronically on phenytoin alone. Because of the low therapeutic index of phenytoin for trigeminal neuralgia it has been replaced as the drug of choice by carbamazepine.

Seventy-five to 80% of patients with tic douloureux respond well to carbamazepine given in the usual anticonvulsant dose range and presumably at usual anticonvulsant blood levels. Since untreated tic tends to wax and wane spontaneously, often disappearing after several months and perhaps not reappearing for years, after the pain has been relieved it is usually not necessary to maintain the patient on medication *ad infinitum*. It is our practice to withdraw carbamazepine slowly after a patient has been pain-free for 3 months.

Neither the pathophysiology of the pain in trigeminal neuralgia nor the mechanism by which phenytoin or carbamazepine produces relief is well understood. On the basis of the observation that trigeminal neuralgia often appears to be due to extrinsic pressure on the fifth nerve, it has been suggested that the paroxysmal pain is due to a transaxonal short-circuiting of the action current secondary to an artificial synapse set up by long-standing pressure. It has been demonstrated in a variety of experimental preparations that pressure on a nerve can result in demyelination and loss of the insulating function of myelin. In such a nerve, action potentials traveling along a single fiber can trigger action potentials along adjacent fibers. This does not occur in normal peripheral nerves. This pressure effect is somewhat analogous to a short circuit and is often referred to as cross talk. Such a mechanism could be involved in trigeminal neuralgia, and the efficacy of anticonvulsants could be related to their ability to act as membrane stabilizers. A variety of other mechanisms has been proposed and recently reviewed by Fields and Raskin (8).

OTHER DISORDERS

Glossopharyngeal neuralgia is closely related to trigeminal neuralgia in both the character of the pain and the presence of trigger points, although nocturnal pain is much more common in the former. Both phenytoin and carbamazepine have been reported to be effective in this disorder, but controlled studies have not been carried out.

Lightning pains of tabes dorsalis have been reported to improve during treatment with phenytoin or carbamazepine in a few patients. The same is true for postherpetic neuralgia. From clinical experience it appears that the efficacy of phenytoin and carbamazepine in either of these conditions is quite limited, but once again because of the lack of alternatives, a clinical trial is probably warranted. The same situation exists in relation to painful diabetic neuropathy. In all of these, carbamazepine is probably more likely to be helpful than phenytoin, although this is unproven. Both

TABLE 1. *Pain syndromes that have been reported to improve with anticonvulsant therapy*

Disorder	Anticonvulsant	Reference
Trigeminal neuralgia	Phenytoin	Iannone et al. (11)
Trigeminal neuralgia	Phenytoin	Braham and Saia (2)
Trigeminal neuralgia	Carbamazepine	Blom (1)
Trigeminal neuralgia	Carbamazepine	Killian (12)
Glossopharyngeal neuralgia	Carbamazepine	Ekbom and Westerberg (5)
Tabes dorsalis	Phenytoin	Green (10)
Tabes dorsalis	Carbamazepine	Ekbom (4)
Post-herpetic neuralgia	Phenytoin	Reeve (14)
Diabetic neuropathy	Phenytoin	Ellenberg (6)
Diabetic neuropathy	Carbamazepine	Rull et al. (15)
Postsympathectomy neuralgia	Phenytoin	Raskin et al. (13)
Postsympathectomy neuralgia	Carbamazepine	Raskin et al. (13)
Multiple sclerosis	Carbamazepine	Espir and Millac (7)
Multiple sclerosis	Carbamazepine	Shibasaki and Kuroiwa (16)
Thalamic pain	Phenytoin	Cantor (3)

agents have been reported to have great efficacy in the relief of postsympathectomy neuralgia. Certain episodic pains in multiple sclerosis, aside from trigeminal neuralgia, have been successfully treated with anticonvulsants. These include transient episodes of limb pain and severe painful tonic spasms. Thalamic pain, however, only rarely responds to anticonvulsant therapy.

Hemifacial Spasm

Hemifacial spasm is predominantly a disorder of the aging population. It usually begins as a frequent unilateral twitching of the orbicularis oculi. These involuntary bursts of muscle contractions progress to involve other muscles on the same side of the face. Later in the disease, mild facial weakness may occasionally be observed as well as prolonged contracture of the involved facial musculature.

Like trigeminal neuralgia, hemifacial spasm is often thought to be due to pressure on the affected nerve. Because of this similarity, we have employed carabamazepine with good success in the treatment of this disorder (9).

As in the treatment of trigeminal neuralgia, after the complete cessation of abnormal discharges, as manifested by symptomatic relief, carbamazepine can be withdrawn without immediate recurrence of the spasms.

BIBLIOGRAPHY AND *SELECTED REVIEW

1. Blom, S. (1962): Trigeminal neuralgia: Its treatment with a new anticonvulsant drug (G-32883). *Lancet*, i:839–840.
2. Braham, J., and Saia, A. (1960): Phenytoin in the treatment of trigeminal and other neuralgias. *Lancet*, ii:892–893.
3. Cantor, F. K. (1972): Phenytoin treatment in thalamic pain. *Br. Med. J.*, 3:590–591.
4. Ekbom, K. (1966): Tegretol, a new therapy for tabetic lightning pains: Preliminary report. *Acta Med. Scand.*, 179:251–252.
5. Ekbom, K. A., and Westerberg, C. E. (1966): Carbamazepine in glossopharyngeal neuralgia. *Arch. Neurol.*, 14:595–596.
6. Ellenberg, M. (1968): Treatment of diabetic neuropathy with diphenylhydantoin. *N.Y. State J. Med.*, 68:2653–2655.
7. Espir, M. L. E., and Millac, P. (1970): Treatment of paroxysmal disorders in multiple sclerosis with carbamazepine (Tegretol). *J. Neurol. Neurosurg. Psychiatry*, 33:528–531.
*8. Fields, H. L., and Raskin, N. H. (1976): Anticonvulsants and pain. In: *Clinical Neuropharmacology, Vol. 1*, edited by H. L. Klawans, pp. 173–185. Raven Press, New York.
9. Friedman, P., Sklaver, S., and Klawans, H. L. (1971): Neurological manifestations of Pagets disease. *Dis. Nerv. Syst.*, 32:809–817.
10. Green, J. B. (1961): Dilantin in the treatment of lightning pains. *Neurology (Minneap.)*, 11:257–258.
11. Iannone, A., Baker, A. B., and Morrell, F. (1958): Dilantin in the treatment of trigeminal neuralgia. *Neurology (Minneap.)*, 8:126–128.
12. Killian, J. M. (1961): Tegretol in trigeminal neuralgia with special reference to hematopoietic side effects. *Headache*, 9:58–63.
13. Raskin, N. H., Levinson, S. A., Hoffman, P. M., Picket, J. B., III, and Fields, H. L. (1974): Postsympathectomy neuralgia: Amelioration with diphenylhydantoin and carbamazepine. *Am. J. Surg.*, 128:75–78.
14. Reeve, H. S. (1961): Phenytoin in the treatment of trigeminal neuralgia. *Lancet*, i:404.
15. Rull, J. A., Quibrera, R., Gonzalez-Millan, H., and Castaneda, O. L. (1969): Symptomatic treatment of peripheral diabetic neuropathy with carbamazepine (Tegretol): Double-blind crossover trial. *Diabetologia*, 5:215–218.
16. Shibasaki, H., and Kuroiwa, Y. (1975): Painful tonic seizure in multiple sclerosis. *Arch. Neurol.*, 30:47–51.

Chapter 20

Paroxysmal Kinesigenic Choreoathetosis

A variety of terms including paroxysmal choreoathetosis, paroxysmal dystonic choreoathetosis, periodic dystonia, reflex epilepsy, familial paroxysmal choreoathetosis, and paroxysmal dyskinesia have all been used to describe this rare disorder that was first reported in 1940. The disorder or group of disorders is characterized by sudden abnormal movements and posturing of the limb, trunk, and face. While often referred to as choreatic or athetotic, the movements always result in some degree of sustained posture and by strict definitions are really dystonic in character. They can be either unilateral or bilateral, last usually 15 to 30 seconds, and are often associated with dysarthria and a sustained facial grimace. Consciousness is not lost (1). The paroxysmal movements are invariably precipitated by sudden movements.

The disorder is often familial, apparently inherited as an autosomal recessive. It usually begins in childhood or early adolescence. EEGs done during the attack are usually normal. Pathologic study has failed to reveal any significant lesion of the extrapyramidal system, but most investigators feel that the pathophysiology of the movements involves the basal ganglia.

Favorable responses have been reported with a variety of anticonvulsants. Their use was based on the concept that this disorder may represent a form of reflex epilepsy. This concept has been seriously questioned and the mechanism whereby anticonvulsants improve this disorder is unknown. The anticonvulsants that have been used include phenytoin (2), carbamazepine (1), phenobarbital, and primidone. The former two have had the greatest efficacy and are used in their usual anticonvulsant dose range.

A single patient also responded to treatment with levodopa (3).

REFERENCES

1. Kato, M., and Arki, S. (1969): Paroxysmal kinesigenic choreoathetosis. *Arch. Neurol.*, 20:508–513.
2. Kertesz, A. (1967): Paroxysmal kinesigenic choreoathetosis. *Neurology*, 17:680–690.
3. Loong, S. C., and Ong, Y. Y. (1973): Paroxysmal kinesigenic choreoathetosis. *J. Neurol. Neurosurg. Psychiatry*, 36:921–924.

Chapter 21

Affective Disorders

The starting point for most of the recent theories of the biochemistry of affective disorders is a pair of accidental observations reported in the early 1950s. First it was noted that iproniazid, used in the treatment of tuberculosis, produced significant elevation of mood in many patients. Isoniazid, which soon replaced iproniazid because of the greater hepatic toxicity of the latter, did not cause the same degree of mood elevation. It was soon proposed that the mood elevation produced by iproniazid was related to the ability of iproniazid to inhibit the enzyme monoamine oxidase (MAO). During the next 10 years, numerous agents capable of inhibiting MAO were tested and found to be of value in the treatment of depression. Since the ability to inhibit MAO is the only property shared by all these agents, and since their antidepressive activities largely parallel their potency as MAO inhibitors, their efficacy is widely accepted to be directly related to their ability to inhibit MAO.

MAO is an enzyme found within neurons that synthesize dopamine, norepinephrine, and serotonin. Its role in the degradation of all three neurotransmitters is shown schematically in Fig. 1. MAO inhibition by iproniazid or other inhibitors results in increased levels of dopamine, norepinephrine, and serotonin in the brains of various experimental animals. This finding suggests that the efficacy of MAO inhibitors in treating depression could be related to their effects on one or more of

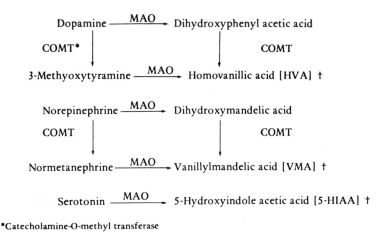

*Catecholamine-O-methyl transferase

FIG. 1.   Role of MAO in catabolism of monoamines.

these neurotransmitters. Historically norepinephrine and serotonin were implicated since at the time there was no evidence that dopamine played any role in the brain other than to act as an intermediary in the synthesis of norepinephrine.

The second observation leading to speculation on the biochemical basis of depression followed the introduction of reserpine in the treatment of hypertension. This agent produced depression in a small but significant number of patients in the same manner as it produced parkinsonism. Reserpine had been shown in animals to deplete the brain of dopamine, norepinephrine, and serotonin by blocking their uptake into presynaptic storage vesicles. Like the observation about iproniazid MAO inhibition, the reserpine-induced depression suggested that one (or more) of these neurotransmitters plays a role in depression. The fact that reserpine-induced depression does not correlate well with reserpine-induced parkinsonism suggests that dopamine is not primarily responsible.

These two observations gave rise to two hypotheses on the biochemistry of depression: a serotonin and a catecholamine, or norepinephrine, hypothesis. These "mass action" theories suggest that depression is associated with a functional central deficit of one or more brain neurotransmitters, whereas mania is correlated with a functional central excess of one or more of these amines.

Much of the work since carried out has been directed toward trying to establish the single neurotransmitter that is primarily involved in the initiation and maintenance of affective illness. As a result, there arose an indoleamine theory (implicating serotonin as the principal neurotransmitter involved in affective illness) and a catecholamine theory. The latter originally implicated norepinephrine alone but later became divided into norepinephrine and dopamine theories, supporting norepinephrine and dopamine, respectively, as the major neurotransmitters altered in a mania and depression. The dysfunctions hypothesized by each theory are summarized in Table 1.

The major methodologic approaches utilized in testing of mass action hypotheses have included the following: (a) animal studies involving manipulation of neuro-

TABLE 1. *Mass action theories of affective illness*[a]

Mass action theory	Hypothesized level of neurotransmitter and major metabolite		
	In mania	In depression	In normals
Serotonin	Increased serotonin	Decreased serotonin	Normal serotonin
(Major metabolite—5-HIAA)	Increased 5-HIAA	Decreased 5-HIAA	Normal 5-HIAA
Norepinephrine	Increased norepinephrine	Decreased norepinephrine	Normal norepinephrine
(Major metabolite—MHPG)	Increased MHPG	Decreased MHPG	Normal MHPG
Dopamine	Increased dopamine	Decreased dopamine	Normal dopamine
(Major metabolite—HVA)	Increased HVA	Decreased HVA	Normal HVA

[a]Reprinted from ref. 23.

transmitter systems, sometimes correlated with behavioral and biochemical effects; (b) measurements of monoamine neurotransmitters and their metabolites in postmortem brain specimens from suicide victims assumed to have suffered from depression; (c) studies of amine-related enzymes in peripheral tissues of affectively ill individuals; (d) pharmacologic studies evaluating the effects of certain agents on clinical affective states, as correlated with simultaneous effects on monoamine neurotransmitters; (e) clinical trials in manic and depressed patients with monoamine precursors (i.e., precursor load studies) and other substances (most often inhibitors of enzymes in monoamine synthetic and metabolic pathways) that alter the levels of neurotransmitters; and (f) assays of the levels of amines and their metabolites in the urine and cerebrospinal fluid (CSF) of manic and depressed patients.

Comprehensive reviews by Goodwin and Murphy (12) and Goodwin and Post (13) evaluate the limitations, reliability, and potential of each of these research strategies and present the detailed findings relating to monoamine neurotransmitter levels in mania and depression. The highlights of the serotonergic and catecholaminergic hypotheses are discussed below, followed by a presentation of the possible role of other neurotransmitters.

THE SEROTONIN HYPOTHESIS

The serotonin hypothesis of affective disorders states that there is a causal relationship between cerebral serotonin deficiency and depression and a similar relationship between excess serotonin and mania. Successful treatment of depression would depend on increasing serotonin activity at some cerebral receptors, whereas successful treatment of mania would depend on decreasing its activity. The serotonin neurons that might be involved in depression and mania are the midbrain raphe neurons. These neurons with cell bodies in the midbrain have diffuse synaptic (serotonergic) synapses throughout both the limbic cortex and the neocortex. Traditional anatomic considerations suggest that the limbic lobe plays a role in emotion, and that the tracts from the mesencephalon (median raphe and dorsal raphe nuclei) to the limbic forebrain may be of prime importance in the pathophysiology of the disorders of affect; those to the neocortex may also play a role.

The first biochemical data relating serotonin deficiency to depression were presented by Aschroft and his associates (3), who reported decreased levels of 5-hydroxyindoles in the CSF of patients with depressive psychoses. Other studies confirm the presence of decreased levels of 5-hydroxyindoleacetic acid (5-HIAA) in the CSF of depressed patients as a presumed reflection of decreased cerebral serotonin turnover. No study, however, has demonstrated both decreased CSF 5-HIAA in depression and increased CSF 5-HIAA in mania. In fact, studies report decreased CSF 5-HIAA in psychotic depression as well as in mania and in depressed patients after recovery from depression (9). These reports of reduced levels of 5-HIAA in CSF from both depressed and manic patients support the notion of a serotonin deficit in patients with affective disorders. However, the persistence of reduced 5-HIAA levels in patients following successful drug and electroconvulsive treatment (ECT) is not consistent with a primary mass action type relationship between the depressed state and serotonin depletion. A more reasonable hypothesis is that indoleamines play a permissive role; some primary alteration in serotonin may be necessary to permit affective abnormalities to occur, but the alteration in serotonin alone neither produces the clinical state nor predicts the direction of mood change, i.e., depression or mania.

Attempts have also been made to document deficiencies in regional concentrations of serotonin in the brains of suicides. Both Lloyd et al. (20) and Gottfries (15) examined serotonin and its metabolite 5-HIAA in discrete regions of postmortem brain specimens of suicide victims. Previous studies suggested a deficiency of serotonin but had been limited to the examination of the whole lower brainstems as homogenous units. Gottfries (15) found normal levels of serotonin and 5-HIAA in various brain regions; Lloyd et al. (20) found decreases in serotonin in the raphe nuclei dorsalis and centralis inferior of the lower brainstem, although 5-HIAA remained comparable to controls. In the higher brainstem regions and telencephalon, serotonin was found to be normal. In the mammillary bodies of the limbic system, 5-HIAA was found to be increased. Lloyd et al. (20) concluded that alterations of serotonin metabolism in depressed patients in fact may be discrete, affecting only specific functional systems rather than the whole brain or gross subdivisions. This proposal represents a second departure from standard mass action theories, in that only selective serotonergic pathways are involved in depression. This would be analagous to parkinsonism, in which one dopaminergic pathway is significantly altered. Not all norepinephrine, dopamine, or serotonin systems may be critical in determining affective normality or pathology. If serotonergic mechanisms are significant in affective disorder, agents that alter affect may work by altering serotonin.

Because of greater efficacy and safety, tricyclic antidepressants, such as imipramine and amitriptyline, have virtually replaced MAO inhibitors. The tricyclic antidepressants do not alter cerebral serotonin concentrations; rather, they block the reuptake of serotonin into presynaptic neurons. Active reuptake into the presynaptic neuron is the most important process in terminating the effect of serotonin, norepinephrine, and dopamine at their respective receptors, whereas inhibition of active reuptake into the presynaptic neuron prolongs the activity of the neurotransmitter at its receptor. It is thus possible to attribute the efficacy of tricyclic antidepressants to prolonging activity of serotonin at its receptor, much as the efficacy of amantadine in parkinsonism may be related to its ability to block the presynaptic uptake of dopamine and thereby prolong activity at dopamine receptors.

If the analogy to parkinsonism is pursued, serotonin precursors may be valuable in the treatment of depression. The pathway for serotonin synthesis is shown in Fig. 2. Both tryptophan and 5-hydroxytryptophan (5-HTP) have been used in man. Although some investigators claim that tryptophan is as effective as ECT in the treatment of depression (8), most studies show that its efficacy is more limited; some have failed to show any clinical improvement (26).

Attempts have been made to extend the serotonin hypothesis to mania and to treat the latter disorder with the serotonin antagonist methysergide. The efficacy

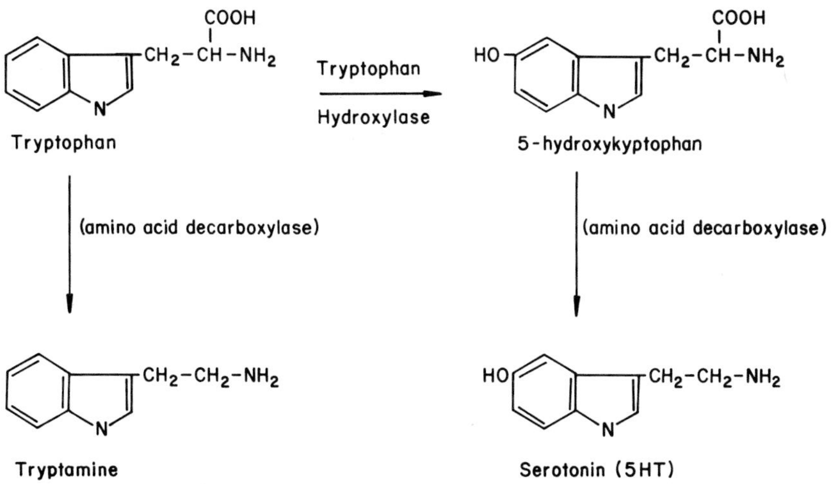

FIG. 2. Synthesis of serotonin.

of this approach remains unproven. If serotonin plays a primary role in the expression of mania, methysergide would be expected to demonstrate significant efficacy; if serotonin plays a permissive role, methysergide may not be expected to abate mania.

THE CATECHOLAMINE HYPOTHESIS

At the time of the original observations that MAO inhibitors ameliorated, and reserpine occasionally caused, depression, dopamine was thought to exist only as a precursor of norepinephrine and not to act as a neurotransmitter. Consequently, the catecholamine hypothesis of the biochemical aspects of depression was in actuality a norepinephrine hypothesis, and the two terms often were used interchangeably. More recent work suggests that dopamine might have an independent role in affective disorders.

The catecholamine (norepinephrine) hypothesis suggests a causal relationship between cerebral norepinephrine activity and affective disorders. Decreased cerebral norepinephrine activity is thought to be causally related to depression, whereas increased activity is the cause of mania. According to this hypothesis, successful pharmacologic treatment of depression must result from increasing the activity of norepinephrine at its cerebral receptors, whereas successful treatment of mania depends on decreasing its activity.

As in the serotonin hypothesis, scant biochemical data support the norepinephrine hypothesis; most deal with urinary catecholamine metabolites. Since most of these metabolites are derived from sources other than brain, and since there is no evidence that urinary output truly reflects cerebral norepinephrine, dopamine, or serotonin metabolism in man, no attempt is made to review this information. The one possible exception is the norepinephrine metabolite 3-methoxy-4-hydroxyphenylglycol (MHPG), formed by the partial oxidation and reduction of norepinephrine or normetanephrine (Fig. 3). MHPG is the principal product of brain norepinephrine catabolism, and 50% or more of the urinary MHPG in subhuman primates may be derived from cerebral sources.

The first studies of CSF catecholamine metabolites in depression and mania measured the concentration of homovanillic acid (HVA). As the final and major metabolite of dopamine, HVA in no way reflects cerebral norepinephrine catabolism (Fig. 1). The analogous catabolite of norepinephrine is vanillylmandelic acid (Fig. 1), which is not found in CSF in measurable quantities. CSF studies of HVA levels reflect only cerebral dopamine turnover. Data on CSF concentrations of MHPG in affective psychosis are conflicting. One group of investigators reported that MHPG is decreased in depression and normal in mania, whereas another group found an increase in mania and no alteration in depression (27). The significance of such studies is questionable, since we do not know how well CSF MHPG levels reflect cerebral norepinephrine concentrations or turnover in man. The studies on urinary output of MHPG in mania and depression are again conflicting; some studies show decreased MHPG in depression, and others find no significant alteration.

As previously stated, MAO inhibitors increase cerebral norepinephrine concentrations and are valuable in combating depression. The tricyclic antidepressants do not raise cerebral norepinephrine concentrations but instead block reuptake of norepinephrine in presynaptic neurons, thereby prolonging activity at the norepinephrine receptors. This is similar to their effect on cerebral serotonin reuptake and can be easily interpreted to support both hypotheses.

The biochemicopharmacologic study of Maas et al. (22) lends additional support to the norepinephrine hypothesis. These investigators described decreased urinary levels of MHPG in a subgroup of depressed patients. These patients responded better to treatment with imipramine than did those patients with normal urinary MHPG. This finding supports the concept that decreased norepinephrine metabolism is causally related to depression in these individuals, and that increasing the activity of norepinephrine at its receptors by treatment with imipramine is beneficial to such patients.

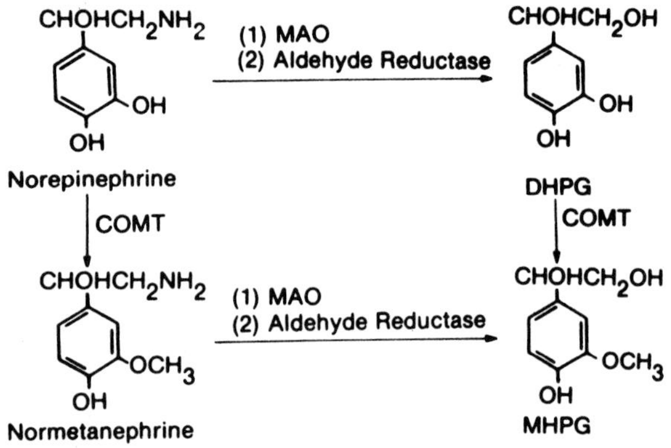

FIG. 3. Formation of MHPG.

Reserpine can cause depression and has a more profound effect on cerebral norepinephrine than on either serotonin or dopamine. Serotonin and dopamine are synthesized from the appropriate precursor by L-amino acid decarboxylase before being taken up into storage granules. Synthesis of these two neurotransmitters continues unabated in the reserpinized brain. The enzyme that catalyzes the synthesis of norepinephrine from dopamine is also located within the storage granule. As a result, dopamine must be taken up into the granule in order for norepinephrine synthesis to occur. Since reserpine blocks this uptake, norepinephrine synthesis is disrupted; this raises the possibility that norepinephrine is of primary importance in reserpine-induced depression.

If decreased norepinephrine activity causes depression, mania should be a manifestation of increased norepinephrine activity; decreasing the activity at its receptors should then improve mania. Although specific cerebral norepinephrine receptor site antagonists have not been tested in mania, attempts have been made to study the effect of blocking norepinephrine synthesis in both mania and depression. α-Methyl-p-tyrosine, a tyrosine hydroxylase inhibitor that blocks cerebral catecholamine synthesis without altering cerebral serotonin synthesis, has been given to several patients with affective psychosis. It is reported to produce marked improvement in mania and marked worsening in depression (5). Although these studies involve only a few patients, they support the role of catecholamines in affective disorders. It is hypothesized that the norepinephrine neuronal system ascending from the locus ceruleus and medullary reticular formation to the limbic forebrain, hypothalamus, and neocortex is involved in affective disorders.

Neuroleptic agents are of value in the treatment of acute mania. They act as dopamine receptor site antagonists and decrease dopamine activity at its receptors. The activity of these drugs in mania, however, seems less specific than the effect of lithium; the former are more effective in decreasing motor activity in manic patients than in altering mood elevations.

Investigations of CSF HVA in affective disorders may relate to the role of dopamine in mood disorders. Numerous studies report decreased CSF HVA concentration in depression, especially in patients with retarded depression. Levodopa has been used in the treatment of depression with some beneficial results. Its efficacy, although limited, raises the possibility that dopamine may play a therapeutic role in affective disorders. Apparently beneficial results are achieved only in patients with retarded depression, and the agent is of no value in agitated depression (14). Thus in a subgroup of patients with retarded depression, decreased dopamine activity may play a role. Also, in depressed patients with a history of mania, levodopa regularly induced hypomania, usually without relieving depression (25), raising the possibility that dopamine may play a role in the induction of mania in susceptible individuals. These data are complicated by the fact that motor activity alters CSF concentration. Degree of exercise is most strongly reflected by CSF HVA levels and to a lesser extent by 5-HIAA and MHPG concentrations (28). It is then likely that decreased levels of CSF HVA in patients with retarded depression may reflect the motor retardation and not the mood depression.

The pharmacologic data lend only partial support to a dopamine hypothesis. MAO inhibitors increase cerebral dopamine concentration, but the more effective tricyclic antidepressants do not block dopamine reuptake and do not increase the activity of dopamine at dopamine receptors. Furthermore, there is no correlation between reserpine-induced depression and reserpine-induced parkinsonism, a finding that suggests that dopamine may not be pivotal in the production of reserpine-induced depression.

THE CHOLINERGIC APPROACH

The monoamines are not the only putative neurotransmitters implicated in affective disorders. Acetylcholine, the first discovered transmitter, has been receiving significant attention, based on concepts of the behavioral implications of neurotransmitter balance as seen in movement disorders. The application of a model of catecholamine–acetylcholine balance in affective disorders was first suggested by Janowsky et al. (16). Specifically, these workers propose that affective states may be based on a balance between central cholinergic and adrenergic neurotransmitter activity in those areas of the brain that regulate affect. Depression is then conceptualized as a disease in which balance is shifted toward cholinergic dominance; mania is hypothesized to be the pharmacologic opposite.

In support of these contentions, Janowsky et al. (17) studied the effects of the reversible cholinesterase inhibitor physostigmine on patients with symptoms of hypomania. In a double-blind study, the administration of physostigmine caused a rapid and dramatic decrease in manic symptomatology in all patients, with simultaneous induction of depressive symptomatology in more than half. Despite the limitations of this study (i.e., the more consistent effect of physostigmine on motoric activity as compared to its less consistent effects on mood and thought disturbance), additional experimental data support the concept of an adrenergic–cholinergic balance theory of affective illness. These include animal studies demonstrating antagonistic cholinergic (inhibiting) and adrenergic (activating) central behavioral effects. Additional pharmacologic speculations attribute the depressive effects of reserpine to its central cholinomimetic properties. Many tricyclic antidepressants are strong anticholinergic agents, and their efficacy might be related in part to their central anticholinergic properties (10). Since not all antidepressants are anticholinergic agents, this mechanism cannot account for all the efficacy of these drugs. It must be kept in mind, however, that acetylcholine may play a secondary rather than a primary role in the proposed homeostatic balance controlling affective states analogous to the secondary role it plays in the balance controlling striatal function. This would help explain the partial efficacy of cholinergic and anticholinergic agents in treating the affective disorders.

IDENTIFICATION OF SUBGROUPS

In the last few years, mass action theories have been further modified by attempts to delineate subgroups of patients with affective disorders who may be biochemically and therefore pharmacologically different. At least three such approaches have been explored: (a) unipolar versus bipolar, (b) presynaptic versus postsynaptic, and (c) serotonergic versus catecholaminergic (noradrenergic). In consideration of the numerous classifications of affective illnesses, and depressions in particular, the strongest support exists for the bipolar-unipolar dichotomy. Numerous clinical, genetic, biochemical, and pharmacologic correlates suggest that unipolar and bipolar affective illness may represent biologically distinct entities.

Clinically, the unipolar patients have a later age of onset than the bipolar patients, and their depressions have mixed features of agitation and retardation accompanied by a significantly greater occurrence of anger, anxiety, and somatization. The depressed phase of bipolar illness tends to be characterized by seclusiveness, non-verbalization, and increased sleep. Studies by several groups have also suggested that bipolar and unipolar affective disorders are genetically independent. Several biologic variables have been noted to differ in unipolar and bipolar groups. These include cortical evoked potentials, urinary 17-hydroxycorticosteroids, platelet MAO activity, and red cell catechol-o-methyltransferase activity. Although urinary excretion of MHPG has been shown to demonstrate clear unipolar-bipolar differences, no consistent unipolar-bipolar CSF metabolite differences (either baseline or in response to probenecid) have been established. These differences have been reviewed by Moskowitz and Klawans (23) and by Murphy (24).

Finally, different responses to certain pharmacologic agents distinguish unipolar from bipolar illness. A significantly higher percentage of bipolar than unipolar depressive patients respond to lithium with remission of depressive symptomatology. Lithium prophylaxis of recurrent depression is more successful in bipolar than in unipolar patients. Bipolar patients tend to respond less well to imipramine than do unipolars and are more susceptible to tricyclic-induced manias. They are also more susceptible to MAO inhibitor-induced manias. Bipolar depressives also tend to be significantly more susceptible to levodopa-induced hypomania. Finally, evidence exists for a differential response to L-tryptophan in bipolar versus unipolar depressed patients.

Attempts to correlate depression with decreased activity of some neurotransmitter at its receptor is analogous to parkinsonism, raising the possibility that both pre- and postsynaptic problems could result in clinically identical depression (19).

In most instances of parkinsonism, the pathophysiology is believed to consist of a decrease of available dopamine at striatal dopamine receptors secondary to degeneration of dopaminergic neurons of the substantia nigra. In other words, there is a deficiency of neurotransmitter at a hypothetically normal dopamine receptor; the disorder, therefore, is presynaptic. This presynaptic dopamine deficiency should be reflected biochemically by decreased CSF HVA (assumed to represent decreased dopamine turnover) and pharmacologically by response to levodopa therapy (leading to increased dopamine turnover and, thereby, to increased activity of dopamine within the striatum). Most but not all parkinsonian patients hold true to these criteria.

As discussed in Chapter 1, there are other forms of parkinsonism that are characterized not by a deficiency of dopamine but by a loss of striatal responsiveness to dopamine, i.e., a postsynaptic receptor site dysfunction. The normal dopamine turnover and limited efficacy of levodopa therapy that characterize this group are logical only in light of a receptor site disorder. Despite the disparity in the actual site of dysfunction in pre- and postsynaptic disorder, the two forms of parkinsonism have identical clinical manifestations.

The concept that dysfunction may exist presynaptically (as consistent with the various mass action hypotheses) or postsynaptically may be applied to the study of affective illness. Van Praag took preliminary steps toward a theory encompassing both pre- and postsynaptic levels of dysfunction by stating that central monoamine deficiency occurs in only a proportion of individuals suffering from affective illness (32). Although biochemically distinct, Van Praag's two subgroups of depressed patients (with and without central monoamine deficiencies) were clinically identical, as the analogous two categories of parkinsonian patients. The author speculated that the responsiveness to antidepressants is related to the presence or absence of disorders of monoamine metabolism. A positive response would be consistent with a presynaptic disorder and a negative response with a postsynaptic one. Aschroft and Glen (2) proposed the existence of a low output subgroup of depression (with low output of amine transmitters) and a low sensitivity subgroup (with low sensitivity of amine receptors) that are clinically indistinguishable. These categories are synonomous to pre- and postsynaptic subdivisions.

These speculations concerning pre- and postsynaptic categories of dysfunction are strongly supported by the work of Maas et al. (21,22). These investigators found that depressed patients demonstrating decreased urinary excretion of MHPG (reflective of decreased CNS norepinephrine) prior to treatment with imipramine or desimipramine had a better response to medication and excreted greater quantities of normetanephrine and MHPG (both metabolites of norepinephrine) during the period of tricyclic therapy than did clinically similar patients without decreased urinary MHPG. The group of patients who excreted greater quantities of urinary MHPG prior to treatment tended to be nonresponsive to treatment with imipramine or desimipramine and demonstrated marked decrements in the quantity of MHPG excreted during the period of pharmacotherapy. The possibility that the imipramine responders may constitute a subgroup whose disorder is presynaptic, and the nonresponders a subgroup whose disorder is postsynaptic, is consistent with the above data. No postsynaptic adrenergic agent is presently available to test this.

Parallel evidence has been found from studying central serotonergic activity in depressed individuals treated with the serotonin precursor 5-HTP (34). It has been shown that pretreatment 5-HIAA accumulation after probenecid tended to be subnormal in responders but normal in nonresponders. Although the limited size of the population in this study makes any conclusions tenuous, the results are not inconsistent with a differentiation of pre- and postsynaptic sites of dysfunction.

Application of these findings and speculations may help unify seemingly conflicting data pertaining to normal or abnormal levels of a particular neurotransmitter. Affective illness should be conceived in terms of not only neurotransmitter excesses and deficiencies (presynaptic) but altered receptor site sensitivity (postsynaptic) as contributory to the basic pathophysiology of at least some categories of depression and mania.

Much of the above evidence, however, may not differentiate pre- from postsynaptic affective disorders but may separate serotonin- from norepinephrine-related clinical disease. This view has been reviewed by Maas (21), wherein depressive disorders may be divided into two groups using specific biochemical and pharmacologic criteria. The criteria used combine observation of clinical efficacy of different tricyclic antidepressants, differential effects of these tricyclic antidepressants on biogenic amine reuptake, and levels of various urinary metabolites. Most of the available tricyclic antidepressants inhibit the membrane reuptake of both serotonin and norepinephrine *in vitro* but not equally (see Table 2). One assumption of this theory is that these *in vitro* animal data apply to man *in vivo*.

One group of depressed patients (serotonergic) is characterized by (a) a normal or high urinary MHPG level, (b) a favorable treatment response to amitriptyline, (c) a lack of mood change during a trial of dextroamphetamine, and (d) a failure to respond to imipramine. That serotonin is pharmacologically significant in at least a subgroup of patients is further supported by the observation that clomipramine, a relatively specific inhibitor of serotonin reuptake, is potentiated as an antidepressant by tryptophan and itself potentiates 5-HTP; there is a negative correlation between CNS serotonin turnover as reflected by CSF HIAA and clinical response to clomipramine (34,35).

The second group of depressed patients (noradrenergic) can be characterized as follows: (a) low pretreatment MHPG level, (b) a favorable response to treatment with imipramine or desipramine, (c) a brightening of mood following a trial of dextroamphetamine, and (d) a failure to respond to amitriptyline.

Since depression is a biochemically heterogeneous illness, it is likely that significant differences will be obscured when depressed subjects are compared as a group with normal individuals. This might account for the variable reports of CSF MHPG levels in depressed versus normal subjects.

CLINICAL PHARMACOLOGY OF TRICYCLIC ANTIDEPRESSANTS

The structure of the major tricyclic antidepressants is shown in Fig. 4. These agents are structurally similar to phenothiazines. The synthesis of imipramine, the prototype of all tricyclic drugs, involves replacing the sulfur atom in the phenothiazine molecule with a dimethyl bridge. This relatively minor structural alteration produces a critical difference in pharmacologic activity.

TABLE 2. In vivo *effect of some antidepressants and dextroamphetamine on biogenic monoamine membrane reuptake*

Drug	Serotonin	Norepinephrine	Dopamine
Clomipramine	4 +	0	0
Amitriptyline	4 +	1 +	0
Nortriptyline	2 +	2 +	0
Imipramine	3 +	2 +	0
Desipramine	0	4 +	0
Dextroamphetamine	0	3 +	4 +

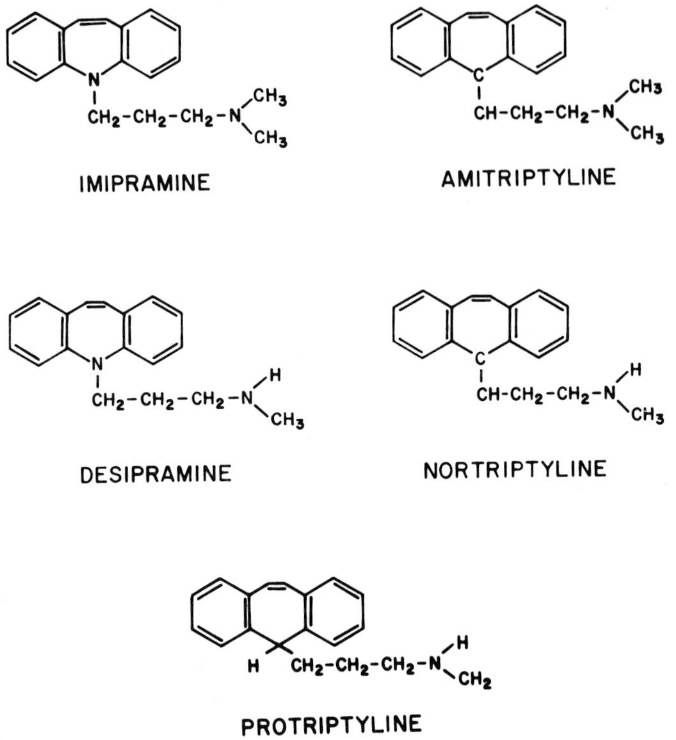

IMIPRAMINE

AMITRIPTYLINE

DESIPRAMINE

NORTRIPTYLINE

PROTRIPTYLINE

FIG. 4. Chemical structures of the major tricyclic antidepressant drugs.

The tricyclic antidepressants are readily absorbed from the gastrointestinal tract. In humans, imipramine and amitriptyline are partially metabolized to their desmethyl derivatives (desipramine and nortriptyline). Knowledge of this process led to the synthesis of desipramine in the hope that it would exert its antidepressant action more rapidly than does its parent compound. Clinical studies, however, demonstrate no difference in speed or action of the newer compounds. The desmethyl derivatives are said to be less sedating than their parent compounds. Amitriptyline is reported to be more sedating than imipramine; protriptyline is less so.

The principal tricyclic antidepressants—imipramine, amitriptyline, nortriptyline, desipramine, protriptyline—constitute the most effective class of antidepressants and are beneficial to approximately 70% of depressed patients within 3 to 4 weeks. Because of their relatively greater therapeutic effectiveness, and because they have the least risk of side effects, the tricyclic drugs are probably the drugs of choice for most depressive illness.

In general, it is the severe psychotic or endogenous depressive patient who responds best to tricyclic drugs, whereas the chronic characterologic depressive patient responds less well. The therapeutic response, when it occurs, develops after a lag period of 3 to 14 days and results in marked improvement in behavior and a striking decrease in depression. Patients who remain unresponsive after 3 weeks of treatment at adequate dosage levels probably will not respond at all; they should be shifted to another drug or receive ECT. The possibility that all depressed patients may not be biologically the same and that the various tricyclics may be different should be considered when changing agents; e.g., a patient unresponsive to desipramine may do best on amitriptyline.

Since depression is frequently a recurrent disorder, the role of maintenance therapy in preventing relapses is of great practical importance. Except for the fact that patients with incomplete response relapse more frequently, there are no adequate predictors as to which patients require tricyclics. Davis (11) suggests that once remission is achieved, patients should be continued at full dosage for 1 month. The dosage is then reduced by approximately 50% for maintenance treatment. Extended medication with tricyclic agents or lithium may be indicated for unipolar patients prone to frequent recurrences. Maintenance lithium is of course the agent of choice for bipolar patients to prevent the recurrence of both aspects of this disorder (29).

Some nonresponders may not respond for pharmacokinetic reasons. Under ordinary circumstances, as the tricyclic agents are administered, blood levels build up until they reach a fairly constant level within about 1 week. There are considerable individual differences in plasma levels. Some patients have a metabolic defect that results in the accumulation of unusually high plasma and brain levels. Consequently, they may fail to improve clinically because they are receiving a toxic dose. Others metabolize the tricyclic drugs with unusual rapidity; as a result, they fail to develop adequate blood levels and hence have low brain levels. These patients may prove especially slow in responding to the medication and are likely to remain unresponsive to lower dosages. Studies with nortriptyline have shown a curvilinear relationship between clinical improvement and plasma nortriptyline levels (18).

The prototype of these studies was done by Asberg and her colleagues (1). Among those patients who failed to respond were two subgroups with very high and very low blood levels of nortriptyline. Several patients were found to have relatively high plasma levels of nortriptyline and yet responded poorly. After their dose was reduced, some of these patients responded rapidly and were discharged from the hospital within 1 week, suggesting that their initial unresponsiveness to the drug was attributable to an excessively high plasma concentration. This curvilinear relationship, in which there is a therapeutic window for clinical efficacy, applies to nortriptyline and other secondary (e.g., protriptyline and desmethylimipramine) but not tertiary (e.g., imipramine, amitriptyline, and doxepin) amine tricyclics. These latter agents seem to be characterized by a linear relationship between clinical efficacy and blood level without a therapeutic window other than the one imposed on all drugs by clinically evident dose-related toxicity.

The use of the tricyclic antidepressants is accompanied by a variety of side effects. The most common are related to the antimuscarine activity and include dry mouth, palpitations, tachycardia, loss of accommodation, postural hypotension, vomiting, constipation, edema, and aggravation of narrow-angle glaucoma. This is the same profile seen with anticholinergic treatment of parkinsonism. Occasionally, urinary retention and paralytic ileus leading to serious or even fatal complications have been reported. These are more likely to occur when the tricyclic drugs are combined with other anticholinergic agents. Autonomic effects tend to be mild and usually grow less distressing after the initial weeks of treatment (tolerance). These side effects may require readjustment of the dosage level.

Since the tricyclic antidepressants inhibit the reuptake of released norepinephrine, thereby potentiating its function, additive drug interactions may occur with guanethidine-type drugs. Guanethidine and related antihypertensive medications are taken into the peripheral noradrenergic neuron by the membrane pump in order to exert their hypotensive effects. When this pump is blocked, the uptake of guanethidine is prevented, and thus its antihypertensive effect is abolished. Other rare problems include rashes, cholestatic jaundice, and blood dyscrasias. A possible cardiovascular effect, with flattened T-waves, prolonged Q-T interval, and depressed S-T segments, has been described.

These agents can also produce CNS effects, including (a) postural and intention tremor, either as an exacerbation of preexisting benign essential tremor or eliciting the same type of tremor de novo in susceptible individuals; (b) insomnia, especially in elderly patients; (c) precipitation of mania; and (d) anticholinergic-mediated speech arrests.

Severe toxic reactions and extreme hyperpyrexia, often leading to death, may result when tricyclic antidepressants and MAO inhibitors are used in close conjunction. Therefore, MAO inhibitors should be discontinued at least 1 week prior to the initiation of tricyclic therapy. Overdosage of tricyclic antidepressants may result in life-threatening consequences. The clinical picture is characterized by temporary agitation, delirium, myoclonus, convulsions, hyperreflexive tendons, disturbance of temperature regulation, mydriasis, and progression to coma, accompanied by shock and respiratory depression. Cardiac rhythm may be disturbed, resulting in tachycardia, atrial fibrillation, ventricular flutter, and atrioventricular or intraventricular block.

Management of cardiac function is critical during coma, as death can result from cardiac arrhythmia. If the patient survives this period, vigorous resuscitative measures, cardioversion, continuous cardiac monitoring, and chemotherapy to manage arrhythmias should be applied in an intensive care unit. Physostigmine (0.25 to 4 mg i.v. or i.m.) is useful to counteract anticholinergic toxicity and tachycardia; propranolol is helpful in preventing arrhythmias. The patient must be kept under constant medical supervision for several days to permit immediate attention to any delayed cardiac difficulties that may arise. Finally, because ingestion of several grams can be fatal, care must be exercised to prevent suicidal depressed patients from gaining access to large numbers of antidepressant tablets.

LITHIUM

Lithium salts were first used to treat acute mania by Cade in 1949 (7). The more than 80 reports that have since been published are unanimous in their endorsement of this agent in the treatment of mania (31). Lithium is more specific in its effect on pure mania than are the neuroleptic agents. Chlorpromazine and other neuroleptic compounds may be more rapid in controlling manic activity, but their effect is less specific; they rapidly decrease agitation and overt motor activity in manic patients without altering mood. Lithium decreases agitation and motor overactivity more slowly, but the effect is associated with a definite normalization of mood.

Long-term lithium therapy for the prevention of recurrent mood disorders is of greater theoretical interest. Lithium salts were initially used prophylactically to prevent recurrent episodes of mania and were found to be effective. It was soon recognized that lithium prophylaxis also significantly prevented depressive episodes in patients with cyclic manic-depressive disorders. Some evidence now supports the view that long-term lithium salt therapy can prevent or at least decrease episodes of depression in patients with recurrent depressions without mania. Lithium is also of value in the treatment of acute depression.

The clinicopharmacologic observations that this single salt is of value in treating mania, preventing recurrent mania, ameliorating recurrent depression, and perhaps treating acute depression do not fit well with the biochemical theories of affective disorders. There is no clear understanding of the effect of lithium on cerebral monoamine metabolism or activity nor how any such single effect might prevent both mania (a reflection of increased monoamine activity) and depression (a possible reflection of decreased monoamine activity). The most intriguing suggestion may be that lithium modulates receptor site responsiveness, thereby preventing periodic increases or decreases of monoamine activity.

The clinical efficacy and side effects of lithium correlate well with the drug serum levels. On the average, a dose of 300 mg lithium carbonate increases serum lithium level by 0.2 to 0.4 mEq/liter. Studies indicate that serum lithium levels of 0.9 to 1.4 mEq/liter are adequate for the treatment of most patients with acute mania; levels of 0.7 to 1.2 mEq/liter are recommended for maintenance therapy. Levels exceeding 1.5 mEq/liter should be used with caution, and levels of 2.0 mEq/liter warrant immediate reduction.

The majority of patients on lithium therapy experience side effects. These reactions are usually mild and rarely require discontinuation of medication. Most side effects occur during the first few weeks of treatment and include gastrointestinal irritation (nausea, vomiting, abdominal pain, and diarrhea), renal symptoms (polyuria, often accompanied by thirst), and weakness, fatigue, and drowsiness. These reactions are usually transient and disappear within a few weeks, although polyuria and thirst may persist for long periods, even at low doses. Edema and weight gain may occur later in treatment. These reactions appear to be fully reversible and disappear when lithium is withdrawn. The most common, most annoying, and most likely to persist is a fine postural and intention tremor that occurs in the vast majority of patients; it can be quite disabling. In such individuals, this appears to be either an exacerbation of preexisting benign essential tremor or a precipitation of a similar tremor in susceptible individuals. Usually, reduction of dosage will either eliminate the tremor or significantly reduce its intensity. The beta-adrenergic blocker propranolol has proved beneficial in some cases. Weight gain is another annoying reaction. Approximately 10% of the patients who receive lithium over a long period report weight gains exceeding 5 kg; weight gains of 15 kg or more are not uncommon. The mechanism of weight gain during lithium therapy is not known. Other complications not related to dosage level include (a) leukocytosis, (b) mild transient hypothyroidism, (c) progressive renal damage, (d) diabetes insipidus-like syndrome, and (e) EEG changes (increased amplitude and decreased frequency). These are reviewed by Prien (29). Lithium-induced kidney damage is more common at higher serum levels. The frequency and significance of this side effect are still unclear.

Toxic confusional states may occur in the absence of other signs of toxicity and at relatively low serum lithium levels. These reactions resemble early organic brain syndrome and are characterized by disorientation, confusion, lack of continuity of thought, memory loss, lability of mood, and reduced comprehension. The symptoms are usually preceded by a steady or precipitous rise in lithium dosage, often within the first few weeks of treatment, but may occur at serum lithium levels as low as 1.0 mEq/liter. The condition usually remits within a few days following reduction or withdrawal of the dosage. It has been suggested that patients with schizophrenia or organic brain disorders are particularly susceptible to this complication because of a decreased tolerance of the CNS to lithium.

Once the therapeutic or maintenance level of lithium has been established, it is necessary that the kidneys be able to excrete as much lithium as is administered. If the kidneys cannot handle lithium intake (owing to excessive dosage or undetected renal insufficiency), accumulation and intoxication may result. Prodromal symptoms include nausea, vomiting, diarrhea, coarse tremor, drowsiness, ataxia, muscle twitching, and slurred speech. These symptoms may be present for 4 or more days before more severe problems occur and are easily reversed by reduction of dosage or discontinuation of medication.

As intoxication advances, increased neurologic complications lead to impaired consciousness, ataxia, and, eventually, coma and occasionally seizures. Although most cases of lithium intoxication occur at serum levels exceeding 2.0 mEq/liter, some patients may become toxic at serum levels considered to be within safe limits.

There is no specific antidote for severe lithium intoxication. Effective treatment must result in increased lithium excretion. This is complicated by the fact that lithium passes relatively slowly through neural cell membranes. Administration of aminophylline and osmotic diuresis using mannitol or urea are reported to increase lithium excretion, although results have been inconsistent. Hemodialysis has been employed successfully in a few cases. If treatment is delayed or inadequate, death may result, usually from pulmonary complications.

Until recently, it was thought that patients who survived severe lithium intoxication suffered no permanent neurologic damage. However, reports during the past few years indicate that patients may suffer irreversible brain damage following acute intoxication. The basal ganglia and cerebellum are affected. Symptoms include ataxia, nystagmus, choreoathetoid movements, and hyperactive deep tendon reflexes. The most frequent complication is ataxia.

The best way to manage lithium intoxication is to prevent its occurrence by careful screening of patients, proper regulation of dosage, and adequate clinical and biochemical monitoring during treatment. Any condition that might impair adequate elimination of the lithium ion is a relative contraindication to lithium therapy; significant renal disease is an absolute contraindication.

CARBAMAZEPINE

Based on its psychotropic effects, carbamazepine has been used in acute mania with significant efficacy. This agent has also shown significant short-term prophylactic effects. Its long-term efficacy and exact role in affective disorders are not well defined.

MAO INHIBITORS

The MAO inhibitors have been almost completely replaced by tricyclic antidepressants, which usually have greater efficacy and safety. Side effects include (a) conversion of retarded depression into an agitated or anxious depression, (b) precipitation of hypomania, (c) autonomic effects, such as orthostatic hypotension, delayed micturition and ejaculation, dry mouth, and constipation, and (d) hypertensive crises, usually associated with severe headache and occasionally resulting in intracranial hemorrhage. Such syndromes are seen in patients on MAO inhibitors who ingest food containing the pressor amine tyramine. Tyramine is normally destroyed by MAO. Foods with high tyramine content include some cheeses, especially cheddar and camembert, beer, chianti, chicken liver, yeast products, chocolate, and pickled products, such as herring. A variety of pharmacologic agents can also produce such episodes. These include amphetamines, tricyclic antidepressants, ephedrine, and levodopa.

REFERENCES AND *SELECTED REVIEWS

1. Asberg, M., Cronholm, B., Sjoqvist, F., and Tuck, D. (1971): Relationship between plasma levels and therapeutic effect of nortriptyline. *Br. Med. J.*, 3:331–334.
2. Aschroft, G. W., and Glen, A. I. M. (1974): Mood and neuronal functions: A modified amine hypothesis for the etiology of affective illness. *Adv. Biochem. Psychopharmacol.*, 11:335–339.
3. Aschroft, G. W., Crawford, T. B. B., and Eccleston, D. (1966): 5-Hydroxyindole compounds in the cerebrospinal fluid of patients with psychiatric or neurologic disease. *Lancet*, 2:1049–1052.
4. Beckmann, H., and Goodwin, F. K. (1975): Antidepressant responses to tricyclics and urinary MHPG in unipolar patients. *Arch. Gen. Psychiatry*, 32:17–21.
5. Brodie, H. K. H., Murphy, D. L., Goodwin, F. K., and Bunney, W. E. J. (1971): Catecholamines and mania: The effect of alpha-methyl-p-tyrosine on manic behavior and catecholamine metabolism. *Clin. Pharmacol. Ther.*, 12:218–229.
6. Bunney, W. E. J., Goodwin, F. K., and Murphy, D. L. (1972): The switch process in manic-depressive illness. *Arch. Gen. Psychiatry*, 27:312–317.
7. Cade, J. F. J. (1949): Lithium salts in the treatment of psychotic excitement. *Med. J. Aust.*, 36:349–353.
8. Coppen, A. (1967): The biochemistry of affective disorders. *Br. J. Psychiatry*, 113:1237–1244.
9. Coppen, A., Prange, A. J., Jr., Whybrow, P. C., and Noguera, R. (1972): Abnormalities of indoleamines in affective disorders. *Arch. Gen. Psychiatry*, 26:474–479.
10. Davis, J. (1975): Critique of single amine theories: Evidence of a cholinergic influence in the major mental illnesses. In: *Biology of the Major Psychoses*, edited by D. X. Freedman, pp. 333–342. Raven Press, New York.
*11. Davis, J. (1976): Tricyclic antidepressants. In: *Drug Treatment of Mental Disorders*, edited by L. L. Simpson, pp. 127–146. Raven Press, New York.

*12. Goodwin, F. K., and Murphy, D. L. (1974): Biological factors in the affective disorders and schizophrenia. In: *Psychopharmacological Agents*, edited by M. Gordon, pp. 9–31. Academic Press, New York.

*13. Goodwin, F. K., and Post, R. M. (1975): Studies of amine metabolites in affective illness and in schizophrenia. In: *Biology of the Major Psychoses*, edited by D. X. Freedman, pp. 299–332. Raven Press, New York.

14. Goodwin, F. K., Murphy, D. L., Brodie, H. K. H., and Bunney, W. E. J. (1976): L-dopa, catecholamines, and behavior. A clinical and biochemical study in depressed patients. *Biol. Psychol.*, 2:341–366.

15. Gottfries, C. G. (1974): Paper read at World Congress of Psychiatry, section on Biological Psychiatry. Munich, Germany.

16. Janowsky, D. S., El-Yousef, M. K., Davis, J. M., and Sekerke, H. J. (1972): A cholinergic/adrenergic hypothesis of mania and depression. *Lancet*, 2:632–635.

17. Janowsky, D. S., El-Yousef, M. K., Davis, J. M., Hubbard, B., and Sekerke, H. J. (1972): Cholinergic reversal of manic symptoms. *Lancet*, 2:1236–1237.

*18. Kinard, C. O., Chang, S. S. and Davis, J. M. (1978): Plasma levels of antidepressant and clinical response. In: *Clinical Neuropharmacology, Vol. 3*, edited by H. L. Klawans, pp. 103–112. Raven Press, New York.

19. Klawans, H. L. (1975): Amine precursors in neurologic disorders and the psychoses. In: *Biology of the Major Psychoses*, edited by D. X. Freedman, pp. 259–272. Raven Press, New York.

20. Lloyd, K. G., Fasley, I. J., Deck, J. H. N., and Hornykiewicz, O. (1974): Serotonin and 5-hydroxyindoleacetic acid in discrete areas of the brainstem of suicide victims and control patients. In: *Advances in Biochemical Psychopharmacology, Vol. 11, Serotonin—New Vistas*, edited by E. Costa, G. L. Gessa, and M. Sandler. Raven Press, New York.

21. Maas, J. W. (1975): Biogenic amines and depression. Biochemical and pharmacological separation of two types of depression. *Arch. Gen. Psychiatry*, 32:1357.

22. Maas, J. W., Fawcett, J. A., and Dekirmenjian, H. (1972): Catecholamine metabolism, depressive illness, and drug response. *Arch. Gen. Psychiatry*, 26:252–262.

*23. Moskowitz, C., and Klawans, H. L. (1977): Theoretical aspects of the pharmacology of affective disorders. In: *Clinical Neuropharmacology, Vol. 2*, edited by H. L. Klawans, pp. 55–84. Raven Press, New York.

*24. Murphy, D. L. (1976): Neuropharmacology of depression. In: *Drug Treatment of Mental Disorders*, edited by L. L. Simpson, pp. 117–125. Raven Press, New York.

25. Murphy, D. L., Goodwin, F. K., Brodie, H. K., and Bunney, W. E. J. (1973): L-dopa, dopamine, and hypomania. *Am. J. Psychiatry*, 130:79–82.

26. Murphy, D. L., Baker, M., Goodwin, F. K., Miller, H., Kotin, J., and Bunney, W. E. J. (1974): L-tryptophan in affective disorders: Indoleamine changes and differential clinical effects. *Psychopharmacologia*, 34:11–20.

27. Post, R. M., Gordon, E. K., Goodwin, F. K., and Bunney, W. E. (1972): Cerebral norepinephrine metabolism in affective illness: MHPG in the cerebrospinal fluid. *Science*, 179:1002–1003.

28. Post, R. M., Kotin, J., Goodwin, F. K., and Gordon, E. (1973): Psychomotor activity and cerebrospinal fluid metabolites in affective illness. *Am. J. Psychiatry*, 130:67–72.

*29. Prien, R. F. (1978): Lithium in the treatment of affective disorders. In: *Clinical Neuropharmacology, Vol. 3*, edited by H. L. Klawans, pp. 113–130. Raven Press, New York.

*30. Schildkraut, J. J. (1969): Neuropsychopharmacology and affective disorders. *N. Engl. J. Med.*, 281:197–201.

31. Schou, M. (1968): Lithium in psychiatric therapy and prophylaxis. *J. Psychiatr. Res.*, 6:67–95.

32. van Praag, H. M. (1974): Toward a biochemical classification of depression. *Adv. Biochem. Psychopharmacol.*, 11:357–368.

*33. van Praag, H. M. (1977): Significances of biochemical parameters in the diagnosis, treatment, and prevention of depressive disorders. *Biol. Psychiatry*, 12:101–131.

34. van Praag, H. M., Kort, J., Dols, L. C. W. and Schut, T. (1972): A pilot study of the predictive value of the probenecid test in application of 5-hydroxytryptophan as an antidepressant. *Psychopharmacologia*, 25:14–21.

35. Walinder, J., Skott, A., Nagy, A., Carlsson, A., and Roos, B. E. (1975): Potentiation of antidepressant action of clomipramine by tryptophan. *Lancet*, 1:984.

Chapter 22

Schizophrenia

Schizophrenia is a symptom complex consisting of disturbances in thinking and feeling, including withdrawal, detachment from reality, disruption of interpersonal communication, and, often, hallucinations and delusions. Neither the pathogenesis nor the pathophysiology of schizophrenia is understood. In most discussions of schizophrenia, these two separate processes are not clearly differentiated. The pathogenesis of schizophrenia consists of the primary defect, either genetic or environmental; the pathophysiology consists of the manner in which this defect alters normal neuronal function, resulting in the abnormal behavior known as schizophrenia. Current research in schizophrenia has been focused almost entirely on pathogenesis and has been concerned primarily with finding a biochemical abnormality in known schizophrenics (17).

The theories of the pathogenesis of schizophrenia fall into one of three broad categories, each of which involves a different mechanism. The first maintains that schizophrenia results from the action of an abnormal small molecule (neurotransmitter or psychotomimetic compound). The second suggests that schizophrenia involves an abnormal large molecule (structural protein or enzyme). The third proposes that schizophrenia involves abnormal environmental influences. We have proposed a pharmacologic model of schizophrenia that is consistent with and helps to explain all three mechanisms of pathogenesis. This model is based on the premise that a small molecule (drug, neurotransmitter) acts on a large molecule (receptor site) in order to produce a specific effect (excitatory or inhibitory) on the postsynaptic membrane. The sum of all the individual excitatory and inhibitory influences on a given neuron at any time will determine whether or not the neuron fires. The complex pattern of similar influences on a large number of neurons will determine the behavior of the organism, and alterations in any step of this process can participate in the production of abnormal behavior (18).

SMALL MOLECULE HYPOTHESIS

Much of the biochemical research is based on the model of drug-induced psychosis and focuses on finding an abnormal neurotransmitter-like molecule in schizophrenics. If the organism produces, or is exposed to, this psychotomimetic compound, schizophrenia results.

The small molecule hypothesis raises several questions. The most obvious are related to the existence of such a compound, its site of action, and its mechanism of producing abnormal behavior in schizophrenics (14). The small molecule theories are based on the assumption that the brains of schizophrenics are normal and that the schizophrenic is therefore "poisoned" by an endogenous toxin. The mechanism of action of a structurally abnormal small molecule might involve one or more of the following:

a. The abnormal molecule may be a more effective agonist at the specific receptor site than may the normal molecule. Theoretically, the former can also act as a partial agonist or antagonist of the normal transmitter. Because the most effective treatment of schizophrenia involves drugs that act as antagonists at specific receptor sites, however, the abnormal small molecule most likely acts as an agonist.

b. The abnormal molecule may not be readily detoxified by normal enzymatic processes, thus allowing action at the specific receptor site for a prolonged period.

c. There may be no effective reuptake mechanism, so that the small molecule (false transmitter) acts for a longer time than does the normal transmitter.

d. There may be no effective feedback control on the synthesis of the abnormal small molecule; thus overstimulation of the receptor site would not decrease concentrations of the false transmitter.

Speculations about the role of small molecules are derived from the observation that most hallucinogens structurally resemble normal neurotransmitters. Although the state produced by these agents does not resemble schizophrenia, it is a true psychosis. In 1962, Osmond and Smythies (24) suggested that abnormal metabolites of epinephrine might have a mescaline-like structure and effect and thus be responsible for schizophrenia. They suggested that 3,4-dimethoxyphenyl-ethylamine (DMPEA), which differs from mescaline only in the absence of a methoxy group in the 5-position of the phenol ring, might result from the abnormal methylation of epinephrine and have psychotomimetic properties.

If DMPEA production is the primary abnormality in schizophrenia, then it must act at a normal specific receptor site to elicit schizophrenia. Because of the structure of DMPEA, it is likely but not certain that it acts at a receptor site that normally responds to either dopamine or norepinephrine. Furthermore, DMPEA should then exist in the brains of patients with schizophrenia and not in the brains of normal individuals, and when administered to either schizophrenics or normal individuals, it should elicit a schizophrenic reaction. In 1962, Friedhoff and Van Winkle (7) claimed to find DMPEA in the urine of schizophrenic patients but not controls. Other investigators have not been able to consistently reproduce this finding.

In 1966, Hollister and Friedhoff (10) administered DMPEA, mescaline, and placebo in a double-blind study to 13 volunteers, 12 of whom were recovered psychiatric patients; the authors concluded that DMPEA had no psychotomimetic effect. Johnson et al. (13) gave a structurally similar and presumably more potent compound, N-acetyldimethoxy-phenglethylamine (NADMPEA), to four volunteers and concluded that this compound also had no psychotomimetic effect. If DMPEA is related to schizophrenia, its significance is not as a psychotomimetic; this may indicate that abnormally methylated compounds are present in schizophrenics.

A similar and equally inconclusive argument has been made about the possible role of adrenochrome and a variety of other small molecules in the pathogenesis of schizophrenia. Hoffer et al. (9) proposed adrenochrome as an abnormal metabolite of epinephrine in 1954 and ingested some themselves to prove its psychogenic properties. They later suggested that if abnormal epinephrine metabolism produced adrenochrome, causing psychosis, schizophrenia could be treated by administration of a methyl acceptor, such as nicotinic acid, to slow the production of epinephrine. Although efficacious results with this treatment have been claimed, the work has not been consistently replicated in controlled studies.

The concept that schizophrenia is etiologically related to abnormally methylated compounds is supported by the fact that the administration of methyl donors augments schizophrenic manifestations in more than half the cases (25). Initially, methionine was given as a methyl donor in conjunction with a monoamine oxidase (MAO) inhibitor to chronic schizophrenics on the assumption that methylated amines, such as dimethyltryptamine or bufotenin, would result from ingestion of methionine and might have psychotomimetic properties, like those of mescaline or LSD. Since MAO is the enzyme primarily responsible for the degradation of normal neurotransmitters, MAO inhibitors were used to prolong the life of the endogenous amines (norepinephrine, dopamine, and serotonin) to increase the possibility that they would be abnormally methylated. Unfortunately, these experiments could not distinguish between effects of abnormally methylated metabolites and those of abnormal amounts of normal neurotransmitters generated by the simultaneous administration of the MAO inhibitor.

Antun et al. (2) gave methionine alone to 11 diagnosed schizophrenics, seven of whom responded with an "acute schizophrenic psychosis" that disappeared rapidly when the drug was discontinued. This finding suggests that it is not simply an abnormal amount of a normal neurotransmitter that exacerbates schizophrenic manifestations. However, whether the psychotomimetic effect of methionine is a property of a normal or an abnormal receptor site and thus of a normal or an abnormal brain remains unclear, since methionine was not given to normal subjects in any of these experiments. The questions of the identity of the abnormally methylated molecule and where in the brain the abnormally methylated amine may act also remain unanswered.

Saavedra and Axelrod (26) found both tryptamine and an enzyme capable of methylating tryptamine to N-methyl- and dimethyltryptamine (DMT) in rat and human brain. They also reported an inhibitor of this methylating enzyme in normal rat brain. Since DMT is a known psychotomimetic compound, the authors suggested that functional psychosis may be related to the absence of the inhibitor for this transmethylating enzyme or to some defect in the feedback control mechanism for its synthesis. They proposed that dopamine, norepinephrine, 5-hydroxytryptamine, or histamine may normally inhibit the reaction, since they all serve as substrates for that enzyme. Therefore, increased amounts of catecholamines or serotonin, in conjunction with inadequate feedback control, may result in toxic levels of psychotomimetic compounds.

Using a similar approach, Hall and Hartridge (8) reported that catecholamine-*o*-methyltransferase accentuated symptoms of acute schizophrenia in four patients. Since catecholamine-*o*-methyltransferase is a methylating enzyme specific for the catecholamines, these data suggest that an abnormally *o*-methylated catecholamine, such as norepinephrine or dopamine, may be involved in the pathophysiology of schizophrenia.

To prove that an abnormal small molecule acts on normal brain to produce schizophrenia, such a molecule must be clearly demonstrated in patients and be able to elicit appropriate symptoms in both schizophrenics and normal subjects. Neither criterion has been met for any proposed theory.

Amphetamine-induced psychosis may be the most interesting and reproducible example of the small molecule hypothesis. The psychosis associated with chronic amphetamine addiction can mimic acute schizophrenia and has been proposed by many authors as a working model of the disease (15,27). Amphetamine psychosis is characterized by paranoid delusions, auditory and visual hallucinations, and stereotyped behavior. Although it is reported that patients suffering from amphetamine psychosis lack the thought disorder characteristic of schizophrenia, because of the similarity between the two states, they are often indistinguishable, even to trained observers (4). The action of amphetamine is known to involve the dopaminergic system. Amphetamine causes the release of dopamine from nerve terminals in the striatum and elsewhere, thus making more dopamine available to act on the dopamine receptors.

Amphetamine-induced psychosis is important in the theory of schizophrenia because when given chronically to patients with previously normal brains, amphetamine can elicit a schizophrenic-like disorder. This suggests that when given chronically, abnormal amounts of a normal small molecule can cause psychosis and is probably analagous to levodopa-induced psychosis (see Chapter 1).

Neuroleptic drugs are the treatment of choice in schizophrenia. They are preferable to various types of psychotherapy, electric shock therapy, and placebo (20). Neuroleptics have been shown in controlled studies to significantly decrease thought disorder, blunted affect, withdrawal, autistic behavior mannerisms, and uncooperativeness. Hallucinations have been shown to be diminished markedly on phenothiazines in some studies but only slightly in others. How the neuroleptics act to limit schizophrenic behavior is not yet known.

Chlorpromazine, which has been studied extensively, acts to block the dopamine receptor sites in the brain (31), a mechanism of action attributed to all neuroleptics, since they block amphetamine-induced stereotyped behavior in small animals. This effect correlates so well with antipsychotic activity that most new neuroleptics are tested for their ability to block amphetamine-induced stereotyped behavior. The best evidence of this effect of chlorpromazine is based on animal studies in which the administration of neuroleptics greatly increased the amount of homovanillic acid (HVA) in the brain. The increased concentration of HVA suggests a negative feedback system that promotes an increase in the synthesis and turnover of dopamine in response to the blockade of the dopamine receptor sites. Nyback and Sedvall

(23) reported that in rats, chlorpromazine greatly increased the amount of dopamine accumulated in the striatum but not in other brain regions. This last finding is suggestive of the idea that neuroleptics act primarily on the dopamine receptor sites, since the striatum is where they are principally located within the central nervous system (CNS). This hypothesis is also supported by the fact that neither norepinephrine nor serotonin accumulated significantly in the brains of small animals after the administration of neuroleptics (23). Neuroleptics seem to act primarily to block dopamine receptor sites.

The question of how the neuroleptics block the dopamine receptor sites remains unanswered. Janssen (12) has shown that both phenothiazines and haloperidol form monolayers on water-lipid interphases at low concentrations. He suggests that the dopamine receptor sites are coated with the neuroleptic drugs and thus are blocked. Francois and Feher (6) have shown that chlorpromazine limits the usual increase in birefringence of corneal and scleral cell membranes treated with toluidine blue. The authors state that chlorpromazine attaches to the nonlipid portion of the membrane in competition with the dye, thus limiting its optical effect. Neither of these explanations accounts for the apparent specificity of the neuroleptic drugs for the dopamine receptor site. Horn and Snyder (11) have suggested that the molecular structure of chlorpromazine is similar to that of dopamine, and that this similarity might account for the specific ability of chlorpromazine to block the dopamine receptor site. Unfortunately, structural similarity is not an adequate explanation for the specificity of haloperidol and other butyrophenones, which do not resemble the phenothiazines or dopamine. Regardless of the actual mechanism whereby neuroleptics act to block the dopamine receptor sites in the striatum, it is generally accepted that this is their principal pharmacologic property. It is hypothesized that it is this blockade that leads to the attenuation of the signs and symptoms of schizophrenia (14,17,27).

If the blockade of dopamine at the dopamine receptor sites is in fact the essential effect of chlorpromazine on the pathophysiology of schizophrenia, then that pathophysiology might involve (a) an abnormal amount of dopamine acting at a normal dopamine receptor site, (b) an abnormal dopamine or "false transmitter," or (c) an abnormal dopamine receptor site. If an abnormal amount of dopamine acting at the dopamine receptor site were involved in the pathophysiology of schizophrenia, then dopamine turnover in schizophrenia should be either abnormally low, reflecting feedback inhibition of dopamine synthesis, or abnormally high, reflecting increased dopamine synthesis and an inoperative feedback mechanism. Studies of cerebrospinal fluid (CSF) HVA in schizophrenics showed normal concentrations of HVA. These results indicated that dopamine synthesis and turnover are probably not increased in schizophrenia.

If an abnormal type of dopamine were involved in the pathophysiology of schizophrenia, it should be possible to show that this "false transmitter" or its metabolite exists in schizophrenics, preferably in the CNS, that it does not exist in normal individuals, and that when given to either schizophrenic or normal individuals, it produces the symptoms of schizophrenia. These criteria have not been met for any proposed dopamine analog.

LARGE MOLECULE HYPOTHESIS

Kornetsky and Mirsky (21) found a differential effect of chlorpromazine on schizophrenic and normal individuals. Schizophrenic subjects required 20% more of the drug before exhibiting significant effects, whereas normal subjects on the lower dose showed "severe tremor and discomfort" as well as "marked effects" on the continuous performance test. The authors also reported a differential effect on blood pressure with chlorpromazine. Schizophrenics suffered much less postural hypotension than did normals. Less impairment was found on two of four performance tests in schizophrenics than in normals on chlorpromazine. However, there were no significant differences between schizophrenics and normals on any of the four tests with secobarbital. The authors propose that these differences are related to the "central neural loci upon which chlorpromazine acts." The implication of these data is that the dopamine receptor sites in the brains of schizophrenics are abnormal. Chlorpromazine, which is known to act primarily at the dopamine receptor sites, has a different effect on schizophrenics than on normals, whereas secobarbital, which acts nonspecifically in the CNS, has the same effect on both groups.

In animal experiments, chronic amphetamine and levodopa administration result in alterations in dopamine receptors (including increased concentration and affinity). These studies suggest that such alterations in dopamine receptors could be involved in the pathophysiology of amphetamine- and levodopa-induced psychosis and, by analogy, schizophrenia. Attempts have been made to measure dopamine receptor site function in the brains of known schizophrenics. While some evidence of increased numbers of neuroleptic binding sites has been published, the reproducibility and significance of this finding remains unclear.

As discussed above, increasing evidence suggests that at least two different dopaminergic cell populations exist in the striatum. Several clinical observations in schizophrenics support the concept of pharmacologically different dopamine receptors: (a) schizophrenics on chronic neuroleptics often develop tolerance to the parkinsonian but not the antipsychotic effects of these drugs; (b) schizophrenics in whom tardive dyskinesia develops, which is thought to reflect increased dopamine receptor hypersensitivity, do not manifest increased schizophrenia. It remains unclear which dopamine receptors are involved in schizophrenia.

Klawans et al. (17) suggested that striatal dopamine receptors participate in the pathogenesis of schizophrenia, whereas Stevens (29) suggested that the receptors of the nucleus accumbens play the primary role. Most investigators favor the latter explanation, although the site of this structure in man is unclear (22).

Recent work with clozapine provides the best clinical evidence of two types of receptors and that those in the mesolimbic system are more likely to be involved in schizophrenia. Structurally a dibenzodiazepine, clozapine has been reported to decrease the symptoms of schizophrenia without concomitant extrapyramidal side effects. Unlike other drugs with antipsychotic properties, clozapine is not a neuroleptic. It does not produce catalepsy and only mildly inhibits amphetamine- or apomorphine-induced stereotyped behavior in small animals. It does, however, affect dopamine turnover in the brain. Andén and Stock (1) studied dopamine and HVA concentration in rabbit brain after incremental doses of clozapine and haloperidol. They found that neither drug influenced the dopamine concentration, but that both drugs increased HVA to more than 150% of the value for untreated control animals at the maximum doses of the drugs used.

Since significant amounts of dopamine have recently been found in the limbic system, Andén and Stock (1) also looked at the differential effect of clozapine and haloperidol on HVA concentration in the limbic system and the corpus striatum. Both drugs increased the concentration of HVA in both brain regions, but the increase caused by HVA was significantly greater in the limbic system than in the striatum. As these authors note, one possible explanation for the ability of clozapine to decrease the symptoms of schizophrenia without producing rigidity or akinesia might be that clozapine has a greater affinity for the dopamine receptors in the limbic system than in the striatum, and that these two dopamine receptors are different.

Snyder and his colleagues (28) have demonstrated that clozapine has a much greater affinity for the muscarinic receptors in rat brain homogenates than does haloperidol or any of the phenothiazines tested. Haloperidol, which has the highest incidence of extrapyramidal side effects, has the lowest affinity for these cholinergic receptors. Therefore, they felt that the incidence of parkinsonian side effects should be inversely proportional to the ability of the antipsychotic agent to act as an anticholinergic agent. Whereas it is true that the two antipsychotic agents with the lowest incidence of drug-induced parkinsonism (clozapine and thioridazine) are strongly anticholinergic, they also have other differences from standard neuroleptics. Both of these agents are poor blockers of striatal dopamine receptors and might be relatively preferential mesolimbic dopamine receptor site antagonists. Work on various animal models confirms that the anticholinergic property of these two agents is not the only factor that differentiates them from other neuroleptics. In most animal models, the coadministration of an anticholinergic agent with a neuroleptic, such as haloperidol, does not mimic the biochemical and behavioral effects of such agents as clozapine or thioridazine.

The ability of clozapine to act as an antipsychotic agent without producing parkinsonism may be construed as evidence for two or more distinct populations of dopamine receptor sites. If there were only one type of dopamine receptor, clozapine would, of necessity, have to block all dopamine receptors equally. It would be expected to decrease the symptoms of schizophrenia but at the same time to elicit parkinsonism.

ENVIRONMENTAL HYPOTHESIS

The influence of accumulated input derived from experience, environmental stress, or emotional reinforcement has not been considered but appears to be an essential component of schizophrenia. A normal small molecule can act at a normal receptor in the brain and still result in an abnormal effect. Multisynaptic pathways and inputs beyond the initial receptor site will modify the quality and nature of the effect generated by any small molecule acting at its receptor site.

As an example, the effect of the hallucinogen mescaline, as it acts on normal receptor sites, is varied and dependent on cultural expectations. Peyotl, a mescaline derivative, creates an acute religious state in Mexican Indians; in other individuals in other settings, the response is significantly different. It is clear that environment and experience of the individual largely determine the behavior produced by psychotomimetic agents. In the same way, experience must help to determine the behavioral response to normal neurotransmitters. If experience-related cellular functions are altered in a patient, the quality of drug-receptor interactions will be distorted, regardless of the normal state of both the individual receptor sites and the small molecules.

A considerable portion of the literature on schizophrenia is concerned with the role of environment and experience in pathogenesis. Anxiety or disturbed communications are believed to hinder the schizophrenic patient and render him less able to function. The physiologic mechanism is not clear. Under abnormal stress, altered object relationships, or anxieties, a normal brain with normal small molecules and normal receptor sites and membranes may generate abnormal behavioral patterns.

One of the major advantages of viewing environmental influence in terms of a receptor site model is its facilitation of the understanding of the use of chemical agents in the treatment of "functional" psychoses. If the abnormal behavioral pattern is triggered by a sequence of small molecule-receptor site interactions, drugs that antagonize or block the interaction of specific small molecules and receptor sites may modify behavior. It is possible, then, that neuroleptic agents decrease the overtly abnormal behavior of schizophrenia by blocking the access of a neurotransmitter (perhaps dopamine) to a receptor site that, when activated because of altered environmental (social) influences, tends to trigger the abnormal behavior. These drugs will decrease the abnormal effect, regardless of whether the abnormality is the small molecule (neurotransmitter), the large molecule (receptor site), or the environmentally conditioned response.

THERAPY OF SCHIZOPHRENIA

The two major classes of drugs used in the specific treatment of schizophrenia are the phenothiazine drugs and the butyrophenone, haloperidol. Although there are many individual phenothiazine agents, they all have the same basic three-ring structure, in which two benzene rings are linked by a sulfur-and-nitrogen atom. The basic three-ring structure can be modified with additions at the 10 and 2 positions. The development of new antipsychotic phenothiazine neuroleptics has been aimed toward enhancing efficacy and diminishing side effects. The available phenothiazines can be grouped into three chemical categories based on the various additions to the basic three-ring phenothiazine structure (2a,3a). They are the aminoalkyl or aliphatic group, the piperidyl group, and the piperazinyl group. Examples of prototypes for each group are shown in Fig. 1. The phenothiazines act ubiquitously throughout the body and exert actions on most organ systems. As a group they have multiple actions at different levels of the nervous system. The one characteristic that they all share, however, is that they block dopamine mediated synaptic transmission. This blockade appears to be a postsynaptic one since, after acute administration of phenothiazine drugs, spinal fluid HVA levels increase. There has been substantial effort to correlate blood levels of various phenothiazine drugs with therapeutic responses. This work has not met with success since therapeutic antipsychotic response does not bear a simple relationship to blood levels of phenothiazines or their metabolites.

Few conclusions can be drawn relative to the pharmacokinetics and metabolism of the phenothiazine drugs. These agents tend to have erratic and unpredictable patterns of absorption when injested orally. Parenteral administration increases availability of active drugs by 4 to 6 times. These drugs are lipophilic and hence accumulate in brain. The plasma half-life for most agents ranges from 10 to 20 hr, although the higher lipid content of the CNS suggests that clearing from the brain may be slower. Metabolites of some phenothiazine agents have been detected in the urine for as long as several months after the drug has been stopped. It has been suggested that this slow clearing may contribute to the typically slow rate of exacerbation of psychosis after stopping phenothiazine drugs.

The major routes of drug metabolism are oxidative processes. Hydrophilic metabolites of these drugs are excreted in the urine or bile. Most oxidized metabolites are inactive. Importantly, age is a significant determinant of the rate of metabolism and excretion of these drugs. The fetus, infant, and elderly patient have diminished capacity to metabolize and eliminate these drugs.

Two parenteral forms of phenothiazines that have antipsychotic activity for 2 to 4 weeks following injection are now in use: fluphenazine enanthate and fluphenazine decanoate. Both are effective and share a unique advantage: compliance is obviously controlled. In chronic ambulatory or even chronic hospitalized patients known to be resistant to regular antipsychotic drug ingestion, the injection of a long-acting drug every 2 to 4 weeks is clearly more effective than oral medication in keeping the patient free of psychosis. Furthermore, the drug may be administered to ambulatory patients in the home by visiting nurses.

Haloperidol is a member of the butyrophenone group with a chemical structure completely different from the phenothiazine drugs. Like the phenothiazines, however, haloperidol is a dopaminergic receptor site blocking agent and has been an effective agent in the treatment of psychotic behavior. Haloperidol is rapidly and almost completely absorbed so that peak serum levels are reached within 2 hr after oral administration. Although relatively high plasma levels are maintained for only 72 hr after a single dose, significant concentrations of haloperidol are still detectable 1 week, and even 1 month, after the administration. Zingales found the therapeutic response to haloperidol unrelated to the absolute plasma level of free unmetabolized

Basic Structure

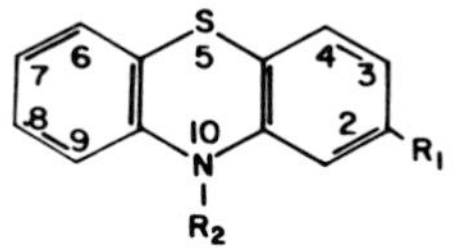

Aminoalkyl (e. g. chlorpromazine)

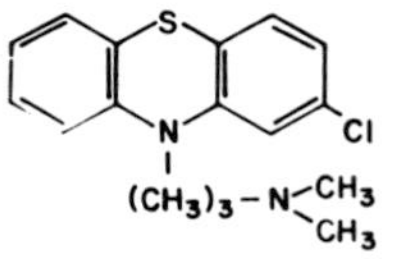

$R_2 = Cl$ $R_2 = (CH_2)_3 - N \begin{smallmatrix} CH_3 \\ CH_3 \end{smallmatrix}$

$R_1 = Cl$
$R_2 = (CH_2)_3 - N$ $N - CH_3$

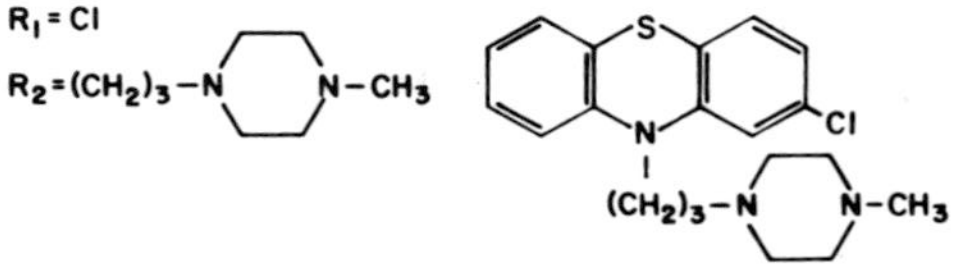

Piperidyl (e. g. prochlorperazine)

$R_1 = Cl$
$R_2 = (CH_2)_3 - N$ $N - CH_2 - CH_2OH$

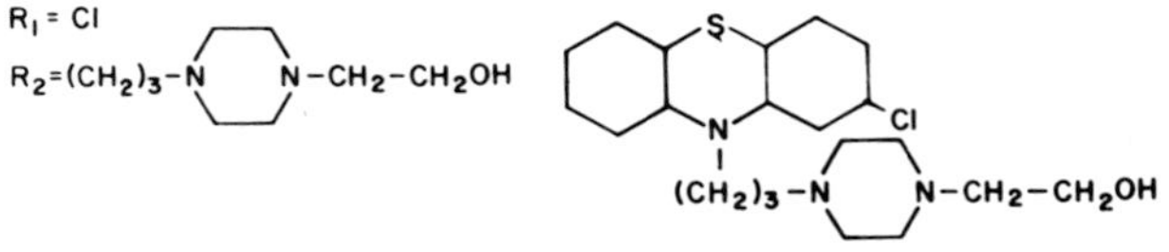

Piperazinyl (e. g. perphenazine)

PHENOTHIAZINES

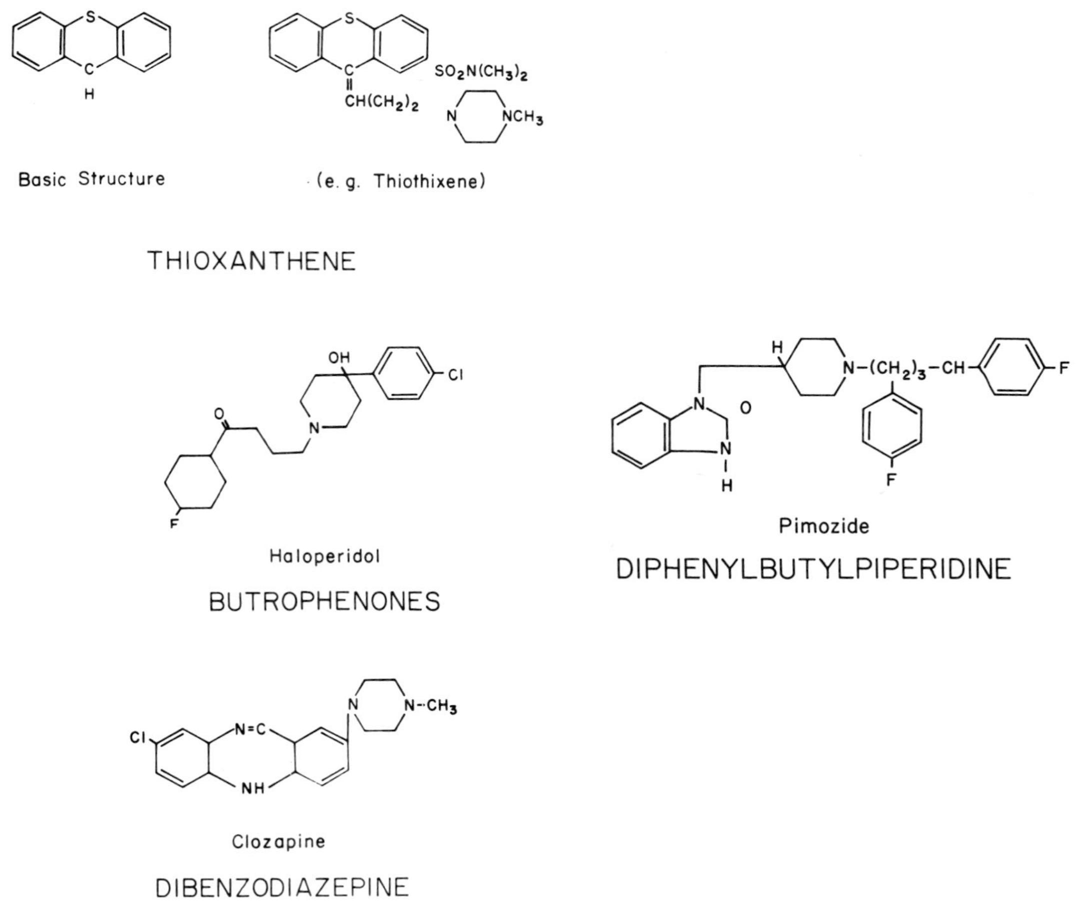
S
C
H
Basic Structure
S
C
CH(CH2)2
SO2N(CH3)2
N
NCH3
(e. g. Thiothixene)
THIOXANTHENE
OH
Cl
O
N
F
Haloperidol
BUTROPHENONES
H
N-(CH2)3-CH
F
N
O
N
H
F
Pimozide
DIPHENYLBUTYLPIPERIDINE
N
N-CH3
Cl
N=C
NH
Clozapine
DIBENZODIAZEPINE

FIG. 1. Major types of neuroleptics.

drug (32). Haloperidol is metabolized predominantly* in the liver so that very little, if any, free drug is excreted into the urine. Dosage information on the major phenothiazines is shown in Table 1. Such information can serve only as a guideline and not as absolute limits, except for the upper limit of 800 mg/day for thioridazine which was established in relation to risk for retinitis pigmentosa. In this we agree with Klein and Davis (20), who have pointed out that individual variation in the biologic characteristics of each patient make absolute guidelines impractical and at times antitherapeutic. This approach contradicts the obvious desire of others to establish extremely firm dosage guidelines for every drug. In fact, there have been increasing indications that government control organizations, such as the Food and Drug Administration (FDA), want the package insert to include absolute dosage limits so that any dosage that exceeds these limits would be considered improper medical care. This is not in the best interest of the patient and may actually deny patients the possible benefits that might result from dosages outside the "approved" range. At present, unfortunately, the manufacturer's package insert is of great and clearly unwarranted legal significance. Often without scientific basis a doctor's liability is greatly increased when the published guidelines are not strictly adhered to.

The situation is of course often without scientific merit. Analogous dosage information for other neuroleptics is given in Table 2. Since most of the side effects of these agents are similar they will be discussed together.

NEUROLOGIC SIDE EFFECTS

Acute dystonia, parkinsonism, and tardive dyskinesia have been discussed previously in detail; a few major points are repeated here. There is clearly a difference

TABLE 1. *Dosages of major phenothiazines[a]*

Phenothiazine	Daily dosage range (mg)	Dosage equivalent to 300 mg chlorpromazine
Aminoalkyl		
Chlorpromazine	100–1,000	300
Triflupromazine	20–150	100
Piperidyl		
Thioridazine	30–800	300
Mesoridazine	50–400	150
Piperazinyl		
Trifluoperazine	2–30	25
Perphenazine	2–64	28
Butaperazine	30–50	30
Prochlorperazine	15–125	60
Thiopropazate	6–30	30
Fluphenazine	0.5–20	6

[a]Adapted from ref. 5.

TABLE 2. *Dosages of major nonphenothiazine neuroleptics*

Neuroleptic	Daily dosage range (mg)	Dosage equivalent to 300 mg chlorpromazine
Thioxanthenes		
Chlorprothixene	50−1,000	300
Thiothixene	10−60	30
Haloperidol	2−40	15
Clozapine	100−1,000	300

in the incidence of dystonia and parkinsonism with different neuroleptics; agents such as haloperidol and fluphenazine have a high incidence, chlorpromazine a middle incidence, and clozapine and thioridazine the lowest incidence. Coadministration of anticholinergics can prevent dystonia and parkinsonism or treat it once it occurs. This effect is not due to lowering circulating phenothiazine levels as was once claimed. It is reasonable to assume that drugs that cause the lowest incidence of parkinsonism may cause the lowest incidence of tardive dyskinesia, but proof of this conjecture is lacking.

Many clinicians endorse the prophylactic use of antiparkinsonian drugs to prevent or minimize the development of dystonia and parkinsonism. Like Cole (5), we do not recommend routine anticholinergics but prefer to use them in patients who develop dystonia (see Chapter 5) and parkinsonism (see Chapter 1). We would recommend their use prophylactically in any patient being restarted on neuroleptics who demonstrated a prior tendency toward dystonic reaction.

Akathisia is manifested by a feeling of acute discomfort in the muscles of the extremities and sometimes of the whole body and can be relieved only by movement. Patients get up and sit down frequently, move their legs and feet up and down, pace to and fro, and appear generally restless and agitated. This is often considered to be an extrapyramidal side effect, although the basis for this supposition is unclear. It often improves with anticholinergic medication and is less common with clozapine and thioridazine. Correct diagnosis is important. Patients sometimes are given increasing doses of the offending phenothiazine drug to relieve this "agitation," but this might worsen the effect. Akathisia probably contributes to outpatient noncompliance. If the treating clinician is in doubt, the diagnosis of akathisia can often be made by a therapeutic test with a single dose of an injectable anticholinergic. This should reduce akathisia but not affect agitation due to the underlying disease (5).

Many patients on chronic neuroleptics manifest more than just akathisia but have a syndrome including restlessness, dysphoria, and agitation (30). These seem to be less common on thioridazine or clozapine and respond to anticholinergics; this is a major cause of noncompliance with subsequent reexacerbation. Sedation often occurs early in the course of therapy and is especially marked with chlorpromazine but also occurs with other phenothiazine and nonphenothiazine neuroleptics.

All neuroleptics can lower the seizure threshold and precipitate seizures. This is not a contraindication to their use in patients with epilepsy. In our experience, this is rarely a problem if a patient's anticonvulsants are monitored properly. The effect of neuroleptics on epilepsy is a result of their influence on cerebral physiology and not related to any influence on the absorption or metabolism of anticonvulsants. Some patients who have been seizure free for some time without anticonvulsants will begin to have seizures when placed on a neuroleptic and again require anticonvulsants.

The autonomic nervous system effects of the neuroleptics include (a) anticholinergic effects, such as dry mouth, blurred vision, and constipation; these can be seen with most if not all agents but may be more common with those with greater anticholinergic propensity (e.g., clozapine, thioridazine); (b) retrograde ejaculation, most commonly seen with thioridazine; and (c) orthostatic hypotension via adrenergic blockade. This latter effect can be seen with all agents but is more common with acute parenteral injection. Tolerance usually develops rapidly.

NONNEUROLOGIC SIDE EFFECTS

Sudden death. While some claims have been made of an increased incidence of sudden death in hospitalized psychotic patients on neuroleptics, recent epidemiologic evidence strongly suggests that this is not true.

Dermatitis. A generalized maculopapular urticarial eruption can be seen within the first month of phenothiazine treatment.

Pigmentary skin changes usually described as a blue-gray discoloration over areas exposed to sunlight and has been seen only with chlorpromazine.

Pigmentary retinopathy can be caused by thioridazine in doses over 1,200 mg/day.

Corneal opacities have been seen with high-dose phenothiazine therapy, especially chlorpromazine.

Cholangiolytic jaundice. This is now rare but at one time occurred in 1% of patients on chlorpromazine.

ECG changes. These have been described with a variety of neuroleptics, especially thioridazine, and consist of alterations in repolarization and in all probability have no clinical significance.

Agranulocytosis is rare except from clozapine. Its occurrence with this agent has prevented its use in the United States. When it occurs, agranulocytosis is quite often acute; it begins during the first 6 weeks of therapy and develops over a few hours.

Klein and Davis summarized the differential side effects of the neuroleptics (20): Promazine had a greater propensity to cause agranulocytosis and jaundice; fluphenazine, perphenazine, and trifluoperazine to cause dystonia and parkinsonism; thioridazine to cause retinopathy and retrograde ejaculation; and chlorpromazine to cause jaundice, sedation, agranulocytosis, and skin photosensitivity.

With haloperidol blood dyscrasias, liver dysfunction, and EKG changes are less common. Early orthostatic hypotension can occur at times, and sedation is usually only mild; dystonia, parkinsonism, and akathisia, however, are common.

Chlorprothixene has a high propensity to cause sedation and autonomic effects but less of a propensity to cause parkinsonism and dystonia. Thiothixene, on the other hand, is associated with a high incidence of both dystonia and parkinsonism.

During the last decade, low dosage-high potency agents have been claimed to be preferred. In our opinion, this concept has no real basis. Therapeutic index, not potency, is the issue in drug selection; and no evidence suggests that the high potency agents have a better therapeutic index.

Except for their neurologic problems, these agents are safe. The incidence of parkinsonism and dystonic reactions on a chronic basis is high, and it is our impression that outpatients treated with these agents have a higher incidence of tardive dyskinesia than outpatients given standard oral neuroleptics. Whether this is due to better compliance or to greater striatal effects of these agents is not known.

BIBLIOGRAPHY AND *SELECTED REVIEWS

1. Andén, N. E., and Stock, G. (1973): Effect of clozapine on the turnover of dopamine in the corpus striatum and in the limbic system. *J. Pharm. Pharmacol.*, 25:346–348.
2. Antun, F. T., Burnet, G. B., Cooper, A. J., Daly, R. J., Smythies, J. R., and Zealley, A. K. (19xx): The effects of L-methionine (without MAOI) in schizophrenia. *J. Psychiatr. Res.*, 8:63–71.
2a. Baldessarini, R. J. (1980): Drugs and the treatment of psychiatric disorders. In: *The Pharmacological Basis of Therapeutics, 6th ed.*, edited by A. G. Gilman, L. S. Goodman, Macmillan, New York, pp. 391–447.
*3. Ban, T. (1971): Current status of chemotherapy of schizophrenia. *Schizophrenia*, 3:116–128.
3a. Ban, T. A., and Pecknold, J. C. (1976): Haloperidol and the butyrophenones. In: *Drug Treatment of Mental Disorders*, edited by L. L. Simpson, Raven Press, New York, pp. 45–60.
4. Bell, D. S. (1965): Comparison of amphetamine psychosis and schizophrenia. *Br. J. Psychiatry*, 111:701–707.
*5. Cole, J. (1976): Phenothiazines. In: *Drug Treatment of Mental Disorders*, edited by L. L. Simpson, Raven Press, New York, pp. 13–30.
6. Francois, J., and Feher, J. (1972): The effect of phenothiazine on the cell membrane. *Exp. Eye Res.*, 14:65–68.
7. Friedhoff, A. J., and Van Winkle, E. (1962): Isolation and characterization of a compound from the urine of schizophrenics. *Nature*, 194:897–898.
8. Hall, P., and Hartridge, G. (1969): Effect of catechol-*o*-methyl transferase in schizophrenia. *Arch. Gen. Psychiatry*, 20:573–575.
9. Hoffer, A., Osmond, H., and Smythies, J. (1954): Schizophrenia: A new approach; result of a year's research. *J. Ment. Sci.*, 100:29–45.
10. Hollister, L. E., and Friedhoff, A. J. (1966): Effect of 3,4-dimethoxy phenylethylamine in man. *Nature*, 210:1377–1378.
11. Horn, A. S., and Snyder, S. H. (1971): Chlorpromazine and dopamine: Conformational similarities and correlation with the antischizophrenic activity of phenothiazine drugs. *Proc. Natl. Acad. Sci. USA*, 68:2325–2328.
12. Janssen, P. A. (1967): The pharmacology of haloperidol. *Int. J. Neuropsychiatry*, 7:10–32.
13. Johnson, G., Friedhoff, A. J., Alpert, A., and Marchitello, J. (1970): Effects of a n-acetyl dimethoxyphenethylamine (NADMPEA) in man. *Psychopharmacologia*, 17:434–438.
*14. Kety, S. (1967): Current biochemical approaches to schizphrenia. *N. Engl. J. Med.*, 276:325–330.
15. Kety, S. S. (1972): Toward hypotheses for a biochemical component in the vulnerability to schizophrenia. *Semin. Psychiatry*, 4:233–238.
*16. Klawans, H. L. (1975): Amine precursors in neurologic disorders and the psychosis. In: *Biology of the Major Psychoses*, edited by D. X. Freedman. Raven Press, New York, pp. 259–276.

17. Klawans, H. L., Goetz, C., and Westheimer, R. (1972): Pathophysiology of schizophrenia and the striatum. *Dis. Nerv. Syst.*, 33:711–719.

*18. Klawans, H. L., Goetz, C., and Westheimer, R. (1976): The pharmacology of schizophrenia. In: *Clinical Neuropharmacology, Vol. 1*, edited by H. L. Klawans, pp. 1–28. Raven Press, New York.

19. Klawans, H. L., Westheimer, R., and Goetz, C. (1975): A pharmacologic model of schizophrenia. *Dis. Nerv. Syst.*, 36:267–275.

20. Klein, D. F., and Davis, J. M. (1969): *Diagnosis and Drug Treatment of Psychiatric Disorders*. Williams & Wilkins, Baltimore.

21. Kornetsky, C., and Mirsky, A. F. (1966): On certain psychopharmacological and physiological differences between schizophrenia and normal persons. *Psychopharmacologia*, 8:309–318.

*22. Meltzer, H. Y., and Stahl, S. M. (1976): The dopamine hypothesis of schizophrenia. *Schizophr. Bull.*, 2:19–76.

23. Nyback, H., and Sedvall, G. (1969): Regional accumulation of catecholamines formed from tyrosine 14-C in rat brain: Effect of chlorpromazine. *Eur. J. Pharmacol.*, 5:245–252.

24. Osmond, H., and Smythies, J. (1952): Schizophrenia. A new approach. *J. Ment. Sci.*, 98:309–315.

25. Pollin, W. (1972): The pathogenesis of schizophrenia. *Arch. Gen. Psychiatry*, 27:29–37.

26. Saavedra, J. M., and Axelrod, J. (1972): Psychotomimetic n-methylated tryptamines: Formation in brain in vivo and in vitro. *Science*, 175:1365–1366.

27. Snyder, S. H. (1972): Catecholamines in the brain as mediators of amphetamine psychosis. *Arch. Gen. Psychiatry*, 27:169–179.

28. Snyder, S. H., Banerjee, S. P., Yamamura, H. I., and Greenberg, D. (1974): Drugs, neurotransmitters and schizophrenia. *Science*, 184:1243–1253.

*29. Stevens, R. R. (1973): An anatomy of schizophrenia. *Arch. Gen. Psychiatry*, 29:177–189.

30. Van Putten, T. (1974): Why do schizophrenic patients refuse to take their drugs? *Arch. Gen. Psychiatry*, 31:67–72.

31. Van Rossum, J. M. (1966): Significance of dopamine receptor blockade for mechanism of action of neuroleptic drugs. *Arch. Int. Pharmacodyn. Ther.*, 160:492–494.

32. Zingales, I. A. (1971): A gas chromatographic method for the determination of haloperidol in human plasma. *J. Chrom.*, 54:15–24.

Chapter 23

Anxiety

Anxiety can be defined as an emotional state that produces an unpleasant feeling of apprehension regarding impending danger. This uncomfortable sensation occurs in the absence of any definable or actual external threat. Anxiety may also be accompanied by somatic symptoms and signs, including palpitations, hyperventilation, pallor, dry mouth, sweating, postural tremor, fatigue, tics, and various other repetitive movements. Psychiatrically, anxiety is considered to result from unconscious or unrecognized intrapsychic conflict. Anxiety is a common human experience, about which there has been considerable interest as a positive force in the learning theory. Levels of anxiety that interfere with function or that cause the patient to seek help are often used to define "clinical anxiety." Tolerable levels, however, like levels of pain, have tremendous variance within the population. It is not surprising, then, that it is difficult to define and to assess possible biochemical correlates of anxiety in those patients who require pharmacologic treatment. Since anxiety is a subjective sensation that may or may not be accompanied by somatic signs, the difficulty of establishing a reliable animal model to investigate anatomic and biochemical correlates is obvious.

Although anxiety is difficult to study, there has been much interest in the use of agents to alleviate it. Bromide salts and ethanol in various concentrations were used as anxiolytics during the last 100 years in the form of both prescription and patent remedies; ethanol is still in use today for similar purposes. The barbiturates also have been employed as anxiolytics and are considered to be valuable in this regard. The modern era of the psychopharmacology of anxiety began with the introduction of the propanediols and the benzodiazepines. This latter class represented the departure from the role of sedation alone in treating anxiety; these agents have been proposed to have a more selective anxiolytic effect.

Klein and Davis (9), in an extensive review of the literature, have detailed the effectiveness of the "minor" tranquilizers in the treatment of anxiety. Although they point out that the treatment populations that have been studied with regard to the anxiolytics often are undefined, these drugs generally are more effective than placebo. In 41 of 44 studies, chlordiazepoxide, diazepam, and oxazepam were superior to placebo in the treatment of anxiety; in 16 of 25 studies, meprobamate and tybamate were also superior to placebo. Meprobamate and the benzodiazepines were compared to the barbiturates, and the former were found to be significantly better in half of the studies. In 11 of 12 studies comparing barbiturates to meprobamate, barbiturates were judged equal to or superior. On the other hand, when the benzodiazepines were compared to meprobamate, only two of seven studies reported these agents to be superior. Finally, when these authors examined the benzodiazepines themselves, and when they reviewed the literature comparing diazepam and oxazepam against chlordiazepoxide, there was no clear indication that any of these drugs was a better anxiolytic than another. The attempt to establish one anxiolytic benzodiazepine as superior continues. As new benzodiazepine derivatives are formulated, claims of superiority must be carefully evaluated (6).

In a more recent review of the clinical results of the effectiveness of the benzodiazepines as anxiolytics, Greenblatt and Shader (5) reported that between 1973 and 1976, 22 of 25 studies indicated that benzodiazepines were more effective than placebo. In addressing the ever-recurring question of whether a single benzodiazepine is most effective, the authors reported that in 21 of 25 studies, little or no difference was found in the effects of the various benzodiazepines. Although these agents are more widely used to treat anxiety than are the propandiols, it is of both historic and theoretical interest that a discussion of the pharmacology of anxiolytics begin with the propandiols.

PROPANDIOLS

In 1946, mephensin was investigated as a muscle relaxant and sedative. It became apparent that its duration of action was too brief to be of practical value. During the next 8 years, more than 1,200 compounds were examined, the best of which was meprobamate, a structural analog of mephensin. Meprobamate was considered to be a new interneuronal blocking agent, primarily effective in blocking polysynaptic pathways (Fig. 1). Although designed as a muscle relaxant, its anxiolytic effect led to widespread clinical use (1). In fact, both its anatomic site(s) and mechanism of action are unknown. It has been suggested that much of its anxiolytic effect is related to mild sedation, and that meprobamate and barbiturates may act by similar mechanisms. In behavioral animal studies designed to promote "conflict," however, there appears to be a greater effect from meprobamate than from phenobarbitol. In these types of studies, the animals are both rewarded (with food) and punished (with electroshock) for performing the same task. In this experimental situation, untreated animals are influenced by the punishment and suppress the response leading to reward. The administration of a pharmacologic agent (e.g., propandiol) that will increase the behavioral response for the rewarding stimulus in this situation is thought to represent an agent that lessens conflict.

Meprobamate also has an effect on the polysynaptic extensor reflex. The locus of this action appears to be supraspinal and leads to the speculation that this drug

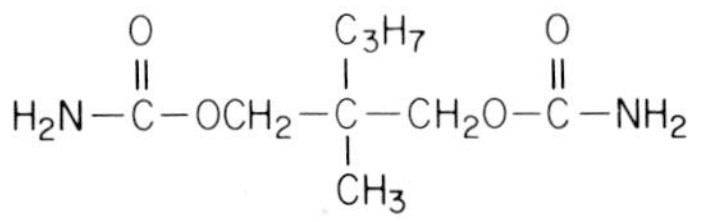

$$H_2N-\overset{\overset{\displaystyle O}{\|}}{C}-OCH_2-\overset{\overset{\displaystyle C_3H_7}{|}}{\underset{\underset{\displaystyle CH_3}{|}}{C}}-CH_2O-\overset{\overset{\displaystyle O}{\|}}{C}-NH_2$$

FIG. 1. The propandiols: meprobamate.

may be an effective muscle relaxant; however, there is little objective evidence for this claim. In fact, the issue of whether or not meprobamate-induced sedation is separable from meprobamate-induced muscle relaxation has been raised. Meprobamate also has been demonstrated to induce high voltage slow waves in the electroencephalogram (EEG) in cats and rabbits. This has been related to its effect on the reticular activating system. It has also been demonstrated to shorten the electrical afterdischarges seen in the limbic regions. The relationship, if anything, between these actions of meprobamate and its anxiolytic effect in man is unclear and tenuous at best.

Tybamate is another anxiolytic propandiol. This compound is similar in structure to meprobamate and represents a butyl group substitution on one of the carbamal nitrogens. Although the two compounds are similar pharmacologically, they can be differentiated by their lipid solubility and effects on spontaneous EEG activity. There is little clinical evidence to recommend tybamate over meprobamate as an anxiolytic. The tendency to develop tolerance to its anxiolytic effect, and the relatively high doses of meprobamate required to be effective—compared to the potentially addicting dose—have caused a decrease in the use of this agent. A full-blown withdrawal syndrome, possibly including delirium and generalized seizures, may develop after chronic treatment with meprobamate.

BENZODIAZEPINES

The benzodiazepines (Fig. 2) are the most widely prescribed drugs in the western world. The two most widely used anxiolytics of this class are chlordiazepoxide and diazepam (Table 1). It was reported that in 1977, 13 million prescriptions for chlordiazepoxide and 54 million for diazepam were written (15). In general, the benzodiazepines are considered advantageous over the barbiturates and the propandiols, although the number of clinical trials to assess the relative efficacy of these drug classes is small. Enough consistent clinical information is available to

TABLE 1. *Common anxiolytic agents*

Drug class	Generic name	Trade name	Dose range up 1,600 mg
Propanediol	Meprobamate	Miltown	to 100
Benzodiazepine	Chlordiazepoxide	Librium, Librax, SK-Lygen, A-poxide, Chlordinium Sealets	to 60
	Diazepam	Valium	to 60
	Oxazepam	Serax	to 120
	Chlorazepate	Tranxene, Azene	to 60
	Prazepam	Verstran	to 60
	Lorazepam	Ativan	to 10
Beta-adrenergic antagonists	Propranolol Solotol	Inderol	

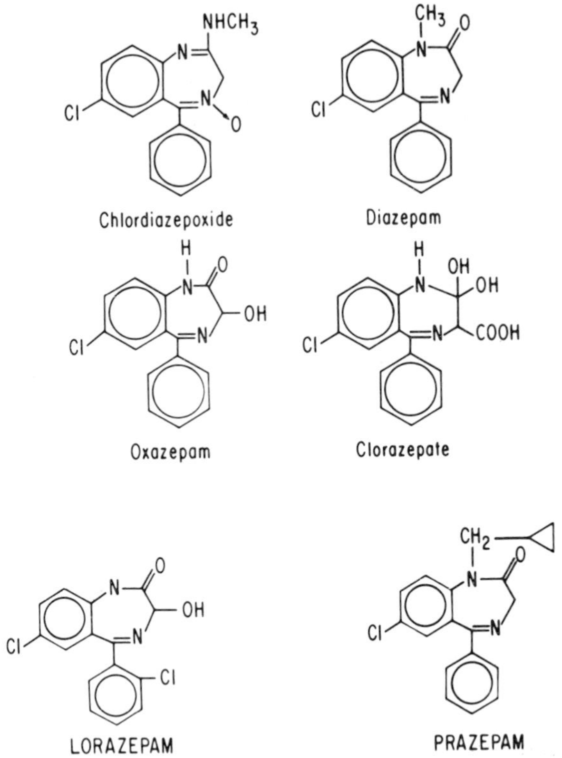

FIG. 2. The benzodiazepines.

establish the benzodiazepines as superior to the barbiturates as anxiolytics and the former are certainly less toxic than the latter. Animal experiments indicate that the benzodiazepines are more potent than meprobamate with respect to their taming influence in aggressive animals. The benzodiazepines also are able to reduce suppressive effects of punishment in conflict experiments. In addition to their anxiolytic effects, these drugs have anticonvulsant, muscle relaxant, and sedative hypnotic effects. The issue of sedation versus selective anxiolytic activity has been raised for the benzodiazepines; however, the anxiolytic dose often may not be sedating.

The benzodiazepines are metabolized by the liver and excreted in the urine. Many of these compounds have pharmacologically active metabolites, which in part accounts for their long half-life. This explains the occasional complaints of a "hangover" feeling the day following administration and the occasional appearance of withdrawal symptoms days after the last ingested dose. The most important clinical-pharmacologic interaction occurs as an additive effect with other CNS depressants, particularly alcohol. However, the benzodiazapines are relatively safe drugs, with high therapeutic-to-toxic ratios. Withdrawal of benzodiazepines can itself cause anxiety. This all too often contributes to markedly prolonged continuation of therapy. In any patient in whom there is a marked exacerbation of anxiety on benzodiazepine withdrawal, the possibility that the anxiety is because of withdrawal and not the patient's initial underlying condition must be considered. The anxiety that is due to drug withdrawal will clear in 7 to 14 days after the withdrawal is completed.

Currently available benzodiazepines useful as anxiolytics include chlordiazepoxide, diazepam, oxazepam, clorazepate, prazepam, and lorazepam. As previously stressed, few studies are available to promote a single one of these agents as the most efficacious anxiolytic. Individual pharmacokinetic properties are briefly discussed. Chlordiazepoxide is slowly absorbed after oral administration and reaches peak plasma levels in 2 to 3 hr; its active metabolites include a lactam and desmethyldiazepam. Diazepam is rapidly absorbed and reaches a peak plasma level in approximately 1 hr; its active metabolites include oxazepam and desmethyldiazepam. Oxazepam reaches a peak plasma concentration at 4 hr and is excreted as a conjugated glucuronide. Clorazepate is almost entirely metabolized to the active compound desmethyldiazepam. Prazepam is a drug precursor, since it is also almost entirely metabolized to its active metabolite, desmethyldiazepam. Although the anxiolytic activities of both clorazepate and prazepam are related to desmethyldiazepam, their rate of conversion differs, clorazepate being more rapidly metabolized than prazepam. Lorazepam resembles oxazepam in molecular structure and in that there are no metabolized active products; it is excreted as the conjugated glucuronide in the urine. Although there is no conclusive evidence that lorazepam is a better anxiolytic than diazepam, it has one advantage in that its intramuscular parenteral administration is more prompt and reliable.

The central biochemical effect of the benzodiazepines remains unclear. In turnover studies, it has been demonstrated that oxazepam reduces serotonin turnover and that chlordiazepoxide reduces norepinephrine turnover. Diazepam has also been shown to reduce turnover of striatal dopamine and hypothalamic and cerebellar norepinephrine. A traditional approach to turnover studies is the attempt to relate altered turnover rates to a known specific action of the drug. An example of this is a study of the relationship of the anticonvulsant properties of diazepam and its depression of norepinephrine and dopamine turnover. It was reported that the diazepam antagonism of pentylenetetrazol-induced seizures might be related to suppression of turnover of striatal dopamine but not to suppression of norepinephrine in the hypothalamus and cerebellum (4). These biochemical results were then used to interpret the effects of diazepam in various animal models of anxiety. This approach is obviously open to serious question.

Whether studies of this type will produce more exact knowledge of the possible transmitter relationships that are altered in the conflict behavioral experiments remains to be seen. Even if a clear understanding of the relationship of transmitter turnover in "conflict" experiments becomes apparent, whether or not this would represent a "good" animal model of anxiety in man remains open to question. This was well illustrated when an attempt was made to study the effect of diazepam on norepinephrine metabolism in man. Smith and colleagues (16) reasoned that since studies of catecholamine turnover using labeled isotope techniques, histochemistry, and amine-depleting agents demonstrated that diazepam decreased central norepinephrine turnover, and since MHPG is considered to be a product of central metabolism of norepinephrine, a study of the effects of diazepam on norepinephrine metabolism in man would also reveal decreased turnover. In contrast to the previous finding in rodents, however, the urinary excretion of MHPG in man after diazepam ingestion shows increased turnover. Since not all MHPG is derived from central norepinephrine, the effect of diazepam on MHPG in man may reflect peripheral activity. This also suggests possible species differences with respect to the behavioral effects of diazepam.

In a recent article, Costa and co-workers (3) examined the mechanism of action of the benzodiazepines. Reviewing several different behavioral models of benzodiazepine activity (anticonvulsant, ataxia, muscle relaxation), biochemical approaches, and neurophysiologic approaches, the authors propose that the benzodiazepines exert their action on the CNS by a facilitation of gamma-aminobutyric acid (GABA-ergic) transmission. They conclude by proposing that since GABA seems to be involved in the behavioral expression of several other benzodiazepine-related behavioral events, it may also be involved in the expression of anxiety.

In a separate review (18), the interrelationship between benzodiazepine action and GABA systems is examined. Presynaptic GABA-mediated inhibition is enhanced by benzodiazepines in the spinal cord, sympathetic ganglia, and cuneate nucleus, whereas postsynaptic GABA-mediated inhibition is enhanced in the substantia nigra, cerebral cortex, hippocampus, and cerebellum. Iontophoretic studies have demonstrated synergism between GABA and benzodiazepines. In addition, benzodiazepines have been reported to antagonize GABA-mediated events. The hypothesis was advanced that "benzodiazepines modulate GABA-mediated synaptic events and that at pharmacologically relevant doses, these drugs potentiate GABA-mediated inhibitions in the CNS." Molecular mechanisms proposed to explain this hypothesis include activation of GABA receptors, increase in presynaptic GABA release, inhibition of GABA removal, and alteration in postsynaptic response to GABA.

The most recent biochemical investigations related to the benzodiazepines is the finding that there are specific benzodiazepine receptor sites in the CNS. A series of publications (11–13) demonstrated a specific diazepam binding site which is highly localized to the synaptasomal preparation of cerebral cortex. In fact, localization of binding sites varied in different anatomic regions, with the highest density of receptors being located in the rat cortex, followed in order by hypothalamus, cerebellum, midbrain, hippocampus, striatum, and medulla.

Mohler and Okada (11–13) also demonstrated a specific diazepam binding site in human brain, the highest density being reported in the cerebral cortex and cerebellum. These investigators suggest that the benzodiazepine binding site represents the site of therapeutic action of this class of drugs. There has been ample confirmation from other laboratories that these sites display characteristics appropriate for receptors, including rapid *in vitro* binding of the ligand, which is reversible, stereospecific, and saturable.

Benzodiazepine receptor sites have also been identified in tissue other than the CNS. These drugs have several different therapeutic effects in man, and whether the diazepam binding site is related to its anxiolytic effect is not known. There appears to be a correlation between the potency of various benzodiazepines to displace the H^3 ligand from the benzodiazepine receptor and the potency of these same benzodiazepines to increase suppressed behavior in conflict experiments and to inhibit pentylenetetrazole-induced seizures. The latter two experimental designs relate to or at least indicate anxiolytic pharmacologic agents. It has even been suggested that there may be an endogenous neurotransmitter substance that normally interacts with the benzodiazepine receptor sites; if there is a functional benzodiazepine receptor in the brain, there should be an endogenous neurotransmitter substance that acts at that site. Employing receptor binding methodology, which may or may not stand the test of time, putative endogenous ligands for benzodiazepine receptors have been identified as the purine nucleosides inosine and hypoxanthine. Other purine compounds have also been reported to exhibit a low affinity inhibition of diazepam binding. Before the purines or any other endogenous substance can be considered to be benzodiazepine-like neurotransmitters, additional evidence is required other than inhibition of diazepam binding, including the ability of the identified substance to produce similar biochemical, behavioral, and physiologic effects and the demonstration that the CNS has the capacity to store, metabolize, and release the agent in question (10). Investigation of the benzodiazepine receptor has sought to parallel and recreate, if possible, the identification of the endorphins and enkephalins and their relationship to the CNS opiate receptor sites. One of the additional difficulties in the case of the benzodiazepam receptors is their widespread distribution throughout the CNS.

As previously indicated, evidence suggests that the activity of benzodiazepines is related to interaction with GABAergic mechanisms. A relationship has been demonstrated between H^3-diazepam binding and GABA. Increased binding of H^3-diazepam is produced when GABA is present. This increase can be prevented by the GABA antagonist bicuculline. Although bicuculline itself can inhibit H^3-diazepam binding, the relationship between GABA and benzodiazepine binding is not simple and likely involves an endogenous modulator of GABA binding and a chloride ionophore. In addition, the lipid environment of the benzodiazepine receptor may also affect the binding characteristics. Evidence exists that benzodiazepine receptor activity may alter phosphatidylcholine synthesis. These complex interactions are not clear, nor is their applicability to the anxiolytic effect of the benzodiazepines known. An endogenous "antianxiety" transmitter (17) remains to be identified.

As the regional biochemical alterations produced by the benzodiazepines must be correlated with specific behavioral models, so must the newly discovered benzodiazepine binding sites. In fact, initial work has demonstrated that seizures induced by either electroshock or pentylenetetrazol in rats transiently increase the number of benzodiazepine binding sites in the cerebral cortex. This suggests that the postictal cerebral cortex may be altered with respect to benzodiazepines, and that part of the anticonvulsant activity of these agents may be related to this (14).

Further investigation of the role of these receptors in relation to known properties of the benzodiazepines includes an attempt to explore possible receptor correlates of tolerance. Since tolerance to both the sedative and anxiolytic effects of the benzodiazepines is known to occur in man, the effect of chronic administration of benzodiazepine on benzodiazepine receptors in rat cortex was examined. After chronic treatment there was decreased binding and it was suggested that this further demonstrates the specificity of the binding and suggests that this may be the mechanism of action that produces tolerance (2). The exact relationship of benzodiazepine binding to anxiolytic or tolerance effects remains unknown.

BETA-ADRENERGIC ANTAGONISTS

A separate class of pharmacologic agents that are being investigated as possible anxiolytics are the beta-andrenergic blocking agents. If these drugs, which are not CNS depressants, can be demonstrated to be anxiolytics, they would represent a theoretical and potential therapeutic advantage over the benzodiazepines. Anxiety can be expressed clinically as both psychic discomfort and somatic disturbances. The psychic discomfort may be expressed as fear, tension, irritability, nervousness, restlessness, and apprehension. This has been called "psychic" anxiety with psychologic symptoms and has been distinguished from "somatic" anxiety, which is expressed clinically with somatic complaints, palpitations, sweating, diarrhea, and tremor. Although this splitting of anxiety into psychic and somatic complaints does not help in defining primary etiologic factors in anxiety, it has proved useful in evaluating the effectiveness of the beta blockers as anxiolytics.

Clinical trials of beta-andrenergic blocking agents in the treatment of anxiety have shown them to be useful in those patients who have primarily somatic symptoms or in those patients in whom the somatic symptoms increase the psychic symptoms. In one study, however, the patients had no preference for the beta-blocking agents, despite the fact that there was definite amelioration of somatic symptoms. In fact, the patients not only failed to prefer the beta blockers to placebo, but they felt no better while taking the beta blockers. A later trial comparing placebo, beta blockers, and diazepam demonstrated that diazepam was better than propranolol in alleviating anxiety (7,19,20).

In some instances, control of somatic beta-andrenergically mediated symptoms could play a major role in the treatment of the patient with anxiety. The effect of those agents, however, is presumably peripheral and not based on CNS action, making them less attractive in terms of understanding the biochemistry of anxiety. On the other hand, it has been postulated that there may be different biochemical forms of anxiety, and while it is true that beta blockers exert a peripheral anxiolytic effect, there may be certain forms of anxiety in which these agents exert a central anxiolytic effect as well (8). At present, this is entirely speculative. Although it is recognized that the clinical use of beta-adrenergic antagonists does result in certain central effects (sleep disorder, hallucinations), these effects, along with the identification of beta receptor sites in the CNS, give additional support to their possible role as central anxiolytics.

NEUROLEPTICS

Several of the neuroleptic agents discussed in Chapter 22 are used clinically as anxiolytic agents. Of these, thioridazine and prochlorperazine are probably most widely employed, with the latter being used primarily as adjunctive therapy in patients with various gastrointestinal disorders. When used as anxiolytic agents the dosages of neuroleptics are much lower than the usual antipsychotic range so that their neurologic side effects are less likely to occur. There has recently been an attempt to ban the use of neuroleptics in anxiety because of the potential risk of tardive dyskinesia (see Chapter 3). The choice of a specific drug for a specific patient always depends on weighing the risk-benefit ratio of available agents. Neuroleptics do cause tardive dyskinesia but in low doses for a short duration (6 months or less) this risk is very low. Neuroleptics do have some advantages over benzodiazepines:

a) Withdrawal does not cause anxiety. Because of this the course of therapy is often shorter.

b) They do not act additively with alcohol to depress CNS function.

c) In elderly patients, especially those with some degree of dementia, neuroleptics are less likely to cause paradoxical agitation than benzodiazepines.

The mechanism of neuroleptics in the treatment of psychosis was discussed in Chapter 22. Whether the anxiolytic effect of these agents is related to their antipsychotic effect or is a different effect is unknown.

THE CHRONIC TREATMENT OF ANXIETY

A number of clinical studies have clearly demonstrated the short-term efficacy of propandiols, benzodiazepines, and to a lesser extent neuroleptics in the treatment of anxiety. Very few long-term studies have been carried out, so we have little information as to the long-term efficacy of these agents that are often taken continuously for many years. The efficacy of these agents in reducing anxiety during such chronic treatment is unproven. Anecdotal data abounds but is complicated by the fact that drug withdrawal, especially of benzodiazepines but also of propandiols, can itself cause anxiety.

BIBLIOGRAPHY AND *SELECTED REVIEWS

1. Berger, F. M. (1954): The pharmacological properties of 2-methyl-2-n-propyl-1,3-propanediol dicarbamate (Miltown), a new interneuronal blocking agent. *J. Pharmacol. Exp. Ther.*, 112:413–423.
2. Chiu, T. H., and Rosenberg, H. C. (1978): Reduced diazepam binding following chronic benzodiazepine treatment. *Life Sci.*, 23:1153–1158.

3. Costa, E., Guidotti, A., Mao, C. C., and Suria, A. (1976): New concepts of the mechanism of action of benzodiazepines. *Life Sci.*, 17:167–185.
4. Doteuchi, M., and Costa, E. (1973): *Neuropharmacology*, 12:1059–1072.
*5. Greenblatt, D. J., and Shader, R. I. (1978): Pharmacotherapy of anxiety with benzodiazepines and B-adrenergic blockers. In: *Psychopharmacology: A Generation of Progress*, edited by M. A. Upton, A. Di Mascio, and K. F. Killum, pp. 1381–1390. Raven Press, New York.
6. Greenblatt, D. J., and Shader, R. I. (1978): Prazepam and lorazepam, two new benzodiazepines. *N. Engl. J. Med.*, 299:1342–1344.
7. Granville-Grossman, K. L., and Turner, P. (1966): The effect of propranolol on anxiety. *Lancet*, I:788.
8. Heimann, H. (1977): Discussion. In: *Beta Blockers and the CNS*, edited by P. Keilholz, p. 244. University Press, Baltimore.
*9. Klein, D. F., and Davis, J. M. (1969): *Diagnosis and Drug Treatment of Psychiatric Disorders*. Williams & Wilkins, Baltimore.
10. Marangos, P. J., Paul, S. M., Goodwin, F. K., and Kolnick, P. (1979): Putative endogenous ligands for the benzodiazepine receptor. *Life Sci.*, 25:1093–1102.
11. Mohler, H., and Okada, T. (1977): Benzodiazepine receptor: Demonstration in the central nervous system. *Science*, 198:849–851.
12. Mohler, H., and Okada, T. (1977): Properties of ^{3}H diazepam binding to benzodiazepine receptors in rat cerebral cortex. *Life Sci.*, 20:2101–2110.
13. Mohler, H., and Okada, T. (1978): Biochemical identification of the site of action of benzodiazepines in human brain by ^{3}H diazepam binding. *Life Sci.*, 22:985–996.
14. Paul, S. M., and Skolnick, P. (1978): Rapid changes in brain benzodiazepine receptors after experimental seizures. *Science*, 202:892–894.
15. Sleeping Pills, Insomnia and Medical Practice Report. (1979): Study of the Institute of Medicine, National Academy of Sciences, Washington, D.C.
16. Smith, R. C., Dekirmenjian, H., Davis, J., Casper, R., Gosenfeld, L., and Tsai, C. (1976): Blood level, mood and MHPG response to diazepam in man. In: *Pharmacokinetics of Psychoactive Drugs*, edited by L. A. Gottscholk and S. Merlis, pp. 141–156. Spectrum, New York.
17. Speth, R. C., Wastek, G. J., Johnson, P. C., and Yamamura, H. I. (1978): Benzodiazepine binding in human brain: characterization using [^{3}H] flunitrazepam. *Life Sci.*, 22:859–866.
18. Tallman, J. F., Paul, S. M., Kolnick, P. S., and Yollager, D. W. (1980): Receptors for the age of anxiety: Pharmacology of the benzodiazepines. *Science*, 207:274–281.
19. Tyrer, P. J., and Lader, M. H. (1973): Effects of beta adrenergic blockade with sotaolol in chronic anxiety. *Clin. Pharmacol. Ther.*, 14:418.
20. Tyrer, P. J., and Lader, M. H. (1974): Response to propranolol and diazepam in somatic and psychic anxiety. *Br. Med. J.*, II:14.

Chapter 24

Minimal Brain Dysfunction

Minimal brain dysfunction (MBD) in children, also termed attentional deficit disorder (ADD), is a heterogeneous behavioral disorder usually characterized by (a) hyperactivity, (b) impulsivity or poor attention, and (c) poor school performance despite normal or near-normal intelligence (5,13). This rather vague triad by itself is not enough to substantiate a definite diagnosis. On the one hand, it clearly segregates from MBD those children who are inattentive and hyperactive and also mentally retarded and who manifest evidence of major cerebral disease. It does not distinguish the child with MBD from a normal child who, because of inadequate parental guidance or inappropriate discipline, is rambunctious and lacks the social skills of his peers. It is for this reason that the diagnosis and management of MBD have become controversial, especially concerning the issue of pharmacologic intervention.

With these limitations clearly in mind, a subgroup of children experience excessive and severe locomotor activity, incessant shifts in attention, and do poorly in school despite scoring adequately on one-to-one testing. These severely disabled children have been diagnosed as having MBD on the premise that an organic and perhaps maturational deficit underlies the pathophysiology of the behavioral problem.

The original descriptions of behavioral abnormalities seen following head injury, encephalitis, and asphyxia in infants were similar to the behavioral patterns observed in some hyperactive children without known specific organic etiology (28). Since these initial behavioral patterns were associated with definite central nervous system (CNS) insults, the hyperkinetic behavioral syndrome was also postulated to have an organic pathogenesis. Some of the early investigators in this field related the abnormal behavioral patterns to a diencephalic disturbance. Laufer and Denhoff (14) proposed an anatomic basis for MBD by demonstrating that abnormal EEG patterns in children with the so-called "hyperkinetic impulse disorder" could be ameliorated by the administration of dextroamphetamine. They concluded that the anatomic substrate was a rostral brainstem and diencephalic abnormality. Although a rostro-caudal pattern of decreasing vulnerability to ischemic insults has long been recognized, recent work has shown that human neonatal diencephalic and rostral brainstem structures are more susceptible to ischemia then originally thought. This may lend credence to the theory of diencephalic dysfunction in the child with MBD. These children may have subtle, unobserved CNS damage during the perinatum, and the behavioral abnormality may be a complex expression of this dysfunction. Since no data are available to corroborate this theory, however, these hypotheses remain conjectural.

The important observation that MBD tends to disappear or at least abate in the vast majority of patients by adolescence suggested that the syndrome may relate to some type of cerebral maturational delay. This concept has prompted a new interest in the biochemistry and pharmacology of child behavior and has led to what is now known as the dopaminergic hypothesis of MBD. This hypothesis offers a reasonable vantage point from which to evaluate biochemical data and suggest new research perspectives. It is derived from three areas of pharmacologic research: (a) animal models of the disorder, (b) neurotransmitter assays in children with MBD, and (c) pharmacologic analysis of centrally active dr gs that are used in the treatment of MBD. Evidence suggests that underactivity of the central dopaminergic system, possibly on the basis of a neurodevelopmental lag, relates to the pathophysiology of the condition.

ANIMAL MODELS

The dopaminergic hypothesis gained its earliest credence from work with experimental animals. Two basic experimental models have been developed, based on the two behavioral aspects of MBD: hyperactivity and poor goal-directed behavior or impulsivity. Neurotransmitter manipulation has led to the induction in animals of behavioral patterns resembling those seen in children with MBD; further manipulation has been shown to ameliorate these behaviors. The two models are compatible with one another in that they both relate to dopaminergic underactivity in young animals.

In rats, there is a predictable period of increased motor activity lasting from approximately day 12 until day 22 (23). This altered behavior correlates with an alteration in catecholaminergic system maturation, since dopamine and norepinephrine levels in newborn rats are approximately 20 to 30% of those of adults, and dopamine and norepinephrine concentrations rapidly increase in the first weeks of life. Adult levels of norepinephrine are reached by 40 days and adult levels of dopamine by 50 days. The greatest concentration increase occurs during the period from 7 to 18 days, roughly when normal hyperactivity is seen. The activity of synthetic enzymes, tyrosine hydroxylase, DOPA decarboxylase, and dopamine β-hydroxylase, parallel these increasing levels. In contrast, the normal cholinergic systems in the striatum, hippocampus, and the frontal cortex mature later, as may the serotonergic system. These studies suggest that a natural model of hyperactivity may relate to adrenergic or dopaminergic predominance over the undeveloped cholinergic and serotonergic mechanisms.

To determine whether dopamine or norepinephrine was primarily responsible for the hyperactivity, Shawitz et al. (23) treated the baby rats with 6-hydroxydopamine and desmethylimipramine to deplete preferentially brain dopamine. They reasoned that if dopamine increases hyperactivity, the rats treated with a dopamine toxin should show no hyperactivity; if the hyperactivity relates to norepinephrine, the rats should still be hyperactive since the toxin would not affect norepinephrine. In fact, neither of these phenomena occurred. Instead, the animals treated with the dopamine toxin became more hyperactive. Since depletion of central dopamine in young rats induced an enhanced and now abnormal hyperactivity, the investigators suggested that in light of the combined data, normal dopamine levels may act to protect against pathologic hyperkinesis.

With this foundation, Campbell and Randall (4) suggested that if decreased dopamine activity relates to hyperactivity, perhaps hyperactive animals could be treated with dopamine agents to abate the hyperactive behavior. They administered amphetamine, a known dopamine agonist, to young animals; this was associated with increased calming behavior. In older animals and adults, amphetamine induces hyperactivity and an increase in nondirected activity. These data suggest that hyperactivity in young animals may relate to a relative decrease in the dopaminergic activity in the CNS, and that the means of abating hyperactivity is to increase dopaminergic activity. By extrapolation to children with MBD, hyperactivity may be related to underactivity of central dopaminergic activity; treatment of such hyperactivity would involve the enhancement of the dopaminergic system.

A second model used in the study of MBD has been that of poor attention or poor goal-directed behavior. Children with MBD demonstrate short attention spans with impulsivity and poor concentration. Some investigators (31) have suggested that these learning difficulties may stem directly from the children's inability to concentrate and direct their attention. Goal-directed behavior has been studied with self-stimulation and conditioned learning experiments in laboratory animals. The findings in this group of experiments confirm the importance of neurotransmitter balance in the physiology of these behaviors and suggest that poor goal-directed behavior correlates with underactivity of the central dopaminergic system.

Experimental animals will self-administer the dopamine agonists amphetamine and apomorphine. Breese and Cooper (2) showed that self-stimulation induced by amphetamine can be counteracted by treatment that interrupts dopaminergic but not adrenergic fibers. Additionally, pimozide, a specific dopamine receptor blocker, suppresses self-stimulation; this inhibition can be reversed by dopamine reuptake blockers, such as cocaine and nomifensine (15). Both serotonin and acetylcholine antagonize self-stimulatory behavior.

These studies demonstrate that goal-directed behavior may be influenced by reciprocal neurotransmitter systems, dopaminergic on the one hand and cholinergic and serotonergic on the other. The same suppressed goal-directed behavior can be elicited by either depressing dopaminergic influence or enhancing serotonergic or cholinergic influences. If these studies are used as a model of MBD in children, the pathophysiology of this disorder would relate to functional underactivity of dopamine in relation to other antagonistic neurotransmitter systems. The relationship of this model to the previous model of hyperactivity in young animals suggests that the most consistent explanation of both behaviors involves a relative underactivity of dopamine.

A final animal model of MBD is that of the telomian-beagle hybrid dog (1). This naturally occurring hybrid exhibits ambient hyperactivity, impulsivity, and high degrees of distractibility. Two subgroups can be identified: one responds to amphetamine with decreased locomotor activity and enhanced learning; and one is resistant to this dopaminergic agonist. These two subgroups have been studied with attention to dopamine, norepinephrine, and serotonin function. Responder dogs have lower levels of dopamine and its major metabolite homovanillic acid (HVA), as well as lower norepinephrine in brain tissue. Cerebrospinal fluid (CSF) measures show lower HVA in the dogs that later respond to amphetamine when compared with the nonresponders. No further studies have been performed on these hybrids. The fact that the responders and nonresponders are behaviorally indistinguishable before amphetamine challenge, both showing hyperactivity and distractibility, makes this model not completely applicable, but it has the advantage of being the first naturally occurring model of MBD to be proposed.

NEUROTRANSMITTER ASSAY

Another approach to identifying specific neurotransmitter involvement in MBD has been the analysis of neurochemical concentrations in various body fluids. Most specifically related to CNS function is CSF. Little work has been performed on the CSF concentration of various neurotransmitters and their metabolites in MBD, but a recent report lends support to the dopaminergic hypothesis. Shawitz et al. (24) examined CSF samples in children with MBD and demonstrated that HVA, the dopamine metabolite, was significantly decreased. The metabolite of serotonin was unchanged. This evidence suggested a possible biochemical alteration in the dopaminergic system, perhaps on a maturational basis, that plays a role in the pathophysiology of MBD. Shetty and Chase (25) found no significant difference in CSF dopamine or serotonin metabolites in children with MBD but noted that changes in HVA levels after amphetamine correlated with clinical improvement. Although this study does not delineate the precise role of dopamine in the pathogenesis or natural history of MBD, it does suggest a relationship between dopamine and MBD.

DRUG STUDIES

The third area of research pertinent to a dopaminergic hypothesis of MBD is the pharmacologic analysis of those agents empirically shown to be of benefit in abating the disorder. The three agents acknowledged to be useful in treating MBD are amphetamine, methylphenidate, and the more recent drug, magnesium pemoline. Although these agents do not share similar chemical structures and affect central neuromechanisms differently, they all enhance catecholamine activity, specifically dopaminergic. That these three drugs are effective in treating MBD and are dopaminergic agents suggests that the pathophysiology of MBD relates to this neurotransmitter system.

Amphetamine is an indirect dopaminergic agonist which causes release of the neurotransmitter from presynaptic terminals (21). It also has direct agonist properties. Amphetamine-induced stereotyped behavior is the accepted and classic animal model of heightened dopaminergic activity in the striatal system (22). Amphetamine has been used to treat Parkinson's disease and is effective although not often used because of its cardiovascular effects in the elderly population. Further clinical evidence suggesting that amphetamine is a dopaminergic agent is the fact that patients exposed to chronic amphetamine develop a characteristic, involuntary choreiform movement disorder. Chorea is felt to relate pharmacologically to an increased activity of dopaminergic systems in the striatum (11).

The pharmacologic mechanism of action of methylphenidate also involves alterations in catecholamine activity (12). Methylphenidate acts primarily on the reserpine-sensitive catecholaminergic neurotransmitter pool (21). Parkinson's disease, a well-defined example of central dopamine deficiency, has been reported to be improved by methylphenidate therapy (9). On the other hand, choreiform movement disorders, regardless of etiology, have been proposed to be related to alterations in striatal dopaminergic mechanisms; methylphenidate therapy has been associated with the induction and exacerbation of choreiform movements (9,19). Methylphenidate also produces gnawing, chewing, stereotyped behavior in laboratory animals, which has a marked similarity to amphetamine-induced stereotyped behavior. The latter behavior is related to striatal dopaminergic mechanisms. These clinical and laboratory reports support the idea that methylphenidate acts by increasing central dopaminergic effects. In fact, Garfinkel and colleagues (8) have proposed that methylphenidate ameliorates the symptoms of MBD by specifically enhancing central dopaminergic effects.

Although preclinical studies with magnesium pemoline have not entirely elucidated its mechanism of action, pemoline has been reported to potentiate central catecholamine activity (20) and has been demonstrated to increase dopamine synthesis and concentration in animal brain (29). This agent has been reported to be useful in the treatment of MBD, but its exact pharmacologic activity remains to be defined. However, since amphetamine, methylphenidate, and pemoline all affect central dopamine systems, it is reasonable to implicate this neurotransmitter in the pathophysiology of MBD.

If dopaminergic underactivity relates to the pathophysiology of MBD, other agents that enhance dopaminergic function may be useful in treating the disorder. Levodopa, the amino acid precursor of dopamine, would be a logical agent to test; in fact, pilot studies have been conducted using levodopa in conjunction with methylphenidate. Jackson and Pelton (10) reported that combined therapy was more efficacious than methylphenidate alone in controlling hyperkinetic and impulsive behavior. Levodopa has not been tested alone, nor has bromocriptine or other direct acting dopaminergic agonists. These agents do not have the risks of addiction or dependency seen with the central stimulants; thus trials may be reasonable in the future.

There have also been reports of controlling MBD with neuroleptic agents, the phenothiazines and the butyrophenone, haloperidol (7). These agents are in fact dopaminergic-blocking agents and, if truly efficacious, would suggest that dopaminergic underactivity is not of pathophysiologic significance to MBD. The distinction must be carefully drawn, however, between sedation and specific improvement in hyperkinesis and inattentiveness. Neuroleptics decrease motor activity but are simultaneously highly sedative. When the parameter of improved attentiveness is measured, the dopaminergic agonists have been shown to be clinically superior to neuroleptic drugs (32).

OTHER NEUROTRANSMITTERS

A number of investigators have studied serotonergic chemistry in relation to MBD. Although reports of lower blood serotonin have been made in hyperkinetic children, CSF determinations have not shown changes in the central serotonin metabolite, 5-HIAA (2,4,16). Alterations in GABA and cholinergic function have been discussed as playing possible modulating roles but not a primary role in the pathophysiology of MBD.

NUTRITIONAL CONSIDERATIONS

Since the early discovery that ketogenic diets can dramatically alter seizure activity in children, pediatric neurologists have been sensitive to possible links between dietary factors and neurologic dysfunction. Many diets and nutritional alterations have been advocated in the treatment of MBD, although few scientific data support them. Animal studies of nutritional deprivation suggest that motoric activity changes when developing animals are malnourished, but these studies do not identify specific deficits (17).

The issue of red dyes has gained attention in relation to the pathogenesis or exacerbation of childhood behavioral disorders. Some investigators have suggested the removal of all foods containing this dye in an attempt to control hyperactive behavior. The cellular and biochemical effects of red dye on dopaminergic activity are being investigated (26).

PHARMACOLOGY OF CENTRAL STIMULANTS

The basic pharmacology of amphetamine and methylphenidate is discussed in detail elsewhere in this volume. The doses of these drugs recommended for use in treating minimal brain dysfunction are: amphetamine, 0.2 to 0.5 mg/kg/day or 5 to 20 mg/day given in divided doses; methylphenidate, 0.3 to 1.0 mg/kg/day or 5 to 40 mg/day given in divided doses. The drugs are rapidly absorbed and induce behavioral changes usually within the first week of therapy. Systemic, neurologic, and psychiatric side effects as well as the issue of drug addiction in the pediatric population are discussed in Chapter 26.

The newest of drugs used in the treatment of MBD is magnesium pemoline. It is a member of the oxazolidine compounds and has a structure that is not related to amphetamine or methylphenidate (see Fig. 1); the empirical formula is $C_9H_8N_2O_2$. Both pemoline and its dione metabolite are pharmacologically active but the latter

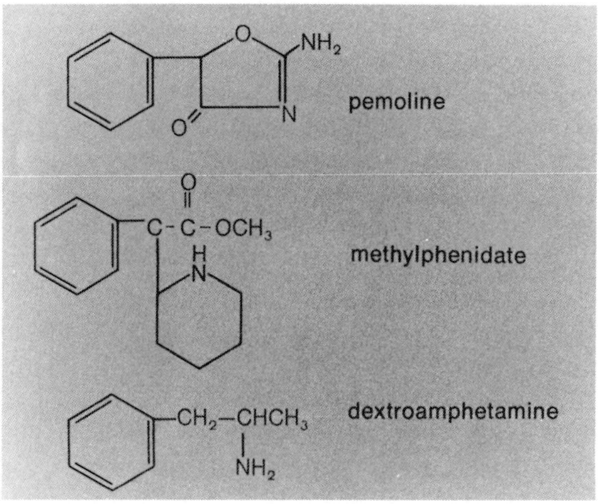

FIG. 1. Structure of pemoline, methylphenidate, and dextroamphetamine.

much less than the parent compound. Drug distribution in the CNS in animals focuses on brainstem structures rather than cortex or cerebellum.

Pharmacokinetic studies indicate the half-life of pemoline to range from 10 to 14 hr; thus midafternoon (i.e., in school) doses of medication are avoided with this drug (6). The behavioral changes are slow to develop, however, and parents and children familiar with amphetamine or methylphenidate must be warned that the onset of action for pemoline may be 2 to 3 weeks. This agent is newer than the other two major drugs, and many side effects reported with the older agents have not yet been seen with pemoline. However, pemoline-associated chorea has now been reported, suggesting that this agent may be associated with the same central dopaminergic toxicity seen with amphetamine and methylphenidate (11). Large growth studies of children receiving pemoline have not been reported. Doses recommended are 37.5 to 112.5 mg (average, 75 mg) given as a single morning dose, with periodic interruptions recommended to reassess behavioral need for the drug. Acute toxicity includes tachycardia, agitation, and restlessness; treatment of an overdose is symptomatic, with induced emesis and lavage.

Nonpharmacologic Considerations

Numerous clinical studies report that nonpharmacologic factors are also important to the pathophysiology of MBD. Pharmacologic manipulation tends to abate abnormal behavior acutely in these children, but the improvement is not maintained without vigorous mobilization of school and family resources. The specifics of these aspects of therapy are beyond the scope of a neuropharmacologic text, but comprehensive reviews are available (3,18,30). The biochemical alterations induced by such behavioral therapy have not been studied in terms of neuropharmacology.

Future Perspectives

MBD has a multidimensional pathophysiology. Pharmacologic evidence derived from numerous research prospectives suggests that dopaminergic underactivity may be significant to aspects of the disorder. Which dopaminergic pathway is involved in MBD is undefined, but the mesorostral system has been suggested (27). This path travels from the midbrain near the reticular activating nuclei, important to arousal and alerting mechanisms, and ends in diffuse cortical projections, important to complex behavioral patterns.

The proposed theory that dopaminergic underactivity is important to the pathophysiology of MBD suggests a number of new possibilities in therapy as well as investigation. Dopaminergic manipulation in the form of agonists other than those already being used may be of potential benefit in children with this disorder. More clinical neurotransmitter data, specifically more CSF assays, may reveal heterogeneous chemical subgroups within the clinical spectrum of MBD. Investigation of these issues may further clarify the specific role of the dopaminergic and other neurotransmitter systems in the pathophysiology of MBD in children.

REFERENCES

1. Bareggi, S. R., Becker, R. E., Ginsburg, B. E., and Gonovese, E. (1979): Neurochemical investigation of an endogenous model of hyperkinetic syndrome in a hybrid dog. *Life Sci.*, 24:481–488.
2. Breese, G. R., and Cooper, B. R. (19   ): Relationship of dopamine neural systems in the maintenance of self stimulation. In: *Neurotransmitter Balances Regulating Behavior*, edited by E. F. Domino and J. M. Davis, pp. 37–56. NPP Books, Ann Arbor, Michigan.
3. Campbell, B. A., and Mabry, P. D. (1973): The role of catecholamines in the ontogeny of arousal. *Psychopharmacologia*, 31:253–264.
4. Campbell, B. A., and Randall, P. J. (1977): Paradoxical effects of amphetamine on preweaning and postweaning rats. *Science*, 195:288–291.
5. Connors, C. K. (1967): The syndrome of minimal brain dysfunction: Psychological aspects. *Pediatr. Clin. North Am.*, 14:749–766.
6. Dodge, P. W., and Celarec, B. (1968): Metabolism of pemoline and pemoline with magnesium hydroxide. *Fed. Proc.*, 27:237.
7. Freed, H., and Peifer, C. A. (1956): Treatment of hyperkinetic emotionally disturbed children with prolonged administration of chlorpromazine. *Am. J. Psychiatry*, 113:22–30.
8. Garfinkel, B. D., Webster, C. D., and Sloman, L. (1975): Methylphenidate and caffeine in the treatment of children with MBD. *Am. J. Psychiatry*, 132:723–728.
9. Holliday, A. M., and Nathan, P. W. (1961): Methylphenidate in parkinsonism. *Br. Med. J.*, 1:1652–1655.
10. Jackson, R. T., and Pelton, E. W. (1978): L-dopa treatment of children with hyperactive behavior. *Neurology*, 28:331.
11. Klawans, H. L. (1973): *Pharmacology of Extrapyramidal Movement Disorders*. Karger, Basel.
12. Kuczenski, R., and Segal, D. S. (1975): Differential effects of D- and L-amphetamine and methylphenidate on rat striatal dopamine biosynthesis. *Eur. J. Pharmacol.*, 30:244–251.
13. Laufer, M. W., Denhoff, E., and Solomons, G. (1957): Hyperkinetic impulse disorder in children's behavior problems. *Psychosom. Med.*, 19:38–49.
14. Laufer, M. W., and Denhoff, E. (1957): Hyperkinetic behavior syndrome in children. *J. Pediatr.*, 50:463–474.
15. Liebman, J. M., and Butcher, L. L. (1973): Effects on self stimulation behavior of drugs influencing dopaminergic neurotransmitter mechanisms. *Arch. Pharm. (Weinheim)*, 277:305–318.
16. Margolin, D. (1978): Hyperkinetic children syndrome and brain monoamines. *J. Clin. Psychiatry*, 39:120–123.

17. Michaelson, I. A., Bornschein, R. L., Lock, R. K., and Rafeles, L. S. (1977): Minimal brain dysfunction hyperkinesis. Significance of nutritional status in animal models of hyperactivity. In: *Animal Models in Psychiatry and Neurology*, edited by I. Hanin and E. Usdin. Pergamon Press, Oxford, pp. 218–226.
18. Millchap, J. G., and Fowler, G. W. (1967): Treatment of "minimal brain dysfunction" syndromes. *Pediatr. Clin. North Am.*, 14:767–777.
19. Palatucci, D. M. (1974): Iatrogenic dyskinesia. *J. Nerv. Ment. Dis.*, 159:73–76.
20. Plotnikoff, N. (1971): Pemoline: Review of performance. *Tex. Rep. Biol. Med.*, 29:467–479.
21. Scheel-Kruger, J. (1971): Comparative studies of various amphetamine analogues demonstrating different interactions with the metabolism of the catecholamines in the brain. *Eur. J. Pharmacol.*, 14:47–51.
22. Scheel-Kruger, J., and Randrup, A. (1967): Stereotyped hyperactive behavior produced by dopamine in the absence of noradrenaline. *Life Sci.*, 6:1389–1398.
23. Shawitz, B. A., Yager, R. D., and Klopper, J. H. (1976): Selective brain dopamine depletion in developing rats: An experimental model of brain dysfunction. *Science*, 194:305–307.
24. Shawitz, B. A., Cohen, D. J., and Malcolm, B. B. (1975): Cerebral spinal fluid amine metabolites in children with MBD. *Pediatr. Res.*, 9:385.
25. Shetty, T., and Chase, T. N. (1976): Central monoamines and hyperkinesis of childhood. *Neurology (Minneap.)*, 26:1000–1002.
26. Silbergeld, E. (1977): Neuropharmacology of hyperkinesis. *Curr. Dev. Psychopharmacol.*, 4:115–123.
27. Snyder, S., and Meyerhoff, J. L. (1973): How amphetamine acts in minimal brain dysfunction. *Ann. NY Acad. Sci.*, 205:310–320.
28. Strauss, A. A., and Lehtinen, L. (1947): *Psychopathology and Education of the Brain-Injured Child*. Grune & Stratton, New York.
29. Tagliamonte, A. P., Taliamonte, J., Perez-Cruet, A., and Greasa, G. L. (1971): Stimulation of brain dopamine turnover by magnesium pemoline. *Fed. Proc.*, 30:223.
30. Weiss, G., and Hechtman, L. (1979): Hyperactive child syndrome. *Science*, 205:1348–1354.
31. Werry, J. S. (1968): Studies on the hyperactive child. IV. An empirical analysis of the minimal brain dysfunction syndrome. *Arch. Gen. Psychiatry*, 19:6–9.
32. Werry, J. S., and Aman, M. G. (1975): Methylphenidate and haloperidol in children. *Arch. Gen. Psychiatry*, 32:790–795.

Chapter 25

Sleep Disorders

Our knowledge of sleep as a complex behavioral state has made great advances in the last two decades. The relationship of sleep stages to specific neurotransmitters has been studied extensively, and the functional role of various anatomic regions of the central nervous system (CNS) in the sleep process has been established (5,29). Despite these advances, our ability to understand and treat commonly encountered sleep disorders remains limited and largely empirical.

The major effect of recent clinical research in the field has been to expand the number of recognized sleep disorders. In some cases, such as sleep apnea, identification of the disorder is straightforward. In other areas, overlap in diagnostic entities is sufficiently great to make the clinical utility of recognizing each variant questionable. We have taken the liberty to group a number of disorders under more general categories when this did not influence the ultimate therapy to be outlined. Similarly, our recommendations for therapy do not include a review of every therapeutic agent reported to be effective in treatment. Every year, reports claim excellent results in a few patients using a novel therapeutic agent, which subsequently fails to show efficacy in larger trials. Our omissions in this area are largely the personal bias of the author and are derived from our own clinical experience. In situations where no universally effective form of therapy is available, we have included various suggestions that are occasionally of benefit.

INSOMNIA

The pharmacologic therapy of insomnia is a relatively simple issue; but successful therapy remains elusive in a large percentage of patients. A discussion of therapy must include guidelines for applying the available sedative agents.

Insomnia is characteristically present in one of three patterns: inability to fall asleep (initial insomnia), inability to remain asleep (early morning awakening), or inability to maintain a prolonged period of sleep (sleep fragmentation). Other features frequently useful in classifying the disorder include its duration, situational dependence, or association with various medical conditions, medications, or additional symptoms (i.e., snoring, daytime hypersomnia, cataplexy, nocturnal apnea, nocturnal myoclonic movements) (22).

On the basis of this additional information, certain groups of insomniacs are readily apparent. A large group has chronic inability to fall asleep; these individuals frequently are high strung, and insomnia is a virtual lifestyle. Frequently, they complain that they lie awake for hours or have not slept for days or weeks at a stretch. Actual all-night studies of these "poor sleepers" indicate that many fall asleep relatively quickly, with sleep latencies only slightly longer than normal volunteers (19). When awakened, they may state that they were in actuality awake; their major problem is related to an abnormal perception of sleep. In isolated cases, electroencephalograms (EEGs) may demonstrate a central rhythm in the 9 to 11 Hz range during sleep (so-called alpha-delta pattern), which has unconvincingly been suggested as evidence of persistent wakefulness during behavioral sleep. The importance of identifying this group lies in the fact that they already are sleeping for "normal" lengths of time. The administration of sedative agents in this group is doomed to failure, and alternative forms of therapy are best employed early in management. Psychologic counselling, exercise regimens, or behavioral modification techniques offer some benefits in motivated patients.

In other cases of chronic insomnia, especially those in which sleep fragmentation is a prominent feature, symptoms of narcolepsy or sleep apnea (9,24) may develop. In the former case, therapy is rarely directed at the insomnia; in the latter, sedative medications worsen the severity of apneic episodes. Identification of the associated condition with an appropriate history and polysomnographic studies should prevent inappropriate therapy directed solely at the complaint of insomnia.

Patients with a history of recent onset insomnia are more likely to benefit from direct forms of therapeutic intervention. The most common etiologies in this group are psychogenic and frequently are associated with either depression or situational anxiety. While not an absolute rule, the traditional association of early morning awakening with depression and inability to initiate sleep with anxiety is consistent enough to direct further lines of inquiry (15,22).

In obtaining the history, it is important to exclude drug-induced forms of insomnia, which frequently follow administration of various phenylethylamine derivatives, xanthines, and corticosteroids. In many cases, dosage reduction, use of shorter acting preparations, or earlier times of administration are curative and obviate the need for sedative therapy. Difficulty in initiating sleep is also a symptom of hyperthyroidism (either primary or iatrogenic) and is observed in Cushing's syndrome and disease. Similarly, sleep disruption is frequently observed in patients with bipolar depression and schizophrenia. In all these situations, a detailed history and physical examination usually provide enough information to direct therapy in an appropriate direction and prevent symptomatic therapy of the isolated complaint of insomnia.

In general, hypnotics are indicated if anxiety appears to be the predominant causative process and seems likely to improve with the passage of time. The critical decision is whether the underlying anxiety is likely to outlive the period of effective sedation, which usually is lost after 2 to 3 weeks, regardless of the agent employed. Where more prolonged periods of sleep disturbance are anticipated, medications can be administered on alternate days in an attempt to delay the development of tolerance (15,22).

The choice of a sedative agent is dictated most by the duration of clinical sedation. Ideally, sedative effects should clear by the time the patient arises in the morning. Other considerations relate to the sleep architectural changes that follow sedative administration, although these probably are not as important as is commonly believed. As a general rule, all agents employed as sedatives are REM suppressant at high dosage. At lower dosages, two patterns of drug effect emerge: barbiturates, chloral hydrate anticholinergics, and ethanol demonstrate REM suppression, while most benzodiazepines decrease deeper stages of slow wave sleep. Flurazepam, L-tryptophan, and triazolam have minor effects on sleep architecture. Insofar as the treatment of insomnia is concerned, all agents appear to decrease sleep latency and the number of spontaneous awakenings (16). Although those agents with the least effect on sleep architecture might offer some advantages on a theoretical basis, clear demonstration that they induce "better" sleep is lacking.

The differences in drug effects have more applicability in situations in which one agent is being used to treat withdrawal from another. In withdrawal from REM suppressants, anecdotal observations suggest that the administration of benzodiazepines at standard dosage is counterproductive in relieving initial insomnia, spontaneous awakenings, and nightmares and seems to exacerbate these complaints. This may be due to slow wave sleep-blocking effects, which may potentiate REM activity. Gradual withdrawl from REM-suppressant medications or substitution of another REM suppressant of lower potency is preferred in this situation. We have avoided the use of benzodiazepines in the treatment of ethanol withdrawal (8), which is probably the most frequently encountered situation in which REM-suppressant withdrawal and REM rebound pose major management problems.

Table 1 summarizes available data on commonly utilized hypnotics. In all cases, except where noted, sleep latency is decreased. Agents that failed to decrease sleep latency are indicated (no significant effect) and are not effective in inducing sleep in normal subjects.

In general, there is no reason to use more than a single agent in the treatment of insomnia. Failure to attain an adequate response on the first night should not signal an immediate need to increase dosage; a trial of 2 to 3 days is indicated. Conversely, especially in older patients, a good therapeutic response in the first days is sometimes followed by excessive morning sedation and even coma (a complication most often encountered with flurazepam).

When initial therapy is unsuccessful, it is desirable to switch to another agent before admitting defeat. A hypnosedative with REM-suppressant effects may appear to be effective when a benzodiazepine is not. An alternative agent frequently employed is L-tryptophan, which is sometimes effective when other agents have failed (10).

In patients with early morning awakening, sedative therapy is rarely effective in the absence of unacceptable morning sedation. If a significant history of depression is encountered, tricyclic antidepressants offer the best results and should be employed as an initial form of therapy (15,22). In these cases, the affective disorder is a better target of therapy than the sleep complaint; improvement in sleep usually

TABLE 1. *Sedatives: dose-related sleep architectural changes*

Medication	Dosage (h.s.)	Major sleep alteration
Barbiturates		
Amobarbital	200 mg	↓ REMS; ↑ REM latency
Heptobarbital	400 mg	↓ REMS
Pentobarbital	100 mg	↓ REMS; ↑ REM latency
Phenobarbital	100 mg	↓ REMS
Secobarbital	100 mg	↓ REMS
Amobarbital +	100 mg	
Secobarbital (Tuinal®)	100 mg	↓ REMS
	3.5 oz	↓ REMS, first half of night
Ethanol	6.0 oz	↓ REMS, entire night
Benzodiazepines		
Chordiazepoxide	50 mg	↓ Stage 4
Diazepam	10 mg	↓ Stage 4
	15 mg	↓ REMS ↓ Stages 2,4
Flurazepam	30 mg	↓ Stages 3,4
Lorazepam	2 mg	↓ REMS
Oxazepam	10 mg	↑ REMS
Triazolam	0.1–1 mg	↓ REMS
Miscellaneous agents		
Chloral hydrate	500–1,500 mg	No significant effect
Diphenylhydramine	50–100 mg	↓ REMS
Glutethimide	500–1,000 mg	↓ REMS
Meprobamate	400–800 mg	No significant effect
Methaqualone	300 mg	No significant effect
Triclofos	1,000 mg	No significant effect
Tryptophan (L-form)	1–10 g	Normal sleep architecture
	> 10 g	↓ REMS

parallels improvement in mood. An occasional pitfall in diagnosis is encountered in patients who begin drinking alcoholic beverages just before retiring. These patients may give a history of some recent event that could potentially lead to depression and may also ave contributed to evening ethanol consumption. While early morning awakening may be related to their underlying affective response, the symptom often clears when bedtime alcohol consumption is halted. This may be related to the REM rebound, which appears in the early morning as the ethanol is metabolized, and leads to disrupted sleep and spontaneous awakening (5,15).

Another area of potential confusion occurs in the patient with sleep fragmentation. This phenomenon is encountered in patients receiving corticosteroids and some Parkinsonian patients receiving levodopa (21). While the complaint is similar to that voiced by patients with early morning awakening, multiple awakenings tend to occur throughout the night. Daytime somnolence and napping also are frequently reported. Response to sedatives or trycyclics is unpredictable, and no satisfactory form of therapy has been found. Administering corticosteroids inthe morning and avoiding evening dosages of levodopa may alleviate the problem and should be attempted where feasible. Other considerations in patients with sleep fragmentation include endocrine disorders that alter cortisol rhythmicity and nocturnal myoclonus (15). The latter disorder is poorly understood and requires all-night polysomnography with electromyogram (EMG) monitoring for diagnosis. No therapy is universally accepted, but some patients respond to the central serotonin-blocking agents cyproheptadine (Periactin) or methysergide (Sansert).

HYPERSOMNIAS

Classification of the various hypersomnias includes disorders characterized by excessively deep sleep, confusion on arising from sleep, excessively long periods of sleep (usually more than 12 hr), persistent lethargy, or episodes of uncontrollable sleep onset (sleep attacks). These symptoms are seen in isolation or in various combinations and may be chronic or episodic in occurrence (15,25). The somnolent states that occur in the context of a variety of systemic disorders or as a result of brain injury are well known to the clinician and do not constitute true "sleep disorders" for the purposes of this discussion. Identification of these secondary forms of hypersomnia is an obvious first step in any evaluation.

When a primary etiology is absent, hypersomnia can usually be related to one of the following: sedative drug abuse, functional disturbances, narcolepsy-cataplexy syndrome, sleep apnea-hypersomnia syndrome, or idiopathic hypersomnia. These are summarized in Table 2. In our own practice, sedative abuse is the most common etiology for hypersomnia and may present as either a chronic or intermittent complaint. Although the use of medications is usually denied, the appearance of drug artifact on EEG studies and positive drug screening examinations of urine and plasma during symptomatic periods establishes the diagnosis.

TABLE 2. *Hypersomnias: Clinical features*

Hypersomnia	Clinical features
Daily	
Sedative drug abuse	+ Urine and plasma drug screen, drug artifact on EEG
Idiopathic	Prolonged nocturnal sleep, frequently familial (40–55%), frequent association of sleep drunkenness, inability to awaken, sleep architecture normal
Functional	Neuraesthenic personality, depression, normal sleep study
Narcolepsy	Sleep "attacks," cataplexy, hypnagogic hallucinations, sleep paralysis, REM onset naps, frequent nocturnal sleep stage shifts
Sleep apnea	Males predominately, snoring, may be hypertensive, obese, multiple apneic episodes during sleep
Cyclic	
Sedative drug abuse	See above
Functional	Association of hypersomnia with emotional stress or symbolic nature of somnolence as part of bipolar depressive syndrome
Kleine-Levin syndrome	Adolescent males, associated hyperphagia and personality changes, may show cyclic temperature elevation

Functional etiologies of hypersomnia often are difficult to establish, and various affective changes are commonly observed in patients with idiopathic hypersomnia, narcolepsy, or sleep apnea. Overall, a history of intermittent episodes of prolonged hypersomnia (days in duration) separated by asymptomatic intervals strongly suggests a functional basis (25). In some cases, continued follow-up suggests a cyclothymic personality disorder or a dissociative state; in others, the psychodynamics underlying the episodes are less obvious. The Kleine-Levin syndrome, characterized by cyclic episodes of hyperphagia and personality changes followed by periods of hypersomnia, is thought to be a psychiatric disorder by some authors, although primary hypothalamic dysfunction has also been suggested (4,25).

Differentiation of idiopathic hypersomnia and functional disturbances in patients with chronic fatigue and somnolence is more difficult. Neurasthenic or depressive personality traits may suggest a functional basis for the complaint but are not infallible. While standard nocturnal polysomnographic studies can be used to exclude sleep apnea and narcolepsy, differentation from idiopathic hypersomnia may be impossible. The absence of short sleep latency times, high awakening threshold, or a clear family history of hypersomnia suggests a functional disturbance (25).

Idiopathic hypersomnia is characterized by excessive daytime drowsiness and frequently is associated with prolonged periods of nocturnal sleep, difficulty in arousal, and sleep drunkenness. A familial incidence is reported in 40 to 55% of cases, and both sexes are affected. Depressive traits are commonly encountered, but more than 50% of patients are psychiatrically normal. Polysomnography demonstrates short sleep latencies, high auditory awakening threshold, excessive sleep duration, and normal cyclic passage through sleep stages. Daytime naps are characterized by slow wave sleep activity; sleep onset REM episodes are not observed. Rarely, patients lack daytime somnolence but manifest other features of the disorder. The pathophysiology of the disorder is unknown, and pathologic studies are lacking (25).

Narcolepsy and sleep apnea-hypersomnia are better defined and more easily recognized causes of hypersomnia (9,15,25). In narcolepsy, daytime sleep tends to occur in irresistible attacks, which occur in inappropriate situations and from which the patient awakens refreshed. Nocturnal sleep is frequently disturbed, and insomnia may precede other symptoms of the disorder. Within a few years, most patients develop additional symptoms; cataplexy, sleep paralysis, and hypnagogic hallucinosis are the best recognized of these and are associated in decreasing order of prevalence. In some patients, episodes of amnesia occur (automatic syndrome); these may be erroneously diagnosed as fugue states or psychomotor epilepsy. In urban centers, a similar constellation of symptoms is not uncommonly offered by central stimulant abusers, and a classic history is not sufficient for diagnosis.

All night polysomnographic studies demonstrate frequent stage shifts, and monitored daytime naps usually demonstrate a rapid appearance of REM sleep. Urine is routinely screened for amphetamine metabolites prior to polysomnographic studies, since acute stimulant withdrawal may be associated with similar sleep events.

In a few patients, similar sleep attacks are not associated with REM onset sleep in what appears to be a variant of the syndrome (25).

The onset of narcolepsy usually occurs in the second or third decade, and a familial incidence is often reported. In almost all cases, the disorder is idiopathic; in some cases, a previous history of encephalitis, or the discovery of an intracerebral tumor, has suggested an association with CNS pathology (25).

Sleep apnea-hypersomnia syndrome has recently emerged as a frequent cause of hypersomnia (9). While the Pickwickian syndrome is the most familiar variant, patients are not necessarily obese. Loud snoring, morning headache, daytime somnolence, and elevated systemic blood pressure are often present. Patients are usually male. Amnestic episodes identical to these observed in narcoleptics may occur. A history of nocturnal apnea usually is not obtained from the patient, but the episodes are frequently noted by other members of the household. Recent publications suggest a familial predilection to the disorder and a possible relationship of sleep apnea to sudden infant death syndrome and high altitude polycythemia (2,9,17).

During sleep, intermittent obstruction of the upper airway occurs secondary to collapse of the oropharynx. Hypoxemia and acidosis rapidly develop, and cardiac arrhythmias may occur. Polysomnographic studies demonstrate an absence of deeper stages of slow wave sleep and frequent awakenings. Simultaneous respiratory monitoring usually demonstrates multiple apneic episodes throughout the night. In addition to obstructive apneic episodes, intermittent respiratory arrest is also frequently noted (central apnea). Increasing weight, intrinsic pulmonary disease, and sedative administration appear to exacerbate symptoms and increase the frequency and duration of apneic episodes (9).

The prevalence of the disorder is probably much greater than earlier reports have suggested, although in many cases the disorder appears to be relatively benign (2). It is unclear whether symptom progression occurs in all individuals with sleep apnea.

HYPERSOMNIA THERAPY

With the exception of those cases in which sedative abuse or a functional disorder is the basis of hypersomnia, therapy with a sleep suppressant is usually required. In some cases, avoidance of sedatives, environmental modification (such as driving with the window open and heater off), or a regular afternoon nap makes continual medical therapy unnecessary. Usually, patients with daytime sleepiness can identify specific times when they are likely to doze off; medications can be timed to control symptoms. In the narcoleptic, sleep attacks are frequently unpredictable. In these cases, coverage for the entire day is required to prevent accidental injury. In all cases, medications should be kept to a minimum dosage and should be given early enough in the day to prevent drug-related insomnia.

The choice of medications available for therapy is large and primarily consists of phenylethylamine derivatives (20). The compounds are classified as amphetamines and nonamphetamines, although all agents act as indirect dopamine agonists and share similar toxicity profiles. The relationship of central dopaminergic activity and central stimulation is controversial, and drug-mediated alterations in central noradrenergic and serotonergic activity may play a role in this effect. Experimental and clinical observations suggest that psychiatric toxicity reactions in the course of chronic therapy are related to the dopaminergic effects of these agents (20).

In general, all the agents currently employed in the treatment of hypersomnia have some sympathomimetic effects and are anorectics. Both these effects tend to be short lived and rarely persist for more than a few weeks. Some reports suggest that alerting effects in the narcoleptic do not undergo tachyphylaxis in the course of chronic therapy; it is more usual to find that dosage requirements increase over time in all forms of hypersomnia. To offset this need for increased medication, we usually instruct patients to discontinue medications at least 2 consecutive days each week (usually over the weekend); this has lessened the need to increase dosage over time. In some cases, sympathomimetic effects tend to recur when medications are restarted following these "drug holidays." In these cases, the administration of propranolol (20 to 40 mg) has proved beneficial in reducing palpitations and transient elevations in blood pressure.

For therapy of intermittent episodes of hypersomnolence or sleep drunkenness, a short-acting stimulant is usually employed. Dextroamphetamine (5 mg), methylphenidate (10 mg), or methamphetamine (2.5 mg) provides an alerting effect which persists for 3 to 4 hr in most patients. In idiopathic hypersomnia with sleep drunkenness, administration 1 hr before the desired time of morning arousal is usually effective (medication being adminstered by a household member). In cases where sleep attacks occur randomly or in patients with persistent debilitating daytime somnolence, an amphetamine may be administered 3 to 4 times per day, or a longer-acting agent may be employed. Pemoline (37.5 mg), phenmetrazine (25 mg), or time-release preparations of methamphetamine (5 and 10 mg) or dextroamphetamine (5 and 10 mg) exerts more prolonged alerting effects and may be effective when administered twice daily. In our own practice, we rarely use time-release preparations, since they frequently exert effects in the late evening, disrupt sleep, and have an uneven behavioral effect.

Dextroamphetamine, methylphenidate, and methamphetamine are controlled substances; other available compounds, marketed as anorectics or decongestants, are classified as nonamphetamines and are available with regular prescriptions. Although governmental classification suggests that these agents differ in their abuse potential and mode of action, no data support this separation. All agents possess central indirect dopaminergic activity, and many of the nonamphetamines have demonstrated a potential for abuse equal to that observed with amphetamine. In practice, all central stimulants should be administered with care, and psychiatric side effects should lead to prompt drug withdrawal. Patients with a prior history of schizophrenia or bipolar depression are particularly prone to psychiatric toxicity reactions and are a high-risk treatment group.

Table 3 lists preparations currently employed in the therapy of hypersomnia. Dosages listed are offered only as a guideline to initial therapy; ultimate require-

TABLE 3. *Medications employed in the treatment of hypersomnia*

Medication	Usual initial dosage (mg)	Available dosage (mg)
Short-acting		
Dextroamphetamine	5	5, 10
Methylphenidate	10	5, 10, 20
Methamphetamine	2.5	2.5, 5
Long-acting		
Phenmetrazine	25	25, 50, and 75 slow release
Pemoline	37.5	18.75, 37.5, 75
Dextroamphetamine	5 slow release	5, 10, 15 slow release
Methamphetamine	5 slow release	5, 10, 15 slow release

ments must be clinically determined. It is unnecessary to employ more than one agent concomitantly. In situations in which psychiatric toxicity emerges, experimental studies suggest crossover between all agents; substitution of an alternative medication is not a solution to the problem (20).

ADJUNCTIVE THERAPY IN HYPERSOMNIA

Narcolepsy

While central stimulants are effective in reducing sleep attacks in narcolepsy, cataplexy, hypnagogic hallucinosis, and sleep paralysis are poorly responsive (25). In patients with these associated symptoms, data suggest that the administration of a tricyclic antidepressant is of value. Imipramine is the best studied agent of this group and is reported to reduce the frequency of all associated symptoms of narcolepsy, with the exception of amnestic episodes (for which no data are available) (12,15,25). Response is obtained with doses as low as 25 mg/day, although 75 mg/day or more may be required. We have found amitryptiline (25 mg) equally effective.

In practice, it is beneficial to begin therapy with stimulants and add a tricyclic agent after a 3- to 4-week period. When both agents are started simultaneously, palpitations are more common, and adverse reactions are difficult to interpret. Dosage of tricyclic agents should be adjusted slowly and therapeutic responses monitored for at least 1 month before a need for increased dosage is established.

Sleep Apnea

Somnolence in the context of sleep apnea is usually manageable with intermittent administration of central stimulants in sleep-provoking settings. Obviously, it would be more parsimonious to treat the underlying respiratory abnormality; considerable interest has focused on this issue. Unfortunately, no currently available form of pharmacotherapy has been found effective in all patients with sleep apnea, and contradictory results with all agents have appeared. In some cases, tricyclic anti-depressants, xanthines, medroxyprogesterone, or progesterone have reduced the frequency and severity of sleep apneic episodes (1,17,18,26,27). Central stimulants are not efficacious in reducing apneic episodes; other respiratory stimulants are not useful (9).

At present, tracheostomy is the only available form of therapy for obstructive sleep apnea, although weight reduction and treatment of underlying pulmonary disorders are often beneficial (6,9,15). In patients lacking clear indications for surgery—which are still rather vague but include life-threatening arrhythmias, in-capacitating somnolence, or pulmonary hypertension—pharmacologic therapy may be indicated. Therapeutic response can be accurately determined only by repeat polysomnography with respiratory monitoring; subjective improvement in somno-lence is frequently unassociated with any detectable improvement in the frequency or severity of apnea. Current studies evaluating the efficacy of tongue-restraining devices in the therapy of sleep apnea are promising and may soon offer a reasonable alternative to surgery.

MISCELLANEOUS SLEEP DISORDERS

Pavor Nocturnus-Nocturnal Terrors

Most commonly encountered in the pediatric age group, nocturnal terrors are characterized by the episodic occurrence of terrifying nightmares shortly after sleep onset, followed by a period of confusion or incomplete arousal. During the period of confusion, affected individuals are frightened and are not immediately able to distinguish reality from the dream-related event. If the subject returns to sleep, there is frequently amnesia for the event the following morning (3,13,15). Subjec-tively, the nightmare lacks the plot development characteristic of normal dreaming and is described as an isolated, threatening situation (i.e., drowning, being trapped in a burning room). Polysomnographic studies have demonstrated that these episodes occur in the deeper stages of slow wave sleep rather than in REM sleep and differentiate the episodes from the usual nightmare (3,15).

In children, the episodes usually disappear with advancing age and, if infrequent, usually do not require treatment. In the adult, similar episodes may occur in patients with hypothalamic lesions but are frequently encountered in patients with a diagnosis of schizophrenia. Patients receiving chronic levodopa therapy may develop noc-turnal terrors after 3 or more years of therapy but usually do so in the presence of major sleep architectural changes (21). Insufficient data have been gathered to justify the conclusion that all these disorders are identical phenomena or are treatable in the same manner.

Low doses of diazepam are reported to abolish the episodes in children, presum-ably by suppressing deeper stages of slow wave sleep (15). A dosage of 2 mg h.s. is frequently adequate. In the adult, appropriate therapy has not yet been defined, although in our own experience, diazepam (5 to 10 mg) at bedtime is sometimes beneficial. Overall, failure on this regimen is associated with a failure to respond at higher dosages or when an alternative stage 3 to 4 suppressant benzodiazepine is substituted. Until more conclusive data become available, it is worth attempting therapy with a variety of benzodiazepines, if the initial response to diazepam is unsatisfactory.

In parkinsonian patients on levodopa in whom nocturnal terrors develop, initial therapy involves administration of medications earlier in the evening (no later than 6 p.m.). This often abolishes the complaint for a number of months, although the symptom tends to recur even when total daily dosage remains stable. In these patients, diazepam is not effective in relieving the episodes and often prolongs the confusional episodes that follow the nocturnal terror. Favorable responses have been obtained following the administration of cyproheptadine (4 to 12 mg h.s.) or methysergide (2 to 6 mg/day) (21). Why serotonin-blocking agents are effective in this disorder remains unclear. Nocturnal terrors in parkinsonian patients are almost always accompanied by nocturnal myoclonic activity. In this respect, the syndrome is unlike the nocturnal terrors seen in children and adults not receiving dopaminergic agents.

Somnambulism

Sleepwalking is not an infrequent phenomenon in the pediatric age group and is often seen in patients who also have nocturnal terrors (3,14,15). It rarely occurs in adults and is sometimes seen in parkinsonian patients on chronic levodopa therapy (21). In those patients who have been studied, the episodes appear to arise out of stage 3 to 4 of slow wave sleep, which may explain the observed association with nocturnal terrors. Differentiation from nocturnal psychomotor epilepsy is sometimes difficult. Therapy is identical to that outlined for nocturnal terrors.

Nocturnal Enuresis

Bedwetting is included in this discussion only because it is thought by many to represent a poorly defined abnormality of sleep (7). The precise pathophysiology of the disorder remains obscure; psychiatric, urologic, and peripheral autonomic etiologies have been suggested. Primary urologic abnormalities should be excluded before assuming that the disorder originates from more obscure causes.

Sleep studies have demonstrated that nocturnal enuresis follows a transition from stages 3 to 4 of slow wave sleep to stages 1 to 2, often in association with a generalized body movement. The physiologic connection between these sleep events and the enuretic episode is unclear. The earlier belief that enuresis occurs during dreaming (REM sleep) has been invalidated.

Most children eventually "outgrow" nocturnal enuresis; in some cases, reassurance (primarily of parents) is a sufficient therapy. Imipramine (25 to 50 mg h.s.) has been reported to be effective in controlling enuretic episodes (11,23), although its mode of action is controversial. Response is usually seen in the first few days of therapy, and the anticholinergic properties of the drug acting on the detrussor and vesicular outlet of the bladder may be more important than any centrally mediated effects. Central stimulants have been advocated in some studies, although most studies have found this form of therapy ineffective. In those patients with frequent nocturnal enuretic episodes in whom the level of psychologic concern is high, a trial of imipramine is usually warranted. In view of the natural course of the disorder, medications should be intermittently withdrawn and the need for continued drug administration reevaluated. In patients in whom drug therapy is ineffective, behavioral conditioning techniques offer an alternative therapeutic possibility (28).

REFERENCES

1. Aranda, J., Cook, C., Gorman, W., Collinge, J., Loughnan, P., Outerbridge, E., Aldredge, A., and Neims, A. (1979): Pharmacokinetic profile of caffeine in the premature newborn infant with apnea. *J. Pediatr.*, 94(4):663–668.
2. Block, A., Boysen, P., Wynne, J., and Hunt, L. (1979): Sleep apnea, hypoapnea and oxygen desaturation in normal subjects. *N. Engl. J. Med.*, 300(10):513–517.
3. Broughton, R. J. (1968): Sleep disorders: Disorders of arousal? *Science*, 159:1070–1078.
4. Critchley, M. (1962): Periodic hypersomnia and megaphagia in adolescent males. *Brain*, 85:627–656.
5. Drucker-Colin, R. R. (1976): Is there a sleep transmitter? *Prog. Neurobiol.*, 6:1–22.
6. Fisher, J. G., de la Pena, A., and Donovan, N. W. (1976): Initial treatment of mixed deep apnea syndrome in an obese patient by starvation. *Sleep Res.*, 5:168.
7. Gastuat, H., and Broughton, R. A. (1965): A clinical polygraphic study of episodic phenomena during sleep. In: *Recent Advances in Biological Psychiatry, Vol. 7*, edited by J. Wortis, pp. 197–221. Plenum Press, New York.
8. Greenberg, R., and Pearlman, C. (1967): Delirium tremens and dreaming. *Am. J. Psychiatry*, 124:133–142.
9. Guilleminault, C., Tilkian, A., and Dement, W. C. (1967): The sleep apnea syndromes. *Annu. Rev. Med.*, 27:465–484.
10. Hartmann, E., Cravens, J., and List, S. (1974): Hypnotic effects of L-tryptophan. *Arch. Gen. Psychiatry*, 31:394–397.
11. Hicks, W. R., and Barnes, E. H. (1964): A double-blind study of the effect of imipramine on enuresis in 100 naval recruits. *Am. J. Psychiatry*, 120:812–814.
12. Hishikawa, Y., Ida, H., Nakai, K., and Kaneko, Z. (1966): Treatment of narcolepsy with imipramine (Trofranil) and desmethylimipramine (Pertofran). *J. Neurol. Sci.*, 3:453–461.
13. Kahn, E., Fisher, C., Edwards, A., and Davis, D. (1973): Mental content of stage 4 night terrors. *Proc. Am. Psychiatr. Assoc.*, p. 499.
14. Kales, A., Jacobson, A., Paulson, M. J., Kalfs, J. D., and Walter, R. D. (1966): Somnambulism: Psychophysiological correlates. *Arch. Gen. Psychiatry*, 14:586–594.
15. Kales, A., and Kales, J. (1974): Sleep disorders. *N. Engl. J. Med.*, 290(9):487–497.
16. Kay, D., Blackburn, A., Buckingham, J., and Karacan, I. (1976): Human pharmacology of sleep. In: *Pharmacology of Sleep*, edited by R. Williams and I. Karacan, pp. 83–210. Wiley, New York.
17. Kryger, M., McCullough, R. E., Collins, D., Scoggin, C., Weil, J., and Grover, R. (1978): Treatment of excessive polycythemia of high altitude with respiratory stimulant drugs. *Am. Rev. Respir. Dis.*, 117:455–464.
18. Lyons, H. A., and Huang, C. T. (1968): Therapeutic use of progesterone in alveolar hypoventilation associated with obesity. *Am. J. Med.*, 44:881–888.
19. Monroe, L. (1967): Psychological and physiological differences between good and poor sleepers. *Abnorm. Psychol.*, 72:255.
20. Nausieda, P. A. (1979): Central stimulant toxicity. In: *Handbook of Clinical Neurology, Vol. 37*, edited by P. J. Vinken and G. W. Bruyn, pp. 223–297. North Holland, Amsterdam.
21. Nausieda, P. A., Kaplan, L. R., Weber, S., Klawans, H. L., and Weiner, W. J. (1979): Sleep disruption and psychosis induced by chronic levodopa therapy. Presented at the 31st Annual Meeting of the American Academy of Neurology, Chicago.

22. de la Pena, A. (1978): Toward a psychophysiologic conceptualization of insomnia. In: *Sleep Disorders: Diagnosis and Treatment*, edited by R. L. Williams and I. Karacan, pp. 101–143. Wiley, New York.
23. Poussaint, A. F., and Ditman, K. S. (1965): A controlled study of imipramine (Trofranil) in the treatment of childhood enuresis. *J. Pedatr.*, 67:283–290.
24. Rechtschaffen, A., Wolpert, E. A., Dement, W. C., Mitchel, S. A., and Fisher, C. (1963): Nocturnal sleep of narcoleptics. *Electroencephalogr. Clin. Neurophysiol.*, 15:599–609.
25. Roth, B. (1978): Narcolepsy and hypersomnia. In: *Sleep Disorders: Diagnosis and Treatment*, edited by R. L. Williams and I. Karacan, pp. 29–59. Wiley, New York.
26. Schmidt, H., and Clark, R. W. (1977): Hypersomnia, narcolepsy-cataplexy syndrome, and sleep apnea: Treatment with protriptyline and pemoline. *Sleep Res.*, 6:179.
27. Shkurovich, Z. M. (1976): The effects of theophylline on the sleep apnea syndrome. *Sleep Res.*, 5:188.
28. Wickes, I. G. (1958): Treatment of persistent enuresis with the electric buzzer. *Arch. Dis. Child.*, 33:160–164.
29. Wyatt, R. J., and Gillin, J. C. (1976): Biochemistry and human sleep. In: *Pharmacology of Sleep*, edited by R. L. Williams and I. Karacan, pp. 239–274. Wiley, New York.

Chapter 26

Toxicity of Central Stimulants

Central stimulants are used therapeutically in several neurologic disorders, especially narcolepsy and minimal brain dysfunction in children, and are also widely self administered. The acute and chronic administration of these agents results in a variety of toxic effects.

ACUTE TOXICITY

Acute nonlethal poisoning with central stimulants is the most commonly recognized manifestation of stimulant toxicity. In general, the clinical picture is dominated by the peripheral sympathomimetic effects of these agents, although various centrally mediated phenomena, including involuntary movements and thought disorders, can occur. Most reports on acute toxicity are limited to amphetamine. The manifestations of intoxication with methylphenidate, phenmetrazine, methamphetamine, and cocaine are essentially identical, with the exception of the more rapid onset of action of cocaine and its local anesthetic, central depressive, and convulsive effects (3).

The dose-response relationships of these agents relative to toxic symptoms vary tremendously (9,11). Marked acute reactions have occurred at dosages of dextroamphetamine as low as 5 mg; other individuals have consumed up to 630 mg of the drug with minimal symptoms of central or sympathetic stimulation. Similar variation in sensitivity occurs with cocaine.

Various authors have divided the clinical picture of sublethal toxicity into categories based on the severity of symptoms encountered (6,12,15) (Table 1). These classifications are relatively arbitrary but have been suggested as guidelines for planning therapy. The definition of toxicity itself is vague in that many of the symptoms classified as mild symptoms of overdosage are utilized as therapeutic effects in various situations. For instance, anorexia may be viewed as a mild toxic effect in situations where increased alertness is the primary objective, while insomnia and anxiety may be undesirable when an anorexic effect is sought.

A review of published cases shows differences in the pattern of toxicity in adults and children, with psychosis being more prominent in adult patients (12).

The higher incidence of psychosis in adults may reflect an age-dependent difference in drug effect or an underlying predisposition to purely psychotic symptoms. While the cases in children reflect accidental overdosage, many of the adult cases

TABLE 1. *Stages of acute intoxication*

Mild	Moderate	Life-threatening
Anorexia	Sweating	Hyperthermia
Motor excitation	Mydriasis	Convulsions
Logorrhea	Hypertension	Circulatory collapse
Insomnia	Premature ventricular contractions	Ventricular fibrillation
Tachycardia	Vomiting	Coma
Tachypnea	Peripheral vasodilatation	Anuria
Anxiety	Panic	Myoglobinuria
	Euphoria	
	Confusion	
	Hallucinations	

of overdosage represent deliberate overdosages, which may reflect underlying psychopathology. Central stimulants have been demonstrated to exacerbate thought disorders in known schizophrenics and may be capable of inducing such thought disorders in otherwise compensated individuals (10).

Certain situations modify the acute toxic properties of central stimulants. Monoamine oxidase (MAO) inhibitors have been reported to potentiate the effects of central stimulants; their concomitant administration may lead to toxic symptoms at otherwise therapeutic dosages. Although the MAO inhibitors are primarily utilized as antidepressants, isoniazide, used in the therapy of tuberculosis, is also active as an inhibitor of MAO and may lead to toxic overdosage when used in conjunction with central stimulants. The potentiation of central stimulant activity by MAO inhibitors is probably related to decreased inactivation of norepinephrine and dopamine. Since the central stimulants act through indirect release and impaired reuptake inactivation of catecholamines centrally and peripherally, impaired enzymatic inactivation further potentiates their pharmacologic activity.

Concomitant administration of thyroid hormone may also potentiate the activity of central stimulants and predispose to acute toxic reactions (2). This potentiation may be primarily peripheral and mimic thyrotoxic crisis or may be manifest in potentiation of central pharmacologic effects.

Toxicity of central stimulant drugs may also be influenced by underlying structural lesions of the CNS. These reactions primarily take the form of hyperkinetic involuntary movement disorders and appear to be related to preexisting pathologic alterations within the basal ganglia and striatum in patients with a history of Sydenham's chorea, chorea due to lupus erythematosis, or other prior cerebral insults (13).

The induction of chorea in response to an acute dosage of a central stimulant is dependent on an underlying structural abnormality of the basal ganglia, which renders the neurons of this area unusually sensitive to exogenous induced dopaminergic stimulation. A similar mechanism to that discussed above may underly the rarely reported appearance of tics or hallucinosis in the acute treatment of childhood hyperkinesis with central stimulants.

Two major subgroups of a stimulant-induced psychosis have been recognized: a relatively pure psychotic thought disorder in the presence of an otherwise alert individual, and toxic hallucinosis in association with drug-induced delirium. The incidence of this phenomenon is difficult to assess but is reported to be very low. In an experimental administration of 10 mg dextroamphetamine to 1,000 volunteers, only one individual suffered a notable psychotic reaction (4). The interpretation of these acute central stimulant-induced thought disorders in some individuals remains unclear. The observation that central stimulants may worsen individually determined symptoms in schizophrenic patients has led to the speculation that latent schizophreniform thought disorders may be precipitated by acute administration of central stimulants (1,10).

TREATMENT

The major methods of treatment rely on removal of the offending agent, blockade of its effects, and general medical support. Elimination of the offending agent may be facilitated by gastric lavage when orally administered stimulants are involved. Usually, however, one must rely on renal excretion as a means of drug elimination. Acidification of the urine markedly enhances the excretion of amphetamine and is recommended in acute overdosage. Cocaine likewise is more rapidly excreted, but to a lesser degree, when urinary pH is acidic. Acidic amphetamine analogs, such as pemoline, would not have their excretion promoted by urinary acidification. Acidification of the urine would also be avoided when rhabdomyolosis is encountered in acute stimulant poisoning, as it may precipitate acute renal failure in such a setting. As an extreme measure, amphetamine may be rapidly cleared from the body through hemodialysis, although with the development of effective pharmacologic treatment, this extreme measure is rarely required (8). Pharmacologic blockade is the most effective treatment of acute stimulant toxicity. Therapeutic measures may be directed at the central or peripheral effects of the central stimulants, as indicated by the clinical setting. Haloperidol or phenothiazines are clinically effective in the treatment of centrally mediated stimulant toxicity (15). In patients presenting with acute psychosis or choreatic movements, these agents are the accepted treatments of choice, regardless of the central stimulant involved in the intoxication.

In cases of acute intoxication in the unaccustomed user, peripheral sympathetic effects may be more dangerous than the associated central manifestations of toxicity. In cases where hypertension and cardiac arrhythmias are encountered, prompt treatment with propranolol, an adrenergic beta-blocker, has been advocated and reported to be effective clinically in cocaine poisoning. Although this treatment rapidly reverses the peripheral sympathomimetic effects of cocaine, it is not reported to reverse centrally mediated effects of this agent. The same observations are probably equally valid for amphetamine. Cases of central stimulant poisoning in which both central and peripheral toxicity are major problems would require both neuroleptic treatment and beta-adrenergic blockade for full reversal.

The above recommendations are valid for mild to moderate toxic reactions. Severe toxicity reactions require additional comment, especially in regard to differential therapy in cocaine poisoning. Since cocaine possesses mixed depressant and excitatory effects, the clinician may be faced with a perplexing picture of convulsions, cardiac arrhythmias, and concomitant respiratory paralysis. Clinical data on the acute treatment of cocaine-induced seizures are not available. Should they be encountered, the use of diazepam or phenobarbital may have additive depressant effects on respiration. The possibility of respiratory arrest should be anticipated in such a setting. Life-threatening cardiac arrhythmias should be initially treated with propranolol, especially when cocaine is suspected as the causative agent. Lidocaine is often used intravenously for the treatment of ectopic ventricular arrhythmias and ventricular tachycardia. Like cocaine, lidocaine is also capable of inducing convulsions in man, suggesting an additional shared central effect. Sufficient data exist to make lidocaine relatively contraindicated in the acute treatment of central stimulant-induced cardiac arrhythmias. If lidocaine treatment is undertaken, dosages should be considerably reduced to avoid possible additive central dysphoric and/or convulsive effects.

FATAL TOXIC REACTIONS

Human data concerning the lethal effects of central stimulants are limited almost entirely to amphetamine. Review of the literature between 1939 and 1972 has disclosed 43 case reports of death subsequent to or associated with amphetamines (11). Examination of the individual case reports shows that death is related to either the direct pharmacologic effects of the drug or secondary complications associated with intravenous administration. Deaths directly attributable to a pharmacologic response to amphetamine were related to (a) hypertensive entracerebral hemorrhage, (b) ventricular fibrillation, (c) left ventricular failure, or (d) hyperpyrexia. In many others, the causes were unclear or difficult to relate to amphetamine use or abuse. Of all deaths clearly related to amphetamine, approximately 50% were the result of a single overdose in individuals not chronically exposed to the drug. In three of these cases, concomitant use of MAO inhibitors probably contributed significantly to the fatal response to amphetamine. This observation is in agreement with the conclusion of Ellinwood (8), who noted that acute fatal drug reactions to amphetamines were far more common in the occasional user but rare in the chronic high dose abuser.

Data on human fatal intoxication from cocaine are limited but differ slightly in some respects from amphetamine. Convulsions are noted far more frequently in association with acute poisoning from cocaine than amphetamine (9). Unlike amphetamine, cocaine is capable of inducing a potentially fatal toxic reaction in those habituated to its use as well as in persons unaccustomed to the drug. Death in cocaine poisoning may reflect direct depression of the medullary respiratory center, which may be heralded by Cheyne-Stokes or ataxic respiratory patterns. As in the case of amphetamine, cerebral hemorrhage, hyperthermia, and acute hypertensive crisis have been reported. The toxic effect of cocaine on the cardiovascular system is similar to that of amphetamine in that hypertension, tachycardia, and ventricular instability are encountered.

CHRONIC TOXICITY

The chronic use of centrally active stimulants has been related to a variety of toxic effects, including (a) thought disorders, (b) movement disorders, (c) possible effects on growth, and (d) possible vasculitis.

THOUGHT DISORDERS

Numerous reports document the occurrence of paranoid psychosis following chronic ingestion of cocaine, methylphenidate, dextroamphetamine, and methamphetamine (14). The psychosis described in most of the published cases is remarkably similar, whether cocaine, diethylproprion, methylphenidate, methamphetamine, or dextroamphetamine was the causative agent. Although an early report claimed a marked similarity between the psychic effects of mescaline and amphetamine, it is now widely accepted that the psychosis induced by cocaine and the amphetamines is virtually indistinguishable and is dissimilar to the effects of the hallucinogens.

Two distinct clinical thought disorders may be encountered. Amphetamine psychosis or central stimulant psychosis should be reserved for nonconfusional paranoid psychoses and is not applicable to those clinical pictures dominated by delirium and confusion, which occur most frequently following acute administration of large dosages of these agents (6,12). The latter syndrome is better described as an acute toxic delirium secondary to central stimulants. This distinction is important, in that different central mechanisms may underlie the two clinical states.

Amphetamine and cocaine psychosis occur most frequently in abusers chronically administering large quantities of these agents (19). The picture is virtually identical to paranoid schizophrenia; without a drug history, differentiation of these entities is impossible (7). While paranoid ideation and hallucinosis are the major features of this syndrome, repetitive meaningless behavioral stereotypes and involuntary movement disorders are integral parts of the overall clinical syndrome (14). Both the psychosis and the abnormal movements are due to increased response of dopamine receptors following chronic stimulation. Drug withdrawal and neuroleptic therapy are the major forms of treatment.

MOVEMENT DISORDERS

Choreatic movement disorders, most often appearing in the form of lingual-facial-buccal dyskinesias, have been reported as additional toxic reactions following the chronic administration of amphetamine in man (16). Similar movements have been reported with methylphenidate and pemoline; they disappear with withdrawal of the offending agents. Like analogous levodopa-induced dyskinesias, these movements are related to chronic agonist-induced hypersensitivity.

POSSIBLE EFFECTS ON GROWTH

There has been some concern that central stimulants may suppress growth rates in children. When placed on central stimulants, children may grow at 60 to 75% of their estimated growth rates; when the drugs are stopped, there is an apparent growth rebound. Safer and Allen (18), in evaluating these growth patterns, found that children on stimulants eventually reach their expected height, although the rate is usually less than in nonmedicated children. It is important to discuss the issue with parents, especially in a family that is genetically short. In such cases, a final height that is even 1 inch less than expected may cause strain on a child's psychosocial development.

VASCULITIS

Systemic vasculitis has been reported following chronic intravenous and oral abuse of amphetamine (5). A similar vasculitic process restricted to the cerebral circulation has been observed in young, central stimulant drug abusers suffering from acute stroke syndromes (17). An additional group of cases in which intracerebral hemorrhage or intracerebral hematoma has occurred in the course of central stimulant abuse may also reflect an underlying vasculitic process rather than a response to acute drug-induced hypertension.

The role of central stimulants in vasculitic disorders is unclear. Some authors have suggested that concomitant infection with hepatitis-B in drug abusers may explain some of the cases of vasculitis.

REFERENCES AND *SELECTED REVIEWS

1. Angrist, B., and Gershon, S. (1970): The phenomenology of experimentally induced amphetamine psychosis. Preliminary observations. *Biol. Psychiatry*, 2:95.
2. Atkinson, J. B. (1954): Factitial thyrotoxic crisis induced by dextro-amphetamine sulfate and thyroid. *Ann. Intern. Med.*, 40:615–618.
3. Bejerot, N. (1970): A comparison of the effects of cocaine and synthetic central stimulants. *Br. J. Addict.*, 65:35–37.
4. Bett, W. R., Howells, L. H., and MacDonald, A. D. (1955): *Amphetamine in Clinical Medicine. Actions and Uses.* Livingstone, London.
5. Citron, B. P., Halpern, M., McCarron, M., Lundberg, G. D., McCormick, R., Pincus, I. J., Tatter, D., and Haverback, B. J. (1970): Necrotizing angiitis associated with drug abuse. *N. Engl. J. Med.*, 282:1003–1011.
6. Connell, P. H. (1958): *Amphetamine Psychosis.* Chapman and Hall, London.
*7. Ellinwood, E. H. (1968): Amphetamine psychosis. *Int. J. Neuropsychiatry*, 4:45–54.
8. Ellinwood, E. H. (1972): Emergency treatment of acute reactions to CNS stimulants. *J. Psychedelic Drugs*, 5:147–151.
9. Gay, G., Inaba, D., Sheppard, C., Newmeyer, J., and Rappott, R. (1975): Cocaine: History, epidemiology, human pharmacology and treatment. *Clin. Toxicol.*, 8:149–178.
10. Janowsky, D., and Davis, J. (1976): Methylphenidate, dextroamphetamine, and levamphetamine: Effects on schizophrenic symptoms. *Arch. Gen. Psychiatry*, 33:304–308.

11. Kalant, H., and Kalant, O. J. (1975): Death in amphetamine users; causes and rates. *Can. Med. Assoc.*, 112:299–304.
12. Kalant, O. J. (1966): *The Amphetamines: Toxicity and Addiction*. Charles C Thomas, Springfield, Illinois.
13. Klawans, H. L., and Weiner, W. J. (1974): The effect of amphetamine on choreiform movement disorders. *Neurology (Minneap.)*, 24:312–318.
*14. Nausieda, P. A. (1979): Central stimulant toxicity. In: *Handbook of Clinical Neurology, Vol. 37*, edited by P. J. Vinken and G. W. Bruyn, pp. 223–297, North Holland, Amsterdam.
15. Ong, B. H. (1962): Dextroamphetamine poisoning. *N. Engl. J. Med.*, 266:1321–1322.
16. Randrup, A., and Munkvad, I. (1967): Stereotyped activities produced by amphetamine in several animal species and man. *Psychopharmacologia*, 11:300–310.
17. Rumbaugh, C. L., Bergeron, R. T., and Fang, H. C. H. (1971): Cerebral angiographic changes in the drug abuse patient. *Radiology*, 101:335–344.
18. Safer, D. J., and Allen, R. P. (1972): Factors influencing the suppressive effects of two stimulant drugs on growth in hyperactive children. *Pediatrics*, 51:660–666.
19. Snyder, S. H. (1972): Catecholamines in the brain as mediators of amphetamine psychosis. *Arch. Gen. Psychiatry*, 27:169–179.

Chapter 27

Migraine

Migraine headache is a common disorder, estimated to affect 15 to 19% of men and 25 to 29% of women at some time in their lives (55). A world estimate of the frequency of migraine headaches has been listed "conservatively" at 6% (about 180,000,000) of the population. The clinical definition is often less clear, and this may account for the high frequency with which migraine headaches are reported. Neither the etiology nor the biochemical pathology of migraine is known, and discussion of the multiple pharmacologic therapies employed in this disorder is often confusing and difficult to interpret. In addition, a wide range of pharmacologic agents have been reported to be successful in the treatment of migraine, although many of the agents have little in common pharmacologically. This chapter briefly reviews the clinical characteristics of migraine headache and its hypothesized pathophysiologic basis. The demonstrated biochemical alteration in patients with migraine is examined, and an attempt to correlate these changes with the pathophysiology is made. Finally, the pharmacologic agents reported to be useful in migraine are reviewed, with special emphasis on the presumed pharmacologic mechanism of these agents in relationship to ameliorating headache.

Since migraine is not associated with any tissue or biochemical abnormality, it is the clinical characteristics of the syndrome that define it. The Ad Hoc Committee on the Classification of Headache (11) delineated the following major vascular headache syndromes: classic migraine, common migraine, cluster headache, hemiplegic, and ophthalmoplegic migraine (Table 1). The migraine headaches that produce the least diagnostic confusion are the complicated and classic migraine. In classic migraine, there is usually a biphasic course. The initial phase is a prodromal stage or "aura," during which transient focal neurologic deficits (e.g., hemianopsia, scintillating scotoma, hemisensory, and/or hemiparesis) occur. The second phase is the occurrence of the headache. This usually begins approximately at the time the aura is resolving. The headache can be unilateral or bilateral and is often described as having a pulsating quality. The headache may last for varying time periods (1 to 2 hr to 2 to 4 days) and may be accompanied by various other disturbances, including irritability, malaise, gastrointestinal disturbances (anorexia, nausea, vomiting, and diarrhea), and autonomic disturbances (altered heart rate, skin pallor, chills, and sweats). Hemiplegic and ophthalmoplegic migraines are examples of classic migraine named for the startling neurologic deficit produced. It is important to recognize that although the biphasic events usually occur in this

TABLE 1. *Major classification of head pain*[a]

Vascular headache of migraine type
  Classic
  Common
  Cluster
  Hemiplegic and ophthalmoplegic
  Lower-half headache
Muscle-contraction headache
Combined headache: vascular and muscle contraction
Headache of nasal vasomotor reaction
Headache of delusional, conversion, or hypochondriacal states
Nonmigrainous vascular headache
Traction headache
Headache due to overt cranial inflammation
Headache due to disease of ocular, aural, nasal, sinusal, dental,
  or other cranial or neck structures
Cranial neuritides
Cranial neuralgias

[a]Ad hoc committee report.

sequence, the focal neurologic deficit may occur after the onset of headache or even following the headache. In these instances, alternate diagnostic possibilities should be considered.

Common migraine is more difficult to diagnose than classic migraine because its diagnostic criteria are less sharply demarcated. There is no aura; the headache can be unilateral or bilateral; the pain can be pulsating, throbbing, or nonthrobbing, and its intensity may vary considerably. The associated autonomic and gastrointestinal disturbances discussed previously may also occur. Following both classic and common migraine, the patient may not feel entirely normal ("washed out," fatigued) for 24 to 48 hr.

Although it has been noted that classic migraine occurs less frequently than common migraine, the diagnosis of classic migraine is better delineated and, because of this, most physiologic and pharmacologic studies have focused on classic migraine. Common migraine deserves considerably more scientific attention (42). In fact, biochemical and pharmacologic approaches to migraine should be defined as to whether the patient population studied consisted of classic or common migraine patients. The two varieties of migraine may not be identical or even closely related. The only way to increase our understanding of common migraine is to study as pure samples as possible of patients with this disorder and not just to lump all patients with various forms of migraine together.

Since the initial demonstration by Graham and Wolff (24) that ergotamine reduced the pain of migraine, the pathophysiology of this syndrome has been related to alterations in vascular tone. The aura of classic migraine has been related to vasoconstriction, and the resolution of the aura and the onset of the headache has been related to a vasodilatory phase. In fact, recent investigation of cerebral blood flow has demonstrated that the prodromal phase of migraine is associated with decreased cerebral blood flow, and that the headache phase is associated with increased cerebral blood flow (18,34,47). Although it was originally postulated that it was the vasodilation of large arteries that produced pain, it is now recognized that more than pressure-induced dilation of extracranial arteries is required for pain. There has been a great deal of interest in the concept that "vasoactive" substances are released in the vicinity of the dilated arteries, and that these substances increase vascular permeability and produce a "sterile inflammatory response." It has been proposed that this combination of vasodilation and sterile inflammation is required for the production of the clinical syndrome of migraine (15). Although it is clear that alterations in cerebral blood flow occur during migraine, it is less certain if it is the large arterial structures that are constricting and dilating. There is some evidence that the small arterioles and capillaries are responsible for the biphasic cerebral blood flow changes associated with the clinical syndrome.

Recent biochemical investigations in migraine have focused on (a) several vasoactive substances, including histamine, serotonin, and prostaglandins, (b) the process of platelet aggregability, (c) the role of sex hormones, and (d) levels of activity of enzymes involved in catecholamine metabolism [monoamine oxidase (MAO)]. Interest in serotonin evolved from the initial report that administration during acute headache would ameliorate pain (3,27). Investigation of serotonin and its metabolites has revealed that there are characteristic changes in the concentrations of serotonin and serotonin metabolites during migraine. Plasma and platelet serotonin levels decrease at the onset and during the attack; the decrease averages about 40% for both free and platelet-bound serotonin (2,51). It has been demonstrated that the urinary concentration of 5-hydroxyindoleacetic acid (5-HIAA), the major catabolic product of serotonin, is increased during the headache attack (13,45). This particular finding has not received universal confirmation (14). Other reports suggest that 5-HIAA did not increase but that urinary serotonin excretion did (1).

No alterations in central serotonin metabolism have been documented during migraine (6,53). The alterations in serotonin peripheral metabolism appear to be specific for migraine, since these changes are not seen in either postpneumoencephalography headache or cluster headache. In the early biochemical migraine literature, reserpine-induced, migraine-like headaches were cited as evidence implicating serotin depletion in the precipitation of the syndrome. The pharmacologic activity of reserpine, however, is more widespread than a sole action on serotonin. It is unsound to relate reserpine-induced depletion of serotonin to migraine on this basis. In addition, although serotonin concentration drops during the initial 12 hr of a migraine attack, it usually normalizes within 24 hr; reserpine-induced depletion of serotonin lasts longer. Although it is clear that serotonin levels are altered in migraine, it is equally clear that precipitation of migraine headache cannot be decisively linked to reducing plasma serotonin to a certain critical level. The decrease in both platelet and plasma serotonin thus far recorded has a wide variability; a given level of serotonin is related to migraine in one patient, but lower levels of serotonin do not produce migraine in another. In fact, Somerville (51) demonstrated that although there was a 43% decrease in platelet serotonin during migraine, the individual patient levels ranged from a 16 to 77% reduction; in one case, platelet serotonin increased 41% during the attack periods. This indicates that altered blood serotonin level is not the primary etiologic factor in precipitating migraine.

The initial finding that serotonin administration relieved migraine provided the impetus for the metabolic studies of serotonin in this syndrome. It would be simple if one could take the clinical accounts of serotonin administration along with the depletion of serotonin in migraine and be confident that serotonin administration replenishes the documented diminished blood serotonin. However, Sjaastad (46) has raised a critical issue: Does the fact that intravenous serotonin relieves migraine necessarily indicate that lack of serotonin is the cause of migraine? A later study raised doubts that serotonin relieves migraine headache (51), and the physiologic role of platelet serotonin in relation to vascular tone is unsure. Lance et al. (29) have proposed that platelet serotonin influences the vasotonic state of the carotid arteries, and serotonin depletion results in dilation of these vessels. The evidence that serotonin plays a physiologic role in the regulation of arterial tone, however, is virtually nonexistent. An explanation for the role of serotonin in migraine is lacking. Is the falling serotonin concentration secondary to other phenomena, or is it part of some unknown cascade of events that produces the well-known physiologic alterations in vascular tone?

Other vasoactive substances that have received considerable interest are the prostaglandins. When injected into nonmigrainous patients, prostaglandin E-1 (PGE-1) produces migraine-like symptoms (8). It is a potent cerebral vessel dilator; in fact, specific PGE-1 vasodilation of the external carotid artery with subsequent reduction in cerebral blood flow in the intracranial distribution has been shown. This action of PGE-1 on blood flow has been used to explain the transient neurologic deficit seen in classic migraine. The pathophysiology of migraine has been stated to be a hereditary hypersensitivity of the external carotid artery to PGE-1 (56). One attractive aspect of this theory is that the release of prostaglandins may be initiated by serotonin, histamine, and tyramine.

Other agents have received attention in an attempt to understand the biochemical basis of migraine. Some unification of multiple theories may be forthcoming. However, no firm evidence establishes a direct link of PGE-1 to migraine attacks. In fact, no difference in blood concentration of PGE-1 has been observed before, during, or after migraine attacks (1). On the other hand, a trial of flufenamic acid in migraine was found to be successful in alleviating acute migraine headaches. Although flufenamic acid is an inhibitor of prostaglandin synthesis (54), there is no evidence that flufenamic acid affected prostaglandin synthesis in these patients. Since aspirin and indomethacin are also prostaglandin synthesis inhibitors, and since aspirin does not acutely relieve migraine, the flufenamic acid effect in migraine may not be related to prostaglandin synthesis inhibition.

Possible dietary triggering factors in migraine led to the postulate that susceptible patients might have a MAO deficiency. This postulate has been explored in successive studies by Sandler and colleagues (23,39–41). These investigations have documented a decrease in platelet MAO activity during the headache. This decrease in platelet MAO activity is significant in relationship to levels in nonmigrainous controls and to levels in the same patient in an attack-free period. It has also been demonstrated that during attack-free periods, migraine patients do not have significantly different MAO levels than nonmigraine patients. This indicates that whatever the significance of the decreased MAO level during the attack, it is not reasonable to raise the question of a primary genetic variation in platelet MAO levels to explain the difference between patients with migraine and those without. Of course, the significance of this finding remains unanswered.

It has been suggested that a decrease in MAO activity is not a precipitating factor in migraine but a secondary event. Since platelet serotonin also falls during the attack, it has been proposed that some nonspecific platelet-damaging agent transiently appears in the circulation and produces the platelet alterations measured. The source of these compounds might be the lungs. Some of the compounds postulated to be involved include prostaglandins and thromboxanes. This is a novel and unproved idea that would make migraine a pulmonary disease (38). Evidence of a serotonin-releasing factor in the plasma of migraine patients has recently been presented (31). Platelets from migrainous patients in an attack-free period were incubated with plasma from other migraine patients during an attack; a 22% drop in serotonin occurred. When these platelets were incubated with plasma from migrainous patients in an attack-free period, no change in platelet serotonin occurred. When platelets from nonmigrainous patients were incubated with the plasma of migrainous patients during an attack, there was no change in serotonin concentration. This supports the hypothesis that a serotonin-releasing factor appears in the plasma during a migraine attack: These results also suggest an abnormality in the platelets of migraine patients; when the platelets of migraine-free patients were incubated in the presence of the presumed "releasing factor," there was no effect.

The role of female sex hormones in migraine attacks has also been explored. Migraine is more frequent in women than in men. Whatever the possible role of sex hormones in migraine, it must be a secondary one, since significant numbers of males do suffer from migraine. The striking association between migraine and the menstrual cycle in some women has led to an examination of the relative roles of progesterone and estrogen in the precipitation of migraine. A large percentage of women with migraine develop the attacks in relation to the premenstrual period or to the menstrual period itself. Initially, it was postulated that migraine occurrence during these times might be related to estrogen-induced water retention; but there is no evidence that water retention plays a role in the production of migraine headaches. In addition, not all women with migraine experience migraine in relation to menstruation; second, not all women who have premenstrual or menstrual migraine experience an attack each month. Although initial measurements of sex hormones implicated progesterone withdrawal in precipitation of the headache, later investigation has implicated estrogen withdrawal as a precipitating factor (48).

Attempts to alter estrogen withdrawal in menstruating women include oral administration of estrogen in the premenstrual period and the use of estradiol implants. These have not had notable practical or theoretical success (49,50), since uterine bleeding difficulties developed, and headache relief was uncertain. The use of oral contraceptives has also been noted to affect the frequency of migraine attacks in some women. The literature suggests that migraines can be precipitated by the use of these agents in nonmigrainous women. In addition, women with migraine may experience exacerbation of both frequency and intensity of headaches. Since the use of oral contraceptives is associated with an increased risk of cerebrovascular accidents, any warning that may have predictive value in patients at risk should be carefully considered. There is evidence that changes in headache frequency, duration, and severity are factors in the months prior to cerebral infarction in women receiving oral contraceptives. In addition, a change in the character of the migraine (common to classic) was also considered to be a premonitory sign (20,21). Patients with these symptoms and signs should not receive oral contraceptives.

A single case of a 27-year-old woman illustrates some of the relationships discussed above. This woman had common migraine headache precipitated by the use of oral contraceptives. After a period of time, these attacks changed into classic migraine episodes. During the time that classic migraine was present, there was evidence of increased platelet aggregability. Oral contraceptives were discontinued, and the patient was treated with antiplatelet aggregability agents. This treatment eventually resulted in cessation of migraine episodes and normalization of platelet response (30). Continuation of oral contraceptives in this case might have had catastrophic consequences. In a small percentage of women, migraine headaches are improved by birth control pills (9,37). Although there are striking case reports of menstrual-related migraine attacks, pharmacologic administration of estrogen has not had therapeutic success. Alterations of estrogen and progesterone in this syndrome will not supply an etiologic answer.

The male sex hormone testosterone has also been examined in migraine patients. The testosterone level in 30 male patients with migraine was compared to the level in 30 males with cluster headache. No difference in level was noted. Four female patients with cluster headache had elevated testosterone levels. This suggestion that testosterone might play a role in cluster headache was discussed (33).

Platelet physiology and function have also been examined in migraine. Although the usually transient focal neurologic deficits that precede classic migraine have been related to decreased cerebral blood flow and vasoconstriction, it is also possible that altered platelet physiology may play a role. This is particularly relevant since migraine occasionally may be associated with cerebral infarction (7,17,32). The role of platelets in transient ischemic attacks and stroke is examined in Chapter 28 on cerebrovascular disease. There are repeated reports that platelet aggregation and adhesiveness are altered in migraine patients (12,16,26). Platelet aggregability appears to be chronically increased in migraine compared to nonmigraine patients, although there is no correlation between severity of prodrome or headache phase and degree of hyperaggregability in migraine patients. In addition, platelet adhesiveness increases in both the prodrome and the headache phase, while aggregation increases during the prodrome and decreases during the headache phase. Since almost all plasma serotonin is directly related to platelet serotonin and since platelets release serotonin when they aggregate, this alteration in aggregation reponse may explain the previously discussed alteration in plasma serotonin concentration seen in migraine. Although the mechanism responsible for altered platelet function is not known, pharmacologic agents that alter platelet functions (aspirin, sulfurpyrizone) may play a role in the chronic treatment of migraine.

Harrington (25) has proposed that migraine is the clinical manifestation of a platelet disorder. This proposal, based on the following general lines of evidence, would make migraine the most common blood disorder: (a) Platelet behavior is genetically influenced, and migraine has definite genetic influences. (b) Platelet aggregation is altered in migraine, and some factors that can precipitate migraine can also alter platelet aggregation (stress). (c) The alterations in plasma serotonin that occur during migraine are related to alterations in platelet serotonin. (d) Alterations in platelet MAO activity occur during migraine episodes. (e) When platelets are activated, beta-thromboglobulin is released; there is a significant rise in this globulin during migraine attacks (22).

The role of histamine in the production of migraine has had cyclic popularity. In 1930, it was shown that intravenous histamine administration to patients without migraine could produce generalized throbbing headache and facial flushing. In ensuing work, it was repeatedly pointed out that there were numerous differences between migraine headache and histamine-induced headache, including the distribution of dilated arterial trees and their pharmacologic responses. Histamine headache is blocked by the prior administration of antihistamine, whereas antihistamines are of no value in the treatment of migraine. On the other hand, ergotamine relieves migraine, but it does not ameliorate histamine-induced headache.

The role of histamine in migraine has been related to its release from mast cells (44). Recently, the association of vascular headaches with Crohn's disease has again raised the question of mast cell release of histamine (5). The demonstration that there are two different populations of histamine receptors has renewed interest in the possible role of histamine in migraine. The H_1 and H_2 receptors have different pharmacologic properties and different anatomic localizations. The clinical question of whether the correct antihistamines had been used in previous studies of migraine was raised. A recent study of cimetidine (H_2 antagonist) alone and in combination with chlorpheniramine (H_1 antagonist) in the prophylaxis of migraine revealed that there was no efficacy for these drugs. This was a double-blind, controlled study of 24 patients with migraine and 20 patients with cluster headache. The authors concluded that although these histamine receptor antagonists were ineffective, this trial did not negate a histamine hypothesis of either migraine or cluster headache (4).

Although these studies demonstrate several interesting biochemical alterations in patients with migraine, how these alterations relate to the production of either pain or focal ischemia remains unclear. The greatest theoretical difficulty in integrating these biochemical findings continues to be the lack of an explanation for the focal neurologic deficit. All the biochemical findings are reflections of some type of systemic dysfunction. Even if the alterations in platelet and plasma serotonin, decrease in platelet MAO, or a myriad of other vascular alterations are etiologic factors in migraine, the question of why transient focal cerebral signs develop is unanswered. These systemic changes are reflected in the circulation, and all blood vessels should be equally susceptible. The alteration in platelet aggregability, particularly the increased adhesiveness and aggregability, at first seems to offer the possibility that several of the known biochemical alterations seen in migraine might be integrated into a single framework. However, there is no evidence that migraine patients have any degree of transient vascular ischemic events caused by platelet emboli in other arterial trees. Why the cerebral circulation should be particularly prone to focal ischemia related to altered platelet aggregation when the iliac vessels, for example, are not is unexplained.

Although this textbook has not been directed primarily at therapeutics, in the case of migraine, an overview of currently employed pharmacologic treatment further illustrates the confusion surrounding both the syndrome and the etiology. There are two general approaches to therapy in migraine: intermittent active treatment and preventive treatment (Table 2). Active treatment of the migraine attack has been directed at the vascular dilation that presumably corresponds with the pain. In this setting, ergotamine, a vasoconstrictor, has been employed. The vasoconstriction produced by this drug is due primarily to its action on alpha-adrenergic receptors, since in most instances it can be inhibited by low concentrations of phenoxybenzamine and phentolamine. In common practice, ergotamine is administered when the aura of the migraine is beginning in an attempt to abort, shorten, or relieve the intensity of the following discomfort. Although the issue of the safety of administering a vasoconstrictor during the prodrome, which itself is a vasoconstrictor phenomenon, has been raised, the action of ergotamine is stronger on the external than the internal carotid arteries. Other pharmacologic activity that may or may not be associated with the usefulness of ergotamine includes inhibition of norepinephrine and serotonin uptake, effects on platelet aggregation, and serotonergic agonist properties.

TABLE 2. *Therapeutic agents in migraine*

Acute	Prophylactic
Ergotamine	Methysergide
Caffeine	Lisuride
Analgesics	Cyproheptadine
Nonnarcotic	Propranolol
Narcotic	Amitriptyline
	Lithium
	MAO inhibitors
	Bromocriptine
	Platelet antagonists
	Prednisone
	Minor tranquilizers

Pharmacologic preventive measures in migraine include a wide variety of agents that appear to be have little in common. Preventive therapeutic measures should be considered when migraine episodes occur at predictable times (e.g., before, after, or during menstruation), when coexisting medical problems prevent the administration of ergotamines, and when the frequency of the attacks exceeds the safety limits for the use of ergotamines (43).

One aspect of the physiology and pharmacology of migraine that has not been dealt with is the well-known association of emotion in the precipitation of migraine. Intense anxiety, anger, fatigue, excessive sleep, and "weekend" letdown of activity have all been related to migraine episodes. The elucidation of the relationship between these states and the pharmacology of migraines awaits further editions of this text. In this context, it can be pointed out that although minor tranquilizers (chlordiazepoxide and diazepam) do not have a known physiologic effect that can be related to migraine, they can be useful as preventive measures in certain migraine-susceptible people. These agents can also be useful in alleviating pain and anxiety during the migraine itself.

Probably the most well-known preventive measure is the use of methysergide. Methysergide is a serotonin antagonist that has been demonstrated to have clinical efficacy in relieving the frequency of migraine attacks. There is no evidence that it is the serotonergic antagonism of methysergide that is responsible for preventing migraine. The important pharmacologic properties of a drug useful in the prophylaxis of migraine need not be directed toward antagonism of vasodilation but toward the initial mechanism responsible for the attack. Since these mechanisms are unknown, there is little justification for choosing any particular property of methysergide or any property of any of the other "prophylactic" drugs to be reviewed as the sole mechanism of prophylaxis (19). Other pharmacologic properties of methysergide include sensitization of smooth muscle, inhibition of serotonin-induced platelet aggregation, and a nonspecific antiinflammatory action. In fact, the latter may play a significant clinical role, since methysergide is able to inhibit serotonin-prostaglandin related inflammatory responses. Another compound said to have antiserotonergic properties is lisuride. Since the use of methysergide in migraine prophylaxis is associated with some uncommon but serious side effects (retroperitoneal fibrosis), an antiserotonergic agent that does not have these effects might be advantageous. Lisuride has been demonstrated to be an effective prophylactic agent in migraine and is not known to cause retroperitoneal fibrosis (52). Whether or not it is the antiserotonergic activity of lisuride that is responsible for decreasing headache frequency is unknown.

Cyproheptadine, another compound reported to be effective in migraine prevention, is clinically less effective than methysergide. It is a potent antagonist of serotonin, histamine, and acetylcholine. Since antihistamines and anticholinergics have never been reliably demonstrated to be effective in preventing migraine, the antiserotonergic action of cyproheptadine may be related to its clinical effectiveness.

The prophylactic value of propranolol in the treatment of migraine was first described in 1966 (35) as a fortuitous finding in a study of angina pectoris and propranolol. Several extensive clinical trials of propranolol in migraine have demonstrated that a significant percentage of patients with migraine have relief with respect to frequency and severity of attacks. Propranolol is a beta-adrenergic receptor antagonist; whether or not this most familiar pharmacologic property is related to its effect in migraine is unknown. Recently, propranolol was reported to affect platelet serotonin uptake. Although the majority of reports of propranolol treatment in the prophylaxis of migraine have been favorable, isolated case reports of recurrent migraine induced by propranolol have been published (36). In contrast to the potential role of beta antagonism in the treatment of migraine, a recent study (28) reported that isoproterenol, a beta agonist, was effective in ameliorating and preventing the visual aura associated with classic migraine (28).

Clinical trials in prevention of migraine have utilized amytriptyline (a tricyclic antidepressant), lithium, MAO inhibitor, bromocriptine (a direct-acting dopamine receptor agonist), and platelet antagonists (aspirin). Chlorpromazine has also been advocated as a prophylactic drug in the treatment of migraine (10). It is unwise to administer this drug in this setting, however, since one of its side effects is the development of a sometimes irreversible movement disorder, tardive dyskinesia.

MANAGEMENT OF THE MIGRAINE PATIENT

From a practical standpoint, the treatment of migraine is often an undertaking that equally utilizes scientific knowledge and the art of medicine. In the usual patient, previous treatment failures are a common feature of the past medical history and any guarantee by the physician that the current presciption will cure the problem is often met with skepticism on the part of the patient.

As a general rule, we assure the patient that the current therapy is likely to relieve symptoms, but we offer the possibility that "individual differences" may make an alternative medication necessary in the future. It has proven unwise to offer a complete "cure" of headaches and a promise of "making the headaches bearable" has a greater chance of being fulfilled.

Initially, an attempt to establish a periodicity to attacks should be made. If the episodes are very infrequent and lack any periodicity, we usually choose to treat each episode acutely. The agents of choice are the ergotamine preparations, which are available as either the tartrate or maleate salts. Dosage schedules and recommended dosages are listed in Table 3. In practice, intramuscular administration is usually confined to the emergency room, though an occasional patient is willing to self administer ergotamine IM as an outpatient. Marketed preparations that combine caffeine and ergotamine do not appear to offer any distinct therapeutic advantage and seem to have greater gastrointestinal toxicity than ergotamine alone. In many patients, however, an episode of emesis seems to signal the end of the headache, and such patients may find these preparations preferable. Ergotamine administration is contraindicated in pregnant women and in patients with coronary or peripheral vascular ischemia or hepatic insufficiency. When taken in excess, normal individuals may experience pallor or cyanosis of the extremities with as-

TABLE 3. *Antimigraine agents*

Drug	Dose	Route	Maximum dose
Ergotamine tartrate	2mg	Oral	2 mg q. 30 min × 3,10 mg q. week max.
	2 mg	Sublingual	Same as above
	2 mg	Rectal supp.	2 mg q. hr × 2, 10 mg q. week max.
	.36 mg	Inhaled	5 doses q. 24 hr, 36 doses q week max.
	.5 mg	Intramuscular	2 doses q. week
Ergonovine maleate	.2 mg	Oral	.6 mg in one day, 1 mg q. week
Propranolol	10 mg	Oral	variable, usual dose 20 to 80 mg/day
Cyproheptadine	4 mg	Oral	variable, usually 4 mg q.i.d.
Methysergide	2 mg	Oral	6 mg/day, not over 6 months continuously

sociated parasthesias or pain. Headache, dizziness, and gastrointestinal symptoms may also occur in this setting and in many ways mimic the symptoms of the migraine attack. Ergotism should be identified on the basis of the patient's history and physical examination and should be treated by prompt drug withdrawal. Antiemetics and vasodilators may be required in extreme cases.

In patients who report a regular periodicity to the headaches, starting medications a few days before they are anticipated is sometimes effective in reducing the frequency and intensity of the attacks. In such patients the daily dosage of ergotamine is reduced to provide the maximum safe dosage in the course of a week. Oral preparations are preferred agents in these situations.

A host of other prophylactic agents has been tried in these patients including minor tranquilizers, tricyclic antidepressants, propranolol, serotonin antagonists, and diuretics. Diuretics were once used regularly for migraines related to menstrual periods, but their efficacy is unclear. In our experience prophylactic ergotamine drugs have the greatest success rate.

In patients with a history of frequent migraine, an attempt is made to "break" the cycle of headaches. Frequently remissions are prolonged, and medications can be discontinued after a 2- or 3-week course of therapy. Ergotamine preparations are utilized initially, again using an oral agent. If this fails to bring the headaches under control, another agent is substituted. Because of the toxicity of methysergide (retroperitoneal and pulmonary fibrosis, though this appears to be rare), propranolol or cyproheptadine are usually administered first. The former agent is contraindicated in patients with asthma or heart failure, whereas the latter agent frequently causes an undesirable amount of sedation. If relief cannot be obtained with any of these regimens (and this may require experience treating a number of headache episodes in the same patient), methysergide is used as a last resort. In any situation, medications are usually tapered in the hope that a "rebound" headache will not be precipitated.

On occasion patients present to the emergency room or office with a treatment-resistant headache, exhausted by pain and recurrent vomiting. In these cases the administration of a narcotic analgesic such as meperidine is often the only recourse available. The chronic administration of narcotic analgesics for migraine, however, is never indicated.

In some cases all attempts at relieving migraine seem to fail and the clinician relying on pharmacotherapy must admit defeat. In these situations, behavioral approaches, using psychological counseling or biofeedback techniques offer an additional avenue of intervention to which the patient may be referred.

OTHER FORMS OF HEADACHE

Cluster Headache (Horton's Cephalgia, Histaminic Headache)

This entity, characterized by bouts of severe unilateral throbbing headache and ipsilateral lacrimation and nasal congestion and flushing, appears in the second to fourth decade and is more common in males (23a). Frequently there is a family history of migraine in patients with this condition, but the relationship of cluster headache to migraine is otherwise unclear. Severe daily headaches tend to occur in "clusters" that may be separated by long symptom-free intervals. Frequently the headache will begin at night, awakening the patient.

Although success has been reported using ergotamine for cluster headache, methysergide is usually the most effective agent in treatment. We usually initiate treatment with methysergide and continue therapy for 2 or 3 weeks after the headaches have ceased. If headaches fail to recur when the drug is discontinued, the patient is advised to keep a supply of the drug available in the event that the headaches recur. Although there is no data to support the belief that early treatment in the course of a headache cluster improves the therapeutic response, clinical experience suggests this may be true.

Chronic Paroxysmal Hemicrania

A headache syndrome bearing many similarities to cluster headache but occurring daily and affecting women has been suggested as a separable entity (46a,53a). In the patients reported, headaches occur on a daily basis for years and are always unilateral. Standard antimigraine drugs do not appear to alleviate the symptoms. Indomethacin has been reported to be curative in this condition, though the mechanism of action is unknown.

REFERENCES

1. Anthony, M. (1974): Patterns of plasma FFA and PGE, changes in migraine and stress. Presented at the Sixth International Migraine Symposium, London, September, 1974.

2. Anthony, M., Hinterberger, H., and Lance, J. W. (1967): Plasma serotonin in migraine and stress. *Arch. Neurol.*, 16:544–552.
3. Anthony, M., Hinterberger, H., and Lance, J. W. (1969): The possible relationship of serotonin to the migraine syndrome. *Res. Clin. Stud. Headache*, 2:29–59.
4. Anthony, M., Lord, G. D. A., and Lance, J. W. (1978): Controlled trials of cimetidine in migraine and cluster headache. *Headache*, 18:261–264.
5. Atkinson, R., and Appenzeller, O. (1978): Mast cells and headache in Crohn's disease. *Headache*, 18:40–43.
6. Barrie, M., and Jowett, J. (1967): A pharmacological investigation of cerebrospinal fluid from patients with migraine. *Brain*, 90:785–794.
7. Boisen, E. (1975): Strokes in migraine: Report on seven strokes associated with severe migraine attacks. *Dan. Med. Bull.*, 22:100–106.
8. Carlsen, L. A., Ekelund, L. G., and Oro, L. (1968): Clinical and metabolic effects of prostaglandin E1 in man. *Acta Med. Scand.*, 183:423–430.
9. Carroll, J. D. (1971): Migraine and oral contraception. *Proc. Intl. Headache Symp.*, Elsinore, Denmark, May 16–18, 1971.
10. Caurness, V. S., and O'Brien, P. (1980): Headache. *N. Engl. J. Med.*, 302:446–450.
11. Classification of Headache (1980): The Ad Hoc Committee on Classification of Headache. *Ann. Neurol.*, 6:173–176.
12. Couch, J. R., and Hassanein, R. S. (1976): Platelet aggregability in migraine and relation of aggregability to clinical aspects of migraine. *Neurology (Minneap.)*, 26:348.
13. Curran, D. A., Hinterberger, H., and Lance, J. W. (1965): Total plasma serotonin, 5-hydroxyindoleacetic acid and p-hydroxy-m-methyoxy-mandelic acid excretion in normal and migrainous subjects. *Brain*, 88:999.
14. Curzon, G., Theaker, P., and Phillip, B. (1966): Excretion of 5-hydroxyindoleacetic acid in migraine. *J. Neurol. Neurosurg. Psychiatry*, 29:85.
15. Dalessio, D. J. (1978): Migraine, platelets, and headache prophylaxis. *JAMA*, 239:52–53.
16. Deshmukh, S. V., and Meyer, J. S. (1977): Cyclic change in platelet dynamics and the pathogenesis and prophylaxis of migraine. *Headache*, 17:101–108.
17. Dorfman, L. H., Marshall, W. H., and Enzmann, D. R. (1979): Cerebral infarction and migraine: Clinical and radiologic correlation. *Neurology (Minneap.)*, 24:317–322.
18. Edmeads, J. (1977): Cerebral blood flow in migraine. *Headache*, 17:148–152.
19. Fozard, J. R. (1975): The animal pharmacology of drugs used in the treatment of migraine. *J. Pharm. Pharmacol.*, 27:297–321.
20. Gardner, J. H., Horenstein, S., and Van Den Noost, S. (1968): The clinical characteristics of headache during impending cerebral infarction in women taking oral contraceptives. *Headache*, 8:108.
21. Gardner, J. H., Van Den Noost, S., and Horenstein, S. (1967): Cerebrovascular disease in young women taking oral contraceptives. *Neurology (Minneap.)*, 17:299.
22. Garvel, M. J., Burkett, R., Rose, F. C., Sandler, M., Glover, V., and Moneada, S. (1978): Platelet function during migraine attack. Second International Migraine Symposium, London (*Abstr.*).
23. Glover, V., Sandler, M., Grant, E., Rose, F. C., Orton, D., Wilkinson, M., and Stevens, D. (1977): Transitory decrease in platelet monamine oxidase activity during migraine attacks. *Lancet*, 1:391–393.
23a. Graham, J. R. (1964): Methysergide for prevention of headache. *N. Engl. J. Med.*, 270:67–72.
24. Graham, J. R., and Wolff, H. G. (1938): Mechanism of migraine headache and action of ergotamine tartrate. *Arch. Neurol. Psychiatry*, 39:737–763.
25. Harrington, E. (1978): Migraine: A platelet hypothesis. *Biomedicine*, 30:65–67.
26. Hilton, B. P., and Cumings, J. N. (1972): 5-Hydroxytryptamine levels and platelet aggregation responses in subjects with acute migraine headache. *J. Neurol. Neurosurg. Psychiatry*, 25:505–509.
27. Kimball, R. W., and Goodman, M. A. (1961): Effects of reserpine on amino acid extraction in patients with vascular headaches. *Neurology (Minneap.)*, 11:116–219.
28. Kupersmith, M. J., Hans, W. K., and Chase, N. E. (1979): Isoproterenol treatment of visual symptoms in migraine. *Stroke*, 10:299–305.
29. Lance, J. W., Hinterberger, H., and Anthony, M. (1967): The control of cranial arteries by humoral mechanisms and its relation to the migraine syndrome. *Headache*, 7:93.
30. Mazal, S. (1978): Migraine attacks and increased platelet aggregability induced by oral contraceptives. *Aust. N.Z. J. Med.*, 8:646–648.

31. Muck-Seler, D., Deanovic, Z., and Duplej, M. (1979): Platelet serotonin and serotonin releasing factors in plasma of migrainous patients. *Headache*, 19:14–17.
32. Murphy, P. J. (1955): Cerebral infarction in migraine. *Neurology (Minneap.)*, 5:359–361.
33. Nelson, R. F. (1978): Testosterone levels in cluster and non-cluster migrainous headache patients. *Headache*, 18:265–267.
34. O'Brien, M. D. (1971): Cerebral blood flow changes in migraine. *Headache*, 10:139–143.
35. Rabkin, R., Stables, D. P., Levin, N. W., and Suzman, M. M. (1966): The prophylactic value of propranolol in angina pectoris. *Am. J. Cardiol.*, 18:370–383.
36. Robson, R. H. (1977): Recurrent migraine after propranolol. *Br. Health J.*, 39:1157–1158.
37. Ryan, R. E. (1978): A controlled study of the effect of oral contraceptives on migraine. *Headache*, 17:250–255.
38. Sandler, M. (1972): Migraine: A pulmonary disease? *Lancet*, 1:618–619.
39. Sandler, M. (1977): Transitory platelet monoamine oxidase defect in migraine. *Headache*, 17:153–158.
40. Sandler, M., Youdim, M. B. H., and Hanington, E. (1974): A phenylethylamine-oxidizing defect in migraine. *Nature*, 250:335–337.
41. Sandler, M., Youdim, M. B. H., Southgate, J., and Hanington, E. (1970): The role of tyramine in migraine: Some possible biochemical mechanisms. In: *Background to Migraine*, edited by A. L. Cochrane, Heinemann Medical Books, London.
42. Saper, J. R. (1978): Migraine—classification and pathogenesis. *JAMA*, 239:2380–2383.
43. Saper, J. R. (1978): Migraine—treatment. *JAMA*, 239:2480–2484.
44. Sicuteri, F. (1963): Mast cells and their active substances: Their role in migraine. *Headache*, 3:86–93.
45. Sicuteri, F., Testi, A., and Anselmi, B. (1961): Biochemical investigations in headache: Increase in hydroxyindoleacetic acid excretion during migraine attacks. *Int. Arch. Allergy Appl. Immunol.*, 19:55.
46. Sjaastad, O. (1975): The significance of blood serotonin levels in migraine. *Acta Neurol. Scand.*, 51:200–210.
46a. Sjaastad, O., and Dale, I. (1974): Evidence for a new treatable headache entity. *Headache*, 14:105–108.
47. Skinhøj, E. (1973): Hemodynamic studies with the brain during migraine. *Arch. Neurol.*, 29:95–98.
48. Somerville, B. (1972): The role of estradiol withdrawal in the etiology of menstrual migraine. *Neurology*, 22:355–365.
49. Somerville, B. W. (1975): Estrogen withdrawal migraine. I. Duration of exposure required and attempted prophylaxis by premenstrual estrogen. *Neurology (Minneap.)*, 25:234–244.
50. Somerville, B. W. (1975): Estrogen withdrawal migraine. II. Attempted prophylaxis by continuous estradiol administration. *Neurology (Minneap.)*, 25:245–250.
51. Somerville, B. W. (1976): Platelet- and free serotonin levels in jugular and forearm, venous blood during migraine. *Neurology (Minneap.)*, 26:41–45.
52. Somerville, B. W., and Herrmann, W. M. (1978): Migraine prophylaxis with isuriole hydrogen moleate. *Headache*, 18:75–79.
53. Southren, A. L., and Christoff, N. (1962): Cerebrospinal fluid serotonin in brain tumor and other neurologic disorders. *J. Lab. Clin. Med.*, 59:320–329.
53a. Stein, H. J., and Rogato, A. Z. (1980): Chronic paroxysmal hemicrania: Two new patients. *Headache*, 20:72–76.
54. Vardi, Y., Rabey, I. M., Streifler, M., Schwartz, A., Lindner, H. R., and Zor, U. (1976): Migraine attacks: Alleviation by an inhibitor of prostaglandin synthesis and action. *Neurology (Minneap.)*, 26:447–450.
55. Waters, W. E. (1975): Prevalence of migraine. *Neurol. Neurosurg. Psychiatry*, 38:613–616.
56. Welch, K. M. A., Spira, P. J., Knowles, L., and Lance, J. W. (1974): Effects of prostaglandins on the internal and external carotid blood flow in the monkey. *Neurology (Minneap.)*, 24:705–710.

Chapter 28

Cerebrovascular Disease

Stroke remains the third leading cause of death in this country, despite a recent report that the incidence is declining in the United States (15). The term stroke encompasses a wide variety of pathophysiologic processes that end in a focal neurologic deficit that persists for more than 24 hr. This chapter is concerned primarily with the pharmacology of thromboembolic cerebral infarction and transient ischemic attacks (TIAs). Intraparenchymal hemorrhage in the central nervous system (CNS) is not discussed since there is no efficacious therapy once the ictus has occurred. The possible role of antifibrinolytic agents in subarachnoid hemorrhage secondary to a ruptured aneurysm will be discussed.

TIA

TIAs are episodes of temporary focal neurologic deficits that begin abruptly and resolve within 24 hr (usually within 5 to 15 min). These attacks leave no residual neurologic findings and can occur in the distribution of either the anterior or posterior cerebral circulation. The importance of TIAs in relation to stroke resides in the fact that they can be a harbinger of stroke. Although the natural history of TIAs is far from clear, patients who experience them are at a higher risk for the development of stroke than are age-matched healthy controls. The literature indicates that the risk of stroke following TIA is approximately 7% per year, with a cumulative incidence of stroke of about 35% after 5 years. The crucial therapeutic issue for patients is the lack of individual applicability of these figures. There is no reliable predicting factor in a given patient to indicate if the patient is in imminent or relative danger of a stroke. Patients with new onset or recurrent TIAs that are occurring in clusters (2 to 3 per day to 2 to 3 per week) are often said to be in greater danger of stroke than those with stable, infrequent TIAs. The first month after the occurrence of an initial TIA has also been associated with a marked increase in stroke incidence (25,37).

The pathogenesis of TIAs can be divided into two broad categories: hemodynamic and thromboembolic phenomena. Hemodynamic factors include any of a variety of cardiovascular dynamic events that produce diffuse cerebral ischemia. Occasionally, the diffuse ischemia will be superimposed on an area of focal pathology (atherosclerotic vessel) which results in focal symptoms as well. Cardiac bradyarrhythmias and tachyarrhythmias, orthostatic hypotension, and vascular compression by musculoskeletal anatomic structures are examples of etiologies in this hemodynamic group. Thromboembolic events in TIA are considered to be more important than the hemodynamic group because the majority of patients have thromboembolic TIAs. In fact, when the relationship between cardiac dysrhythmia and focal ischemic events is examined, it is found to be a rare occurrence. In a survey of 290 patients requiring cardiac pacemakers for either condition or for rhythmic disturbances, only two had focal cerebral symptoms that correlated with the occurrence of the cardiac disturbance. The occurrence of transient symptomatology suggestive of diffuse cerebral ischemia, e.g., syncope, near syncope, and seizures, is more common (31).

The role of thromboembolism is reviewed in greater detail since pharmacologic interference with this process is the basis of its medical management. Recent interest has focused on the etiologic role of atherosclerotic extracranial vascular lesions in TIA. The formation of platelet-fibrin material on these lesions and their subsequent release into the arterial flow as emboli are believed to be the source of the majority of TIAs. The pathogenesis of the initial atherosclerotic lesion is not clear, but this lesion serves as the "vessel wall injury" that is the impetus to bring into activity the interplay between platelets and plasma coagulation factors. This interaction is the mechanism that produces as its end product platelet-fibrin clots and debris (Fig. 1). Although the plasma coagulation system and the platelet activation system are separable processes, the considerable interaction between them results in platelet-fibrin embolic material. Recent emphasis in both the preclinical and clinical literature implicates the platelet aggregation system as being more responsible for stroke and TIA than plasma coagulation factors (6).

Pharmacologic therapy in TIA is based on interference with either plasma coagulation factors or platelet aggregation. Anticoagulants that are used clinically include heparin and warfarin (Coumadin). Warfarin produces anticoagulation by inhibiting the hepatic synthesis of coagulation factors (II, VII, IX, X). Synthesis inhibition is accomplished by interference with the action of vitamin K. Between warfarin administration and suppression of plasma coagulation, there is a time lag.

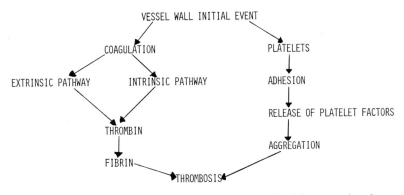

FIG. 1. Mechanism by which platelet-fibrin clots and debris are produced.

Warfarin is used for long-term anticoagulation. It is important to recall that if it becomes necessary to reverse the biologic activity of warfarin by administering vitamin K, there will also be a time lag before the plasma coagulation system returns to normal. Heparin produces immediate anticoagulation and is administered parenterally. Heparin produces no deficiencies of plasma clotting factors; it produces its effect by inhibiting factors related to the conversion of prothrombin to thrombin. When necessary, the anticoagulating effect of heparin can be overcome by the administration of protamine sulfate. This drug is strongly basic and combines with the strongly acid heparin molecule to form a stable complex with no inherent anticoagulant properties.

Interference with platelet function as a means of reducing thromboembolic events is currently receiving considerable attention. Separate physiologic events occur when platelets are activated in the hemostatic system. These include adhesion, release reaction, and aggregation. Adhesion refers to the actual "sticking" of the platelet to the injured and altered vessel wall. When platelets have adhered, structural changes occur within the platelet which result in extrusion of platelet granules. This results in release of adenosine diphosphate (ADP), which promotes aggregation of platelets to one another. Other factors important for platelet aggregation include prostaglandin endoperoxides and platelet factor 3. Assessment of platelet function in cerebrovascular disease indicates increased adhesiveness and aggregation in these patients (1,40).

Drugs that affect platelet function alter both platelet adhesiveness and aggregation. Although a wide variety of nonsteroidal antiinflammatory agents (aspirin, sulfinpyrazone), pyrimidopyrimidine compounds (Persantine), and other miscellaneous agents, including antihistamines, barbiturates, tricyclic antidepressants, and antipsychotics, affect platelet function, the agents that have received the most attention in the therapy of TIA are aspirin, sulfinpyrazone (Anturane), and dipyridamole (Persantine).

A recent review of the early reports of the efficacy of antiplatelet therapy in TIA concluded that there was evidence that aspirin and sulfinpyrazone might reduce the frequency of TIAs, but that there was no efficacy with respect to the important prognostic end points of stroke or death (16). Two important cooperative studies regarding aspirin and sulfinpyrazone in TIA have recently been published.

The Aspirin in Transient Ischemic Attack Cooperative Study (AITIA) followed 178 patients and reported on their prognosis for a 6-month period (11). This study admitted patients with carotid distribution TIAs. Although the patients were randomized, some were selected out in order to undergo endarterectomy. The results of aspirin treatment in these patients revealed that when death, cerebral infarction, retinal infarction, and occurrence of TIAs were grouped together, there was a statistically significant difference in favor of the aspirin group. When the absolute end points of stroke or death were compared, however, there was no statistically significant difference between aspirin and placebo groups. In a separate report, the AITIA group reported the results of aspirin in surgically treated patients (12). This group of patients were those mentioned above who had been selected out of the original study. These patients underwent carotid endarterectomy and then were randomly assigned to aspirin or placebo treatment groups. Again, this study group was unable to demonstrate a statistically significant difference between aspirin and placebo when cerebral infarction, retinal infarction, or death were the end points.

In 1978, the results of the Canadian Cooperative Study Group (8) became available. This study included 585 patients who were followed for an average of 26 months and who were divided into four treatment groups: aspirin, aspirin plus sulfinpyrazone, sulfinpyrazone alone, and placebo. This study reported that aspirin reduced the risk of continuing TIAs, stroke, or death by 19%. Most important, the Canadian group was able to demonstrate that aspirin produced a 48% risk reduction for stroke or death. Unfortunately, this was sex dependent; no significant effect of aspirin was noted in women. Sulfinpyrazone produced a risk reduction of 10% for stroke or death, but this was not considered to be statistically significant. There was no synergism between aspirin and sulfinpyrazone.

In men, the use of aspirin in TIA is an efficacious method to reduce not only frequency of TIAs but also the incidence of stroke or death. This latter finding separates antiplatelet treatment with aspirin from many of the previous reports regarding treatment in TIA with anticoagulants or endarterectomy. These previous studies had demonstrated that these treatment modalities reduce frequency of TIAs but not the incidence of stroke or death.

The Canadian group has not been without its critics. Although complimentary with respect to the time and effort expended, Kurtzke (21) suggests that his own biostatistical analysis of the published data leads him to question the validity of the reported results. In particular, he states that the efficacy of aspirin is not demonstrated, that the true effect of drug therapy may lie in the aspirin-sulfinpyrazone treatment group, and that the sex differences reported are not valid (21). Barnett and colleagues (7) have responded to their critics by restating the original goals of the study and, with their own statistical data, the authors have refuted criticism raised thus far.

The role of anticoagulant therapy in TIA has recently been reviewed by the Study Group on Antithrombotic Therapy. In their analysis of eight separate studies—four randomized (3,4,5,30) and four nonrandomized (13,14,33,38)—which examined the role of anticoagulation in TIA, it was the consistent finding that no benefit was observed with respect to mortality. Evaluation of the other significant end point— stroke prevention—did not yield consistent results. All the nonrandomized studies reported decreased incidence of stroke in patients with TIA when they were treated with anticoagulation; all randomized studies report no reduction in stroke occurrence in anticoagulant-treated TIA patients. Although it is often accepted that anticoagulation therapy can reduce the frequency of TIA, the study group cast doubt on this aspect of anticoagulant therapy. They concluded that the evidence that this form of therapy reduces the frequency of TIA is equivocal. Anticoagulation is associated with increased risk of hemorrhage, including intracerebral bleeding. In fact, in the previously mentioned population study documenting the decrease in stroke, it was determined that during the 1960s, there was a slight increase in intracerebral bleeding. The investigators suggested that the unusual rise in intracranial bleeding in the 1960s might have been related to the widespread use of anticoagulants.

Despite the report by the study group, there continues to be considerable controversy surrounding the use of anticoagulants in TIA. In a recent paper concerned with treatment in TIA, Millikan and McDowell (26) reviewed some of the same reports reviewed by the study group and added some additional nonrandomized studies. They concluded that "anticoagulant therapy decreases the risk of cerebral infarction in patients with transient ischemic attacks" and proposed that anticoagulants were of particular value in a "carefully selected group," although the definition of that group is unclear. It should be noted that even in this setting, the authors recommended continuing anticoagulant treatment for only 6 to 8 months.

Since the Antithrombotic Study Group issued their report, few large studies of TIA patients have examined anticoagulation. One exception is a recent report by Toole et al. (35) which was a prospective nonrandomized study of patients with TIA. These workers found no difference in outcome (continuing TIAs, stroke, or death) in their patients, regardless of which treatment the patients received. Another randomized study of anticoagulation in patients with TIA and/or cerebral infarction was reported by Link et al. (22). These authors concluded that in selected patients with TIA or with mild cerebral infarction in the carotid distribution, anticoagulation was effective in preventing stroke. The patient population, however, was not randomized; also there are several other difficulties, including a selection process that included patients in whom the "biological age was acceptably low" and patients who "were considered able to manage treatment with anticoagulants." In addition, 41 of the 117 patients were selected out of the study when carotid endarterectomy was performed. The conclusion that anticoagulants were beneficial is also drawn from using the patients as their own controls. One interesting aspect of the study was the high rate of cerebral infarction when anticoagulants are stopped. Whether this bears on the question of whether or not anticoagulants are effective in preventing stroke in patients at risk is a different issue.

Another recent report assessing a large number of TIA patients and the role of anticoagulation in prevention of stroke was published in 1978 by Whisnant and co-workers (36). They identified 199 patients with TIA from the record retrieval system at their institution. This was a population study and was not randomized, nor was there any attempt to control treatment parameters initiated by individual physicians. The two major treatment modalities employed were antihypertensives and anticoagulants. The report concluded that patients with vertebrobasilar TIAs had a significant decrease in the incidence of stroke, whereas in patients with carotid TIAs, there was a decrease in number of strokes, but it was not statistically significant. As alluded to above, one of the major complications of anticoagulation therapy is intracranial hemorrhage. This report noted that the overall rate of intracranial hemorrhage was 3.7 times higher for the anticoagulant-treated patients; for the subpopulation of patients aged 55 to 74, the rate of intracranial hemorrhage was more than eight times that of the untreated patients. These authors point out that this increased rate of intracranial bleeding occurred at an institution where both the physicians and laboratories are highly skilled in the use of anticoagulants.

CEREBRAL INFARCTION

The pharmacologic approaches to the patient who has experienced a completed stroke can be divided into those that are designed to (a) affect the thromboembolic mechanism, (b) "protect" the ischemic brain, and (c) lessen the complications of infarction, such as cerebral edema.

A series of studies that have evaluated the effect of anticoagulant therapy in completed stroke has been reviewed and summarized in the report of the Study Group on Antithrombotic Therapy (16). In all of the seven randomized studies, the conclusions are consistent: anticoagulants have no therapeutic benefit in completed stroke. In fact, the possibility is raised that actual danger to the patient may arise from anticoagulant therapy. Of the two nonrandomized studies of anticoagulation in completed stroke, one concluded that there was benefit, and the other concluded that there was no benefit. In view of these findings, it can be concluded that acute anticoagulation in completed stroke is not recommended. The role of antiplatelet agents in completed stroke has not yet been examined in a controlled prospective manner.

Acute treatment of cerebral infarction often involves pharmacologic therapies designed to reduce or limit the extent of infarcted tissue. The rationale for this type of approach is based on the concept that in any cerebral ischemic zone, there may be marginal tissue that can either recover normal function or infarct. The use of vasodilators and barbiturates in stroke are examples of this type of therapeutic approach. Although the use of vasodilators had been common clinical practice in completed stroke, recent investigations have profoundly affected this practice. If cerebral infarction is related in part to ischemia, then producing vasodilation and presumably increasing cerebral blood flow might reduce the extent of a cerebral infarct. Cerebral blood flow is highly regulated to ensure that under a wide variety of conditions, cerebral tissue receives a constant flow. The general mechanisms that play a role in this system include autoregulation, neurogenic input to the cerebral vessels, and tissue acidity.

Although some of the vasodilators in use have been demonstrated in preclinical studies and in patients with cerebral infarction to increase cerebral blood flow, there is no definite evidence that vasodilators are of clinical value in the patient with an acute cerebral infarction (23,24). Probably the most widely employed vasodilator has been papaverine, and not only is there controversy surrounding whether or not there is clinical benefit with cerebral infarction, there is also a controversy with regard to whether papaverine is even capable of increasing cerebral blood flow.

Multiple other pharmacologic agents believed to be vasodilators have also been reported to be without clinical benefit. These include beta-adrenergic blockers, hexobenadine, dihydroergonovine, and nylidrin. In addition to the lack of demonstrated clinical benefit of the vasodilators in cerebral infarction, there is a subtle danger in their use. In the zone of cerebral infarction, many of the mechanisms that normally control cerebral blood flow may be lost or impaired. If a vasodilator is employed, normal areas of brain may respond, while infarcted zones may be incapable of response; blood flow then would be shunted from the infarcted zone to normal tissue.

Recent interest has focused on another vasodilatory agent, pentoxifylline, which is a xanthine derivative with the chemical formula 3,7,-dimethyl-1,5-oxohexyl xanthine. This agent significantly increases peripheral and cerebral perfusion in preclinical animal studies. European clinical studies in patients have demonstrated its beneficial effect in peripheral occlusive arterial disease and in ischemic heart disease. The increase in poststenotic perfusion in these patients appears to be due in part to a direct action of the drug on muscle in the arterial wall via an accumulation of cyclic AMP and in part to an increase of blood flow in ischemic tissue as a result of rheologic effects that modify blood viscosity. Pentoxifylline has been shown to reduce cerebral edema associated with cerebral ischemia in animals; in uncontrolled studies, patients with CNS ischemia have been reported to improve clinically after drug treatment. Central ultrastructural and biochemical changes seen in animals treated with pentoxifylline after ischemia include mitochondrial hypertrophy and enhanced oxygen consumption. These latter effects may offer a potential therapeutic role for this drug; but this remains to be evaluated (17,19,20).

Since the mid-1960s, it has been known that certain anesthetic agents (thiopental, halothane, cyclopropane, chloroform, methoxyflurane, and trichloroethylene) increase survival in animals exposed to hypoxia. Multiple studies of this nature suggest that agents that reduce cerebral metabolism during anoxia and/or ischemia may be clinically useful. In cerebral infarction, it might be possible to suppress metabolic demand in marginal areas of the infarcted zone and thereby have increased survival of cerebral tissue and greater functional recovery. Barbiturates might prove effective in this clinical setting. Several preclinical studies using barbiturates have demonstrated a protective effect in models of cerebral ischemia (18,34,41), but the mechanism of action is unknown. Although depression of metabolic activity has been advanced, the effect may be mediated through other unknown means. Since it has been demonstrated that the barbiturate dose required to reduce cerebral metabolic activity is 10 to 20% of that required to produce narcosis, it may be possible to explore the source of the protective effect more thoroughly (9).

At present, only anecdotal reports have suggested that barbiturates may afford clinical benefit in cerebral infarction. However, as Yatsu et al. (41) pointed out, the issue of whether or not clinical benefits derive from the use of pentobarbital in cerebral infarction will have to be determined by randomized prospective investigations. Some of the methodologic difficulties in a study of this nature have also been delineated. No diagnostic technique allows assessment of the potential viability of cerebral tissue at risk. In other words, how can one distinguish dysfunctioning cerebral tissue that is irreversibly damaged from that which has the potential of being spared? In addition, since barbiturates tend to depress cerebral function, the clinical neurologic picture may be altered, and underlying progression of the original deficit may go unnoticed. Finally, a large patient population is needed in order to study this issue, since associated factors in stroke (e.g., age, diabetes mellitus, hypertension, coronary heart disease) may also influence the outcome of any single ictal cerebrovascular event. The outcome of such a study with barbiturates would be eagerly anticipated.

Another approach to the treatment of cerebral infarction has included the use of ornithine alpha-ketoglutarate (OAKG) (39). OAKG has been used to alter anaerobic glycolysis in hepatic encephalopathy. When cerebral hypoxia occurs, cerebral metabolism turns increasingly to anaerobic glycolysis with increased lactate production; thus a trial of OAKG in cerebral ischemia was undertaken. The investigators studied 50 patients with ischemic stroke in a double-blind, controlled trial. They determined that 5 days poststroke, the level of consciousness of treated patients was better. This effect lasted only while OAKG was administered, however, and at 10 days poststroke, there was no clinical difference between the treated and control groups.

Pharmacologic therapy of ischemic stroke that is directed at one of the major complications of cerebral infarction (cerebral edema) with steroids and/or hyperosmolar agents (glycerol, mannitol) is discussed in Chapter 29 in this volume. The division of cerebral edema into vasogenic and cytotoxic edema has been of considerable usefulness in assessing the role of pharmacologic agents designed to treat this problem. Vasogenic edema is thought to result from an initial disturbance in the blood-brain barrier, with subsequent leakage of osmotic particles and fluid into the extracellular space of the brain. Cytotoxic edema is thought to result from a disruption or dysfunction of the neuronal membrane mechanisms controlling water and electrolyte distribution, which results in the accumulation of intracellular fluid. Corticosteroids have been effective in some models of vasogenic edema but generally have not been effective in cytotoxic edema. The edema that accompanies ischemic cerebral infarction has elements of both vasogenic and cytotoxic edema.

The development of edema appears to be a two-phase event. The early phase is primarily cytotoxic and seems to result from failure of membrane mechanisms, resulting in increased intracellular volume. The later phase occurs when the blood-brain barrier develops leakage. The evolution of these changes may occur over hours to days. Before examining the results of clinical treatment, it is of interest to examine the reasons why corticosteroids might be effective in the treatment of ischemic edema. Anderson and Crawford (2) and O'Brien (28) have listed several potential mechanisms to explain antiedema effects of these agents, including membrane-stablizer effects, mineral corticoid-induced electrolyte alterations, suppression of cerebrospinal fluid (CSF) production, and enhanced CSF reabsorption. Since the concept of ischemic edema is now thought to be a two-phase event which begins not with a leaking blood-brain barrier but with increasing intracellular volume, the membrane-stabilizing effect of steroids in the blood-brain barrier is not of prime importance.

Cerebral edema following ischemic infarction reaches its peak 1½ to 3 days following the ictus. The potential threat of cerebral edema in this setting is particularly obvious in those patients with supratentorial infarcts in whom the advent and progression of the edema results in one of the several intracranial herniation syndromes. Other potential reasons to treat cerebral edema include preventing compromise of the cerebral microcirculation and extension of the infarct and potential salvage of cells in the marginal ischemic zone. As discussed above with respect to demonstrating the efficacy of barbiturate treatment in stroke, there are tremendous difficulties in designing an adequate clinical trial to assess the role of corticosteroids in human infarction. The overall consensus of recent attempts appears to be that their continued use is not efficacious (10,27,29). A recent randomized study of 300 ischemic stroke patients examined whether the routine use of steroids and mannitol differed from routine supportive care. This study concluded that at 10 days postinfarct, there was no clinical difference among the four study groups, which included supportive care, dexamethasome, mannitol, and ergot preparations (Hydergine) (32).

Whether or not a subgroup exists of patients with cerebral infarction in whom corticosteroids should be used remains to be evaluated.

ANTIFIBRINOLYTIC THERAPY

Subarachnoid hemorrhage secondary to aneurysmal rupture is a serious and often fatal cerebrovascular disorder. Unlike many other cerebrovascular events, survival of the initial ictal and peri-ictal period is not necessarily associated with recovery. Whereas the diagnosis and therapeutic decisions (surgical versus nonsurgical) are beyond the scope of this text, the tendency for aneurysms to rebleed with subsequent increases in mortality and morbidity has been approached pharmacologically.

After an aneurysmal rupture, one of the mechanisms responsible for stopping the bleeding into the subarachnoid space is the formation of a perianeurysmal blood clot. It is postulated that this clot not only stops the initial bleeding but may also play a role in preventing rebleeding. The stability of this clot, like all clots, is dependent in part on the activity of the fibrinolytic system. The fibrinolytic activity of CSF increases following subarachnoid hemorrhage, and it is believed that this may result in lysis of the perianeurysmal clot with resultant new aneurysmal bleeding. Aminocaproic acid inhibits fibrinolytic activity by altering the action of plasmin and interfering with the conversion of plasminogen to plasmin. The base of the use of aminocaproic acid in patients with subarachnoid bleeding secondary to aneurysm is its possible ability to prevent lysis of the perianeurysmal clot. This therapy has been particularly advanced as a way of decreasing presurgical mortality in surgical candidates.

Although this therapy remains controversial because of the occurrence of serious side effects (bleeding, deep vein thrombosis, pulmonary emboli, altered mental states), a recent review from the Cooperative Aneurysm Study involving over 1,100 patients suggested that aminocaproic acid may be of some value (1a). This study reported that the incidence of rebleeding in their patients on aminocaproic acid was 10% in the 2-week period following initial hemorrhage compared to reputed rebleeding rates of 18 to 23%. This study also reported that the incidence of serious side effects was low. However, the report was not entirely a prospective randomized study, and the role of this pharmacologic agent in this problem requires further examination.

REFERENCES

1. Acheson, J., Danta, G., and Hutchinson, E. C. (1972): Platelet adhesiveness in patients with cerebrovascular disease. *Atherosclerosis*, 15:123.
1a. Adams, H. P., Nibbelink, D. W., Turner, J. C., and Sahs, A. L. (1981): Antifibrinolytic therapy in patients with aneurysmal subarachnoid hemorrhage. *Arch. Neurol.*,38:25–30.
2. Anderson, D. C., and Crawford, R. E. (1979): Corticosteroids in ischemic stroke. *Stroke*, 10:68–71.
3. Baker, R. N. (1961): An evaluation of anticoagulant therapy in the treatment of cerebrovascular disease: Report of the Veterans Administration cooperative study of atherosclerosis. *Neurology*, 11:132–138.
4. Baker, R. N., Broward, J. A., Fang, H. C., Fischer, C. M., Groch, S. W., Iteyman, A., Karp, H. R., McDevitt, E., Scheinberg, P., Schwartz, W., and Toule, J. F. (1962): Anticoagulant therapy in cerebral infarction. Report on cooperative study. *Neurology*, 12:823.
5. Baker, R. N., Schwartz, W. S., and Rose, A. S. (1966): Transient ischemic attacks. A report of a study of anticoagulant therapy. *Neurology*, 16:841–847.
6. Barnett, H. M. J. (1977): Platelet and coagulation function in relation to thromboembolic stroke. In: *Advances in Neurology, Vol. 16, Stroke*, edited by R. A. Thompson and J. R. Green, pp. 121–140. Raven Press, New York.
7. Barnett, H. M. J., Gent, M., Sachett, D. L., and Taylor, D. W. (1979): Reply to Kurtzke "critique." *Ann. Neurol.*, 5:599–601.
8. Canadian Cooperative Study Group (1978): A randomized trial of aspirin and sulfinpyrazone in threatened stroke. *N. Engl. J. Med.*, 299:53–59.
9. Crane, P. D., Braun, L. D., Cornford, E. M., Cremer, J. E., Glass, J. M., and Oldendorf, W. H. (1978): Dose dependent reduction of glucose utilization by pentobarbital in rat brain. *Stroke*, 6:12–17.
10. Dyken, M., and White, P. T. (1976): Evaluation of cortisone in the treatment of cerebral infarction. *Arch. Neurol.*, 33:69–71.
11. Fields, W. S., Lemak, N. A., Frankowski, R. F., and Hardy, R. J. (1977): Controlled trial of aspirin in cerebral ischemia. *Stroke*, 8:301–315.
12. Fields, W. S., Lemak, N. A., Frankowski, R. F., and Hardy, R. J. (1978): Controlled trial of aspirin in cerebral ischemia. Part II: Surgical group. *Stroke*, 9:309–318.
13. Fisher, C. M. (1958): The use of anticoagulants in cerebral thrombosis. *Neurology*, 8:311–332.
14. Friedman, G. D., Wilson, W. S., Mosier, J. M., Colandrea, M. A., and Nichaman, M. Z. (1969): Transient ischemic attacks in a community. *JAMA*, 210:1428–1434.
15. Garraway, W. M., Whisnant, J. P., Furlan, A. J., Phillips, L. H., II, Kurland, L. T., and O'Fallon, W. M. (1979): The declining incidence of stroke. *N. Engl. J. Med.*, 300:449–452.
16. Gent, E., Barnett, H. J. M., Fields, W. S., Gent, M., and Hook, J. C. (1977): Cerebral ischemia: The role of thrombosis and antithrombotic therapy. *Stroke*, 8:148–175.
17. Hartmann, J. F., Becker, R. A., and Cohen, M. M. (1977): Effects of pentoxifylline on cerebral ultrastructure of normal and ischemic gerbils. *Neurology*, 27:77–84.
18. Hoff, J. T., Smith, A. L., Hankinson, H. L., and Nielsen, S. L. (1975): Barbiturate protection from cerebral infarction in primates. *Stroke*, 6:28–33.
19. Josipovic, V. (1978): Experience with pentoxifylline in the treatment of peripheral and central vascular disease. *Pharmacotherapeutica*, 2:90–93.
20. Kobaladze, S. F. (1978): On the effect of pentoxifylline in ischemic heart disease. *Gehalten Wiesbaden*, 2–6.
21. Kurtzke, J. F. (1979): A critique of the Canadian TIA study. *Ann. Neurol.*, 5:597–599.
22. Link, H., Lebram, G., Johansson, L., and Radberg, C. (1979): Prognosis in patients with infarction and TIA in carotid territory during and after anticoagulant therapy. *Stroke*, 10:529–532.
23. McHenry, L. C. (1972): Cerebral vasodilatory therapy in stroke. *Stroke*, 3:686–691.

24. McHenry, L. C., Jaffee, M. E., Kawamura, J., and Goldberg, H. I. (1970): Effect of papaverine on regional blood flow in focal vascular disease of the brain. *N. Engl. J. Med.*, 282:1167–1170.

25. Meyer, J. S., Guiraud, B., and Bauer, R. (1972): Clinical and pathophysiological considerations of atherosclerotic and thrombotic disease of the carotid arteries. In: *Vascular Diseases of the Nervous System. Handbook of Neurology*, edited by P. J. Vinken and G. W. Bruyn, vol. II, pp. 327–365. Elsevier, New York.

26. Millikan, C. H., and McDowell, F. H. (1978): Treatment of transient ischemic attacks. *Stroke*, 9:299–308.

27. Norris, J. W. (1976): Steroid therapy in acute cerebral infarction. *Arch. Neurol.*, 33:69–71.

28. O'Brien, M. D. (1979): Ischemic cerebral edema—A review. *Stroke*, 10:623–628.

29. Patten, B. M., Mendell, J., Bruun, B., Curtin, W., and Carter, S. (1972): Double-blind study of the effects of dexamethasone on acute stroke. *Neurology (Minneap.)*, 22:377–383.

30. Pearce, J. M. S., Gubbay, S. S., and Walton, J. N. (1965): Long-term anticoagulant therapy in transient cerebral ischaemic attacks. *Lancet*, 1:6–9.

31. Reed, R. L., Siekert, R. G., and Merideth, J. (1973): Rarity of transient focal cerebral ischemia in cardiac dysrhythmia. *JAMA*, 223:893–895.

32. Santambiogio, S., Martinotti, R., Sardella, F., Porro, F., and Randazzo, A. (1978): Is there a real treatment for stroke? *Stroke*, 9:130–132.

33. Siekert, R. G., Whisnant, J. P., and Millikan, C. H. (1963): Surgical and anticoagulant therapy of occlusive cerebrovascular disease. *Ann. Intern. Med.*, 58:637–641.

34. Smith, A. L., Hoff, J. T., and Nielsen, S. L. (1974): Barbiturate protection in acute focal cerebral ischemia. *Stroke*, 5:1–7.

35. Toole, J. F., Yuson, C. P., Janeway, R., Johnston, F., Davis, C., Cordell, R., and Howard, G. (1978): Transient ischemic attacks: A prospective study of 225 patients. *Neurology*, 28:746–753.

36. Whisnant, J. P., Cartlidge, N. E., and Elveback, L. R. (1978): Carotid and vertebral-basilar transient ischemic attacks: Effect of anticoagulants, hypertension, and cardiac disorder on survival and stroke occurrence—A population study. *Ann. Neurol.*, 3:107–115.

37. Whisnant, J. P., Matsumoto, N., and Elveback, L. R. (1973): Transient cerebral ischemic attacks in a community. *Mayo Clin. Proc.*, 48:194–198.

38. Whisnant, J. P., Matsumoto, N., and Elveback, L. R. (1973): The effect of anticoagulant therapy on the prognosis of patients with transient cerebral ischemic attacks in a community, Rochester, Minnesota, 1955 through 1969. *Mayo Clin. Proc.*, 48:844–848.

39. Woolard, M. L., Pearson, R. M., Dorf, G., Griffeth, D., and James, I. M. (1978): Controlled trial of ornithine alpha ketoglutarate (OAKG) in patients with stroke. *Stroke*, 9:218–222.

40. Wu, K., and Hoak, J. C. (1975): Increased platelet aggregates in patients with transient ischemic attacks. *Stroke*, 6:521.

41. Yatsu, F. M., Diamond, I., Graziano, C., and Lundquist, P. (1972): Experimental brain ischemia: Protection from irreversible damage with a rapid-acting barbiturate (Methahexital). *Stroke*, 3:726–732.

Chapter 29

Increased Intracranial Pressure and Cerebral Edema

Intracranial pressure (IP) results from the overall effects of the various intracranial components, including the volume of cerebrospinal fluid (CSF), the blood volume, and the total volume of brain and other tissue. The relationship between the total volume of these components and the resulting IP is defined by the Monro-Kellie hypothesis. Since the volume of the intradural space is virtually constant (nonexpandable), and the contents are nearly noncompressible, any increase in volume of one or more component within the intradural space must result in an increase in IP. Were it not for the fact that some compensation of volume is possible, any increase in volume within the intradural space would cause a linear increase in pressure. Fortunately, some degree of compensation can occur by the following mechanisms: (a) decrease in CSF, (b) decrease of the intravascular volume, especially venous volume, and (c) decrease in brain volume. Obviously, the rate at which changes of intracranial contents occur is a major factor. A rapid increase, such as that caused by a rapidly expanding hematoma, does not allow for compensation by these mechanisms. In contrast, a slowly growing brain tumor may result in alterations in brain and CSF volume without a significant increase in IP. Within the limits of compensation, alterations in the total volume of the intracranial contents do not increase IP; above this, even a small increase in the intracranial contents will cause a large increase in IP. This is illustrated by the pressure-volume graph (Fig. 1), as originally shown by Langfitt (13).

Cerebral edema is only one of the factors that can result in increased intracranial volume and IP. Pharmacologically, this is the most important factor; at times, it can respond to various therapeutic agents. Following the work of Klatzo (11), experimental studies on cerebral edema in a number of models have defined three separate histologic types of cerebral edema: (a) vasogenic, (b) cytotoxic, and (c) interstitial. Vasogenic edema is caused by injury to cerebral blood vessels, especially the blood-brain barrier. The altered function of the blood-brain barrier results in the accumulation of fluid within the brain parenchyma. This type of edema predominantly involves the white matter and is characterized by swelling of both extracellular spaces and cells. The latter occurs primarily in glial components. As a result of the altered permeability of the blood-brain barrier, the edema fluid is essentially a plasma filtrate, which includes serum proteins. Injury to the cerebro-

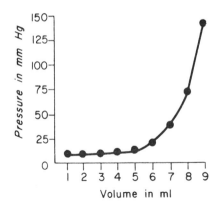

FIG. 1. Effect of volume on pressure in a closed system shows the increase in pressure as water is added to a supratentorial extradural balloon.

vasculature resulting in vasogenic edema is usually seen in focal disease processes and frequently occurs in the vicinity of brain tumors or focal infections.

In contrast, cytotoxic edema is caused by a primary injury to the brain itself and not its vasculature and may involve the gray or white matter, depending on the type of the cytotoxic state. Swelling of various cellular tissue components is characteristic of cytotoxic edema, but the blood-brain barrier per se may be uninvolved. This variant of cerebral edema is typically seen in anoxic injury where diffuse intra- and extracellular accumulation of fluid occurs (plasma or plasma proteins).

Interstitial edema is seen with pseudotumor cerebri (benign intracranial hypertension) and experimental triethyltin intoxication.

There are distinct pharmacologic differences among the three types of cerebral edema. Vasogenic edema, as classically seen with brain tumors, responds well to treatment with glucocorticoids. The mechanism of action of corticosteroids in vasogenic edema is not known. Repair of vascular integrity and the blood-brain barrier, inhibition of lysosomal enzymes, and activation of the Na/K ATPase pump have all been suggested (5). Cytotoxic cerebral edema is not affected by corticosteroid therapy but is improved by the various dehydrating agents. It must be kept in mind, however, that the greatest degree of dehydration occurs in the normal, unaffected brain tissue, not in the tissue swollen by cytotoxic edema. Interstitial edema responds to steroid therapy and to certain diuretics (carbonic anhydrase inhibitors).

CEREBRAL EDEMA AND BRAIN TUMORS

The successful treatment of cerebral edema associated with cerebral metastases was initiated by Kofman and his associates in 1957 (12). In this series, 20 patients with cerebral metastases were treated with prednisolone. Definite efficacy was observed in 14 patients (70%), in whom regression of neurologic symptoms and signs lasted from several weeks to several months. In one patient, clinical improvement lasted for more than 15 months. These investigators attributed the beneficial effect of steroids in these patients to the antiinflammatory effect of these agents, which was thought to reduce the edema. Since this initial study, it is accepted practice to treat patients with steroids for both primary and metastatic tumors of the brain in order to induce regression of associated edema.

The precise mechanism by which glucocorticoids reduced vasogenic cerebral edema associated with primary and secondary tumors is uncertain. Some investigators have suggested that the efficacy of steroids is due to increased urinary output of sodium and chloride; thus steroid therapy is simply another form of dehydration therapy. This is unlikely, as various steroids with different effects on sodium balance have proved to be effective. It has been demonstrated that the administration of dexamethasone before and after production of a subcortical lesion in cats reduces the extravasation of RISA, suggesting involvement of stabilization or maintenance of the integrity of the blood-brain barrier. It has long been known that vascular "leakiness" induced by inflammatory agents, such as histamine and kinins, is prevented by steroids. Steroids are also known to stabilize lysosomal membranes and thereby prevent the lysosomes from releasing hydrolytic enzymes, which would enhance any inflammatory-edematous process. The relevance of these actions of steroids to their beneficial effects in cerebral edema is unclear.

A variety of steroids, including prednisone, prednisolone, methylprednisolone, dexamethasone, and intravenous hydrocortisone have been used effectively in doses equivalent to 60 to 380 mg/day prednisone. Of these, dexamethasone is most widely used in the treatment of acute, severe cerebral edema. A number of different regimens are advocated; but 4 mg i.v. followed by 4 mg i.m. or p.o. every 6 hr for 3 to 14 days is commonly used. Galicich and French (7) and Weinstein et al. (22) have published typical reports of the use of steroids in patients with brain tumors.

The proven effectiveness of steroid therapy for edema seen in association with metastatic tumors has led to their widespread and often indiscriminant use in a variety of circumstances. This should be avoided because of the possibility of significant side effects, including duodenal ulcer, fluid retention, predisposition to infection, diabetes, and psychosis.

Although steroids are frequently employed in head injuries, their value is totally unproven. The lack of definite efficacy here may be related to the fact that steroids are of greatest value in vasogenic but not parenchymal edema, which is the predominant form of edema related to head injury. Alexander (1) studied 110 patients hospitalized because of acute nonmissile head injuries. Half of the randomized patients received dexamethasone. The use of steroids in these acutely head-injured patients, although probably not harmful, was not helpful. In contrast, it is generally accepted that steroids are of value in the treatment of pseudotumor cerebri (18).

CEREBRAL EDEMA IN STROKES

Glucocorticoids are frequently used in the treatment of patients with acute strokes (23). The data supporting the efficacy of steroids within the first 1 or 2 days of stroke are conflicting and for the most part do not demonstrate any steroid-related efficacy (2,18–21). After these first two days, steroids may reduce cerebral edema and simultaneously reduce neurologic deficits. This may be related to the onset of vasogenic edema because of an alteration in the blood-brain barrier. Whether reduction of vasogenic edema and associated clinical improvement preserves brain tissue from ischemic damage is unproven, since typical improvement following a stroke may itself be a result of decreased cerebral edema. Despite these limitations, Yatsu (23) suggests that for patients experiencing apparent progression of neurologic symptoms following the first day or two, not explained by extension of an intraarterial thrombus, steroid use is justified. He has proposed the schema presented in Table 1 for the use of steroids in patients with acute strokes. It must be recognized that the value of steroids in such patients remains unproved.

Patten et al. (17) reported significant improvement in steroid-treated patients in a double-blind study of 31 patients. If the three patients with intracerebral hemorrhage, who are all in the untreated groups, are excluded, there is little difference between treated and untreated patients. Tellez and Bauer (2,21) found no benefit and perhaps a deleterious effect in a double-blind study of steroids in both intracerebral hemorrhage and infarction. Although this was a well-designed prospective study, it includes many patients with massive cerebral insults whose prognosis is poor. While the use of steroids in patients with cerebral infarction whose deterioration seems to be related to cerebral edema (which may in part by vasogenic) may be justifiable, there is no basis for the use of steroids in intraparenchymal hemorrhages.

DEHYDRATING AGENTS

Three hyperosmolar dehydrating agents—urea, mannitol, and glycerol—are used to decrease raised IP, especially when the increased IP is associated with a threat

TABLE 1. *Use of steroids in cerebral infarction*[a]

Indications: To attempt to reduce clinically significant cerebral edema associated with infarction. The occurrence of such edema is suggested by clinical symptoms and signs of elevated IP, increasing neurologic deficits, and herniation syndromes occurring 24 to 72 hr after the initial stroke

Rationale: To decrease the vasogenic component of cerebral edema

Mechanism of Action: Uncertain, but possibly related to restoration of vascular integrity and stabilization of lysosomes

Dosage of Steroids: After first day, at a time of expected blood-brain barrier breakdown, use "long-acting" steroids for sustained effect in doses effective to reduce edema associated with brain tumors: 8 to 10 mg dexamethasone i.v. followed by 4 mg every 6 hr, tapered and discontinued after 7 to 10 days

Contraindications and Cautions: Routine or immediate use of steroids in stroke is not indicated; in the absence of vasogenic edema, clinical studies show no benefit

[a]Adapted with permission from Yatsu (23).

of herniation. These agents dehydrate the brain, as well as other tissues, by creating a rapid and sustained osmolal gradient between the plasma and the various tissues. Each of these agents acts by this same mechanism, although they differ in their distribution and metabolism. All are effective as hypertonic solutions because of their osmotic effect in reducing the water content of the brain. Such agents would be expected to be of greatest benefit in cytotoxic edema. Although these diuretics are effective and generally safe, certain problems must be recognized. There is a variable degree of rebound with these agents, and their efficacy is often of limited duration. The term "rebound" is used to describe an exacerbation of symptoms when the hyperosmolar agent is discontinued. Urea and glycerol are associated with rebound because they readily diffuse into cells. While mannitol is retained extracellularly, it is also associated with similar problems because of idiogenic osmoles. When using hyperosmolar agents on a chronic basis, the dehydrating effectiveness is lost because the brain apparently has mechanisms that increase its cellular osmolality by the creation of what have been termed idiogenic osmoles (8). It is as if brain cells will maintain cellular volume and adjust osmolality in order to preserve function (6).

These agents must be used with caution in many conditions, since rapid reduction in intracranial contents can produce an intracranial space which may then become filled with blood. These agents must be used with extreme caution in patients with renal insufficiency. Despite these precautions, the dehydrating agents may be effective in a variety of disorders that cause generalized increased IP. Table 2 shows the usual dose, route of administration, and time course of effect of these agents.

The basis for the use of hyperosmolar agents in the management of patients with acute strokes, particularly thrombotic infarctions and intracerebral hemorrhages, is the occurrence of cerebral edema, which can be life-threatening. If the patient does not manifest herniation, edema itself does not cause any irreversible brain damage. Since there is no evidence that dehydrating agents are of any value in nonherniating

TABLE 2. *Dehydrating agents*[a]

Drug	Urea	Mannitol	Glycerol
Dose	1.0–1.5 g/kg	1.5–3.0 g/kg	0.5–1.5 g/kg
Mode of administration	q 5–6 hr i.v.	q 4–6 hr i.v.	q 4–6 hr i.v. (10%)
Onset of action	10 min	20–30	Within 30 min
Peak of action	20–30	30–60	30 min (i.v.) 30–60 min (p.o.)
Duration of action	2–6 hr	3–8 hr	24–48 hr (i.v)
Secondary increase IP (rebound)	Yes	See text	Yes
Mechanism of reduction of increased IP	Osmotic gradient	Osmotic gradient	Osmotic gradient
Contraindications	Severe renal or hepatic damage, intracranial hemorrhage	Severe renal or hepatic damage, intracranial hemorrhage	Severe dehydration, intracranial hemorrhage

[a]Adapted with permission from Prockop (18).

stroke syndromes (6), there is no clinical indication for their use in this situation. Overall, the major short-term value of these agents is in rapidly progressive increased IP and herniation associated with mass lesions in which a surgical procedure to remove part of the mass can be carried out following the acute effect of the dehydrating agent.

Urea has been used to reduce increased IP clinically since the initial report of Javid and Settlage (10). The effect of urea is due to its osmotic activity and is dependent on the differential permeability of the blood-brain barrier to water, which is high, and to urea, which is low. As a result of this, urea causes loss of fluid from the brain and from the CSF, which results in a fall in IP (16). Urea is potent in causing a differential osmotic gradient because of its molecular weight of 60, its slow rate of elimination from the blood, and its relatively low permeability through the blood-brain barrier. Since urea eventually does cross the blood-brain barrier and enters cells within the brain, rebound can occur, especially following discontinuation of therapy. When administration is decreased or discontinued, renal elimination will eventually produce a condition in which the concentration of urea is greater in the brain than in the blood; a shift of fluid into the brain with an accompanying increase in IP (rebound) then can occur.

Mannitol has a molecular weight of 182.17. This osmotic disadvantage in relation to urea may be countered, at least in part, by the fact that mannitol does not cross the blood-brain barrier. Theoretically, this should prevent rebound; clinically, however, rebound does occur, probably as a result of the formation of idiogenic osmoles. The rapid renal clearance of mannitol makes its duration of action shorter than that of urea.

Of the dehydrating agents, glycerol has received the most attention in recent years. Despite its efficacy, any advantages of this agent have not been definitely established. Scattered reports of individual patients or small series have shown efficacy often for longer than the few days that can be achieved with mannitol or urea (3). The major toxic side effects are hemolysis, hemoglobinuria, and renal failure, which can be prevented, since they are a function of concentration and are seen only with intravenous administration. Glycerol can be given orally, by nasogastric tube, or intravenously. Oral glycerol is generally considered safe. Nausea and vomiting induced by the sweet taste of glycerol can be severe enough to require its discontinuation. This potential problem can be circumvented by disguising the taste with orange juice or analogous flavored vehicles.

As Prockop (18) has pointed out, glycerol has potential advantages. Urea and mannitol cannot be used chronically. Steroids, while effective in cerebral edema and more effective than glycerol in the edema caused by neoplasm and pseudotumor cerebri, also cause numerous problems which limit their chronic use (3,15). Despite the enthusiasm of many investigators, neither the acute nor the chronic efficacy of glycerol has been definitely proven.

BENIGN INTRACRANIAL HYPERTENSION

Although published data are limited, pharmacologic approaches have for the most part replaced such invasive techniques as serial lumbar punctures, subtemporal decompressions, and various shunting procedures in the treatment of benign intracranial hypertension. The pharmacologic regimen includes glucocorticoids, acetazolamide, and occasionally osmotic agents. We regard dexamethasone, or analogous steroids, as the drug of choice and use acetazolamide only in patients, such as diabetics, in whom the risk of steroids is too great. Acetazolamide does decrease the production of CSF in animals and has proven efficacious in this disorder. We have never had to use any osmotic agents, but oral glycerin has been reported to have efficacy in one series (15). Greer (8) suggests that no pharmacologic therapy is of definite benefit; but since the widespread use of steroids, no patient has required decompressive surgery.

BIBLIOGRAPHY AND *SELECTED REVIEWS

1. Alexander, E. (1972): Medical management of closed head injuries. *Clin. Neurosurg.*, 19:240–250.
2. Bauer, R. B., and Tellez, H. (1973): Dexamethasone as treatment in cerebrovascular disease. 2. A controlled study in acute cerebral infarction. *Stroke*, 4:547.
3. Cantore, G., Guidetti, B., and Virno, M. (1964): Oral glycerol for the reduction of intracranial pressure. *J. Neurosurg.*, 21:278–283.
*4. Fauci, A. S., Dale, D. C., and Balow, J. E. (1973): Glucocorticoid therapy: Mechanisms of action and clinical considerations. *Ann. Intern. Med.*, 84:304.
5. Fishman, R. A. (1974): Cell volume, pumps, and neurologic function: Brain's adaption to osmotic stress. In: *Brain Dysfunction in Metabolic Disorders*, edited by F. Plum, vol. 53, pp. 159–171. Raven Press, New York.
*6. Fishman, R. A. (1975): Brain edema. *N. Engl. J. Med.*, 293:706–711.
7. Galicich, J. H., and French, L. A. (1961): Use of dexamethasone in the treatment of cerebral edema resulting from brain tumors and brain surgery. *Am. Practitioner*, 12: 169–174.
8. Greer, M. (1976): Benign intracranial hypertension. In: *Handbook of Clinical Neurology, Vol. 16*, edited by P. J. Vinken and G. W. Bruyn, pp. 150–168. North Holland, Amsterdam.
9. Guisado, R., Tourtellotte, W. W., Arieff, A. I., Tomiyasu, U., Mishra, S. K., and Schotz, M. C. (1975): Rebound phenomenon complicating cerebral dehydration with glycerol. *J. Neurosurg.*, 42:226–228.
10. Javid, M., and Settlage, P. (1956): Effect of urea on cerebrospinal fluid pressure in human subjects; preliminary report. *JAMA*, 160:943–949.
11. Klatzo, I. (1967): Presidential address. Neuropathological aspects of brain edema. *J. Neuropathol. Exp. Neurol.*, 26:1–14.
12. Kofman, S., Garvin, J. S., Nagamani, D., and Taylor, S. G., III. (1957): Treatment of cerebral metastases from breast carcinoma with prednisolone. *JAMA*, 163:1473.
13. Langfitt, T. W. (1968): Increased intracranial pressure. *Clin. Neurosurg.*, 16:436–471.
*14. Langfitt, T. W. (1973): Summary of First International Symposium on Intracranial Pressure, Hanover, Germany, July 27–29, 1972. *J. Neurosurg.*, 38:541–544.
15. Newkirk, T. A., Tourtellotte, W. W., and Reinglass, J. L. (1972): Prolonged control of increased intracranial pressure with glycerin. *Arch. Neurol.*, 28:95–96.
16. Pappius, H. M., and Dayes, L. A. (1965): Hypertonic urea: Its effects on the distribution of water and electrolytes in normal and edematous brain tissue. *Arch. Neurol.*, 13:395–402.
17. Patten, B. M., Mendell, J., Bruun, B., Curtin, W., and Carter, S. (1972): Double-blind study of the effects of dexamethasone on acute stroke. *Neurology*, 22:377–383.
*18. Prockop, L. (1976): The pharmacology of increased intracranial pressure. In: *Clinical Neuropharmacology, Vol. 1*, edited by H. L. Klawans, pp. 147–172. Raven Press, New York.
19. Rubinstein, M. K. (1965): The influence of adrenocortical steroids on severe cerebrovascular accidents. *J. Nerv. Ment. Dis.*, 141:291.
20. Russek, H. I., Russek, A. S., and Zohman, B. L. (1955): Cortisone in immediate therapy of apoplectic stroke. *JAMA*, 159:102.
21. Tellez, H., and Bauer, R. B. (1973): Dexamethasone as treatment in cerebrovascular disease. I. A controlled study in intracerebral hemorrhage. *Stroke*, 4:541.

22. Weinstein, J. D., Toy, F. J., and Jaffe, M. E. (1973): The effect of dexamethasone on brain edema in patients with metastatic brain tumors. *Neurology*, 23:121–129.
*23. Yatsu, F. M. (1977): Pharmacologic basis of acute stroke therapy. In: *Clinical Neuropharmacology, Vol. 2*, edited by H. L. Klawans, pp. 113–150. Raven Press, New York.

Chapter 30

Toxicity of Centrally Acting Anticholinergic Agents

Literally hundreds of drugs with known anticholinergic properties capable of producing serious neuropsychiatric side effects are presently in use either as prescription or nonprescription (over-the-counter) items. Table 1 lists most of the more commonly used anticholinergic agents. Exposure to a variety of botanical toxins

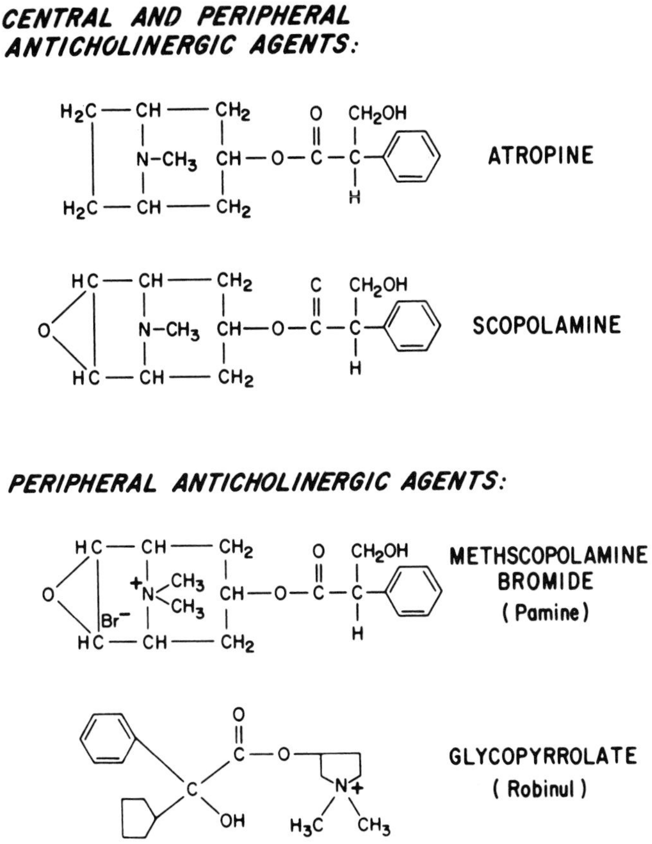

CENTRAL AND PERIPHERAL ANTICHOLINERGIC AGENTS:

ATROPINE

SCOPOLAMINE

PERIPHERAL ANTICHOLINERGIC AGENTS:

METHSCOPOLAMINE BROMIDE (Pamine)

GLYCOPYRROLATE (Robinul)

FIG. 1. Commonly available reversible anticholinesterase inhibitors.

TABLE 1. *Commonly used drugs with central anticholinergic properties*

Antidepressants	Belladonna alkaloids
Amitriptyline	Atropine
Desipramine	Homatropine
Doxepin	Hyoscine
Imipramine	Hyocyamus
Nortriptyline	Scopolamine
Protriptyline	Proprietary drugs (hypnotics, analgesics,
Antipsychotic drugs	antiasthmatics)
Phenothiazines, especially clozapine	Asthma-Dor (belladonna or
and thioridazine	stramonium alkaloids)
Antihistamines	Compoz (scopolamine, methapyriline,
Chlorpheniramine	pryilamine)
Diphenhydramine	Donnagel (belladonna)
Orphenidrine	Endotussin (homatropine)
Promethazine	Excedrin-PM (methapyrilene)
Ophthalmic preparations	Sleep-Eze (scopolamine,
Atropine 1% ophthalmic solution	methapyriline)
Cyclopentolate	Sominex (scopolamine, methapyriline)
Tropicamide	Travalex (scopolamine)
Antispasmodics	Stramonium (frequently used to
Clidinium	adulterate street drugs)
Antiparkinson agents	Numerous other antihistaminics,
Benztropine	antispasmodics, antiparkinson
Biperiden	drugs, ophthalmic preparations, and
Ethopropazine	many proprietary sedatives are
Procyclidine	capable of producing clinical findings
Trihexyphenidyl	of anticholinergic toxicity.

(Table 2) can produce the same syndrome as can stramonium, which is frequently used to cut street drugs. Although the toxicity produced by these agents is directly dose related and therefore on a continuum ranging from mild to moderate to severe, two separate syndromes can be differentiated. The first is seen in patients taking amounts of the offending agents that are fairly close to or within the usual effective dose and also includes the usual presentation of patients using anticholinergics as drugs of abuse. It must be kept in mind that this syndrome can and does occur with therapeutic doses in susceptible individuals. Older patients, especially those with any degree of dementia, are particularly prone to develop toxicity with average or even low therapeutic doses. Toxicity also can result from the additive effects of multiple drugs with antimuscarinic properties.

The syndrome of anticholinergic toxicity usually combines peripheral antimuscarinic (antiparasympathetic) manifestations and central nervous system intoxication. Table 3 lists the common manifestations of central anticholinergic toxicity in their approximate order of increasing toxicity, although exceptions to this order are not uncommon. The peripheral manifestations of anticholinergic toxicity are listed in Table 4. Mydriasis and the various vagolytic manifestations may not be as striking in central anticholinergic toxicity due to tricyclic antidepressants or antiparkinson agents as they are in toxic reactions to belladonna and other naturally occurring alkaloids or ophthalmic preparations, possibly because the former agents have been selected for their central activity.

The second clinical syndrome occurs with massive overdosage. It is usually a result of a suicide attempt using tricyclic antidepressants or accidental overdosage in children. Such patients are frequently comatose with myoclonus, seizures, choreoathetosis, severe cardiac arrhythmias, and respiratory difficulties.

TABLE 2. *Natural sources of anticholinergic toxins*

Amanita muscaria and related mushrooms
Bittersweet (*Solanum dulcamera*)
Black nightshade (*Solanum nigrum*)
Deadly nightshade (*Atropa belladonna*)
Henbane (*Hyoscyamus niger*)
Jerusalem cherry (*Solanum pseudocapsicum*)
Jimsonweed, "locoweed," thornapple, Jamestown weed, cockleburr (*Datura stramonium*)
Fantana, wild sage (*Fantana camara*)
Mandrake (*Mandragora officinarum*)
Potato leaves, sprouts, tubers (*Solanum tuberosum*)
Rabbits and fowl that have fed recently on henbane or other sources
Tomatoes from plants grafted to Jimsonweed
Wild tomato (*Solanum carolinense*)

TABLE 3. *Common signs of central anticholinergic toxicity*

Anxiety	Disorientation
Agitation, restlessness, and insomnia	Delirium
Blocked or arrested speech	Dysarthria
Short-term memory loss	Ataxia
Hallucinations usually visual	Lethargy
Restless, purposeless overactivity	

Reversible anticholinesterase agents have been used successfully to reverse the peripheral muscarinic manifestations. All these agents, with the exception of physostigmine (eserine) salicylate, are charged quartenary ammonium molecules which do not cross the blood-brain barrier. Physostigmine salicylate is a tertiary amine which readily crosses the blood-brain barrier and can increase cholinergic activity both centrally and peripherally. In 1958, Forrer and Miller (3) described the ability of this agent to reverse both the central and peripheral effects of huge doses of atropine. Despite numerous reports of the efficacy of physostigmine in this syndrome, it is still not universally realized that physostigmine can enter the brain to antagonize the central toxicity of anticholinergic agents. Although the use of physostigmine is taken for granted in many teaching hospitals, it is often not used in patients with central anticholinergic toxicity (4,5).

TABLE 4. *Signs and symptoms of peripheral antimuscarinic toxicity*

Dry mucous membranes	Scleral injection
Dilated, poorly reactive pupils with blurred vision and photophobia	Increased temperature
	Urinary retention
Flushed, warm, dry skin	Reduced bowel motility
Tachycardia and tachyarrhythmias	

TABLE 5. *Cholinergic toxicity of physostigmine*

Central: Confusion, seizures, nausea and vomiting, myoclonus, hallucinations; these often occur only after a period of initial clinical improvement of central anticholinergic toxicity.
Peripheral: Bradycardia, miosis, increased mucosal secretions, copius bronchial secretions, dyspnea, tears, sweating, diarrhea, abdominal colic, biliary colic, urinary frequency or urgency.

Physostigmine has been shown to be of value both diagnostically and therapeutically in both mild to moderate and severe central toxicity (1,2,6). The usual test dose in adults is 1 to 2 mg i.m. or slow i.v., which can be repeated if needed after 30 min; in children, it is 0.5 to 1.0 mg. Physostigmine itself can produce both central and peripheral side effects (Table 5). The latter can be prevented or treated by the use of quartenary anticholinergic agents, which do not cross the blood-brain barrier, e.g., methylscopolamine and glycophyrolate.

The relative contraindications to the use of physostigmine include asthma or other respiratory disease, diabetes, gangrene, coronary artery disease, heart block, upper gastrointestinal ulcer, ulcerative colitis, mechanical bowel or bladder obstruction, glaucoma, pregnancy, hypothyroidism, myotonia congenita, and myotonia atrophica. It must be stressed that these are only relative contraindications, and the decision to use physostigmine must be balanced with the potential benefits and risks. The most serious acute complications of excessive or too rapid administration of physostigmine are acute respiratory embarrassment or heart block; the most common acute toxic responses are nausea, vomiting, and diarrhea. Rapid injection of large doses can also induce major motor seizures. Atropine sulfate should be available in case of clinically dangerous cholinergic excess; 0.5 mg can be given by injection to counteract each milligram of physostigmine administered (7). (For further specific details of the therapeutic use of physostigmine see ref. 5.)

BIBLIOGRAPHY AND *SELECTED REVIEWS

1. Burks, J. S., Walker, J. E., Rumack, B. H., and Ott, J. E. (1974): Tricyclic antidepressant poisoning: Reversal of coma, choreoathetosis, and myoclonus by physostigmine. *JAMA*, 230:1405–1407.

2. Duvosin, R. C., and Katz, R. (1968): Reversal of central anticholinergic syndrome in man by physostigmine. *JAMA*, 206:1963–1965.
3. Forrer, G. R., and Miller, J. J. (1958): Atropine coma. A somatic therapy in psychiatry. *Am. J. Psychiatry*, 115:455–458.
*4. Granacher, R. P., and Baldessarini, R. J. (1975): Physostigmine: Its use in acute anticholinergic syndrome with antidepressant and antiparkinson drugs. *Arch. Gen. Psychiatry*, 23:375–380.
*5. Granacher, R. P., and Baldessarini, R. J. (1976): The usefulness of physostigmine in neurology and psychiatry. In: *Clinical Neuropharmacology, Vol. 1*, edited by H. L. Klawans, pp. 63–79. Raven Press, New York.
6. Hollinger, P. C., and Klawans, H. L. (1976): Reversal of tricyclic overdosage-induced central anticholinergic syndrome by physostigmine. *Am. J. Psychiatry*, 133:1018–1023.
7. Rumack, B. H. (1973): Anticholinergic poisoning: Treatment with physostigmine. *Pediatrics*, 52:451–499.

Chapter 31

Use of Steroids in Neurology

Steroid compounds are used in treating a wide variety of neurologic disorders. Indications for their use are often empiric, and sound pharmacologic reasons for prescribing them sometimes cannot be found. In this chapter, the principles of steroid pharmacology are discussed, followed by sections on a number of specific neurologic conditions in which steroids are used. These include inflammatory polyneuropathies, including Guillain-Barré syndrome, Bell's palsy, multiple sclerosis (MS), and polymyositis (PM). The use of steroid drugs in treating cerebrovascular disease, increased intracranial pressure, and myasthenia gravis is discussed in separate chapters.

STEROID PHARMACOLOGY

Adrenocorticotropic hormone (ACTH) is a product of adenohypophyseal secretion and acts on adrenal cortex to release steroids, cortisol, corticosterone, aldosterone, and some weakly androgenic compounds. Naturally occurring sheep, pork, and beef ACTH contain 39 amino acids in a chain, and biologic activity relates to the nitrogen terminal portion of the molecule. In addition to the adrenal stimulatory effect, high doses of ACTH can induce ketosis and insulin resistance. It also induces darkening of skin, since the amino acid 1-13 sequence of ACTH is identical to melanocyte-stimulating hormone (α-MSH). ACTH produces central nervous system (CNS) pharmacologic changes in man; its administration is often associated with mood changes, either euphoria or depression. The chemistry of this effect is unknown. The CNS ACTH pharmacology related to the feedback system for regulation of endogenous ACTH and steroid secretion is better understood (7). Neural pathways converging on the median eminence of the hypothalamus are responsible for stimulating secretion of corticotrypin-releasing factor (CRF), a chemical manufactured in the neural endings of hypothalamic cells. When released, CRF travels in a portal system of vessels to the pituitary gland. Feedback control for CRF secretion may involve all three levels of the endocrine axis: adrenal cortical steroid levels, ACTH levels, and autocontrol from CRF concentrations.

As ACTH is destroyed by gastrointestinal proteolytic enzymes, it must be given parenterally. It is readily absorbed when given intramuscularly but also can be given intravenously. When administered rapidly by intravenous route, the drug is hydrolyzed in minutes; its plasma half-life is 15 min. Slow intravenous administration over 8 to 12 hr is the usual practice; intramuscular gel also is used, where absorption is slow and the drug effect more prolonged. ACTH is used far less than oral steroids in neurology since the latter are easier to administer, and the effect of one is not superior to the other (17). When the MS patient is hospitalized during an exacerbation of the disease, ACTH is still commonly used.

The adrenocortical steroids are derived from cholesterol and fall into three major categories: glucocorticoids, mineral corticoids, and androgenic compounds. Many naturally occurring steroids share properties of more than one category. The steroids used in neurology, except for controlling severe hypotension in conditions like Shy-Drager syndrome, are glucocorticoids; these compounds are the focus of this discussion. ACTH acts on cell membranes of adrenal cortex by stimulating adenyl cyclase and thereby the intermediary, cyclic 3,5-AMP (cAMP). cAMP stimulates steroidogenesis and may act between cholesterol and pregnenolone. As discussed above, under normal circumstances, rates of glucocorticoid secretion are controlled by ACTH levels in circulating blood.

The pharmacology of corticosteroids is complex and multidimensional. These drugs influence carbohydrate, protein, fat, and purine metabolism. They also alter water and electrolyte balance in various tissues via mild mineral corticoid effects. The steroid effects most pertinent to a neuropharmacology discussion are the activities of these agents on the muscular and nervous systems, as well as their antiinflammatory effects.

Steroids clearly alter muscle function, and wasting or diminished work capacity are prominent features of Addison's disease, where there is adrenocorticoid deficiency. This effect of steroids on muscles is not related to electrolyte or carbohydrate alterations but may be related to the important vasoactive aspects of steroid pharmacology via aldosterone. No primary steroid effect on normal muscle cell function or on neuromuscular transmission has been demonstrated (17). Steroid hypersecretion is also associated with muscle weakness, but again the pharmacologic basis for this phenomenon is secondary. Primary hyperaldosteronism is associated with marked hypokalemia, which leads to muscle fatigue. Myopathy associated with Cushing's disease or with high-dose chronic steroid medication is discussed below.

Clinical, electroencephalographic (EEG), and laboratory evidence suggests that steroids effect a number of CNS alterations (32). Patients with Addison's disease exhibit apathy and depression, effects usually reversed with steroid supplements. In patients treated with steroids for therapeutic reasons, elevation in mood that is not necessarily coincident with resolution of their medical problem is characteristic. In some patients, euphoria, restlessness, and insomnia with hyperkinesis are seen; a small percentage display depression or anxiety. Psychosis is rare but may be seen when the patient has a prior history of psychotic behavior. Cushing's syndrome is associated with a high percentage of neurotic and psychotic behavior patterns. That these behaviors are characteristic and reversible when steroid physiology is corrected suggests that these agents have CNS activity. The locus of such pharmacologic activity is not determined.

TABLE 1. *Relative antiinflammatory effects of various steroids*

Compound	Potency
Hydrocortisone (cortisol)	1
Tetrahydrocortisol	0
Prednisolone (Δ^1-cortisol)	4
6α-Methylprednisolone	5
9α-Fluorocortisol	10
11-Desoxycortisol	0
Cortisone	0.8
Corticosterone	0.35
Triamcinolone (9α-fluoro-16α-hydroxyprednisolone)	5
Paramethasone (6α-fluoro-16α-methylprednisolone)	10
Betamethasone (9α-fluoro-16β-methylprednisolone)	25
Dexamethasone (9α-fluoro-16α-methylprednisolone	25

Similarly, EEG changes usually involving diffuse slow wave abnormalities are seen in patients who are hypo- or hypercorticoid (49). These brain wave alterations resolve when the steroid physiology is corrected. Seizure threshold has been lowered in animals treated with cortisol; high-dose cortisone and ACTH have been associated with reversible seizures. Whether these effects relate to primary drug activity on CNS excitability or to secondary electrolyte and carbohydrate alterations in these patients is unclear.

The mechanism of steroid-induced CNS activity may relate to changes in cerebral blood flow, electrolyte changes, or primary interactions between drug and diffuse neural elements. No firm evidence suggests the latter, although the existence of the hypothalamic-pituitary-adrenal axis demonstrates that some CNS cells have specific sensitivity to steroids. Investigators are currently studying the issues of steroid receptors in an attempt to identify and characterize specific drug-membrane inter-action in the CNS. Whether steroids alter peripheral nervous system function is addressed below.

The major effect whereby steroids abate human neurologic disease relates to antiinflammatory effects. ACTH and steroids prevent or suppress the development of local heat, redness, swelling, and tenderness. Microscopically, this change is associated with an inhibitor of the early aspects of inflammation (edema, fibrin deposition, capillary dilatation, and phagocytic activity) as well as the later effects (capillary proliferation and collagen deposition). The steroid antiinflammatory effect is seen regardless of whether the causitive agent is mechanical, immunologic, or chemical; thus steroid response is not diagnostic of a specific etiology or even class of etiologies. Steroids stabilize membranes of lysosomes, and it has been hypoth-esized that this stabilization is the source of their antiinflammatory activity. The relative antiinflammatory effects of various steroids are listed in Table 1.

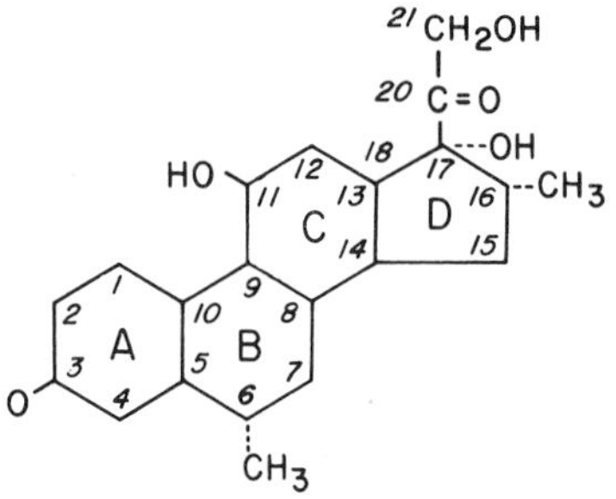

FIG. 1. Structure-activity relationship of adrenocorticosteroids (17).

Immunologically, steroids do not greatly inhibit antibody production in man. The union between antigen and antibody is not prevented by steroids, nor is histamine release. Although delayed T-cell hyperactivity is suppressed with high-dose steroids, the bulk of evidence suggests that steroids induce clinical benefits in neurologic disease because of generalized antiinflammatory effects not specifically immunologic in nature (37).

Cortisol and its analogs, with the exception of desoxycorticosterone, are absorbed by mouth. Prolonged effects can be achieved by intramuscular injections of suspensions or gels. Steroids exist in plasma in two forms: protein bound and free. Under normal circumstances, 90% or more of plasma cortisol is protein bound. Inactivation occurs with reduction of the 4-5 double bond hepatically or extrahepatically. Almost all steroid metabolites are excreted in the urine, with virtually no pulmonary, fecal, or biliary excretion.

Important structure-activity relationships exist for the steroids, based on the four constituent rings (Fig. 1). In ring A, 4-5 double bond and 3-ketone are essential for typical adrenocorticosteroid activity. Introduction of a 1-2 double bond enhances carbohydrate-regulating potency and diminishes relative sodium-retaining properties (prednisone). In ring B, 6α-methylation in man enhances antiinflammatory effects (6α-methylprednisolone). The presence of an oxygen at C-11 in ring C is indispensible for significant antiinflammatory effects. In ring D, 16-methylation enhances relative antiinflammatory effects. The potent antiinflammatory agents paramethasone and dexamethasone are both 16-substituted congeners. As a rule, all presently available antiinflammatory steroids are 17α-hydroxy-compounds.

IDIOPATHIC POLYNEUROPATHIES

Idiopathic inflammatory polyneuropathies are classified clinically into two general groups: those that remit and those that do not (31). Although sequential demyelination in peripheral nerves is common to all these conditions, the homogeneity of each subgroup and the difference in prognosis warrant their division. The pathophysiology underlying these conditions is relatively uniform, as is the presumed pharmacologic basis of steroid treatment.

Of remitting polyneuropathies, acute inflammatory polyradiculoneuropathy (AIPN), also known as Guillain-Barré syndrome, is the most common, estimated to occur at a rate of 1.5/100,000 persons (22). AIPN occurs most commonly in young adulthood and early middle age, preceded in almost half the patients by an antecedent infectious illness, which usually clears before neurologic dysfunction begins (6). The hallmarks of the syndrome are progressive, often severe, ascending weakness, complete tendon areflexia, high spinal fluid protein, possible cranial nerve and respiratory compromise, and substantial or complete spontaneous recovery. Weakness develops over hours or days but should not progress longer than 3 weeks; otherwise, alternate diagnoses should be considered. The severe motor compromise and short duration of progression are the features that distinguish this syndrome from others and hence indicate likely recovery. Only rarely do patients with this specific pattern have more than one episode; but if they do, they are considered as recurrent polyneuropathies.

Because natural recovery is anticipated to be substantial or complete, as long as respiratory and autonomic compromises are treated, pharmacologic intervention has aimed to hasten rate of recovery rather than to specifically alter final outcome. High-dose daily or alternate day steroids, 60 to 100 mg prednisone, have been advocated by some investigators. Others feel that because the medical side effects are hazardous, careful monitoring and symptomatic treatment of respiratory and autonomic dysfunction are sufficient (31,33). To address this controversy, controlled studies have been performed to evaluate the efficacy of corticosteroids in AIPN. Swick and McQuillen (38) showed that the time from onset of illness to recovery was significantly less in ACTH-treated than in nontreated patients with AIPN. Dosage was 100 U for 10 days; however, final extent of improvement could not be shown to be significantly better in patients receiving ACTH when compared to nontreated patients. Frick and Angstwurm (13) confirmed that rate of improvement was augmented by steroid administration.

A recent study, however, is contrary to these positive reports of steroid efficacy. Hughes et al. (20) reassessed 21 Guillain-Barré patients after prednisone treatment at intervals of 1, 3, and 12 months, comparing their resolution to that seen in 19 untreated patients. The control group showed consistently greater improvement at all time intervals. Six drug-treated patients were left with considerable disability, compared to only one control patient. The authors suggested that drug treatment may delay and/or limit improvement and warned against too-rapid acceptance of steroid benefit. While the number of reports favoring steroids far outweigh those opposed, the latter study emphasizes the importance of careful reevaluation of this syndrome and a continued search to understand the pharmacologic mechanism of action of steroids.

It is recommended that steroids be started early in the clinical course of AIPN and that they be tapered within 1 to a few weeks; protracted drug courses are unjustified (31).

Relapsing polyneuropathy initially appears similar to AIPN but is marked by the pattern of multiphasic disability (28). Epidemiologic studies suggest that antecedent illness is atypical for this group, and that the onset of disability tends to be slower (over several weeks), in contrast to the rapid progress of the former condition. Generally, during a new attack, old symptoms reappear, in contrast to the development of new focal signs; some patients, however, show a markedly varied clinical picture from one attack to another. As with AIPN, motor signs are prominent, areflexia is the rule, and cranial nerve lesions can be seen. CSF protein is raised during each attack. It is not well established whether protein levels return toward normal during remission.

Steroids in the dose range discussed above have been used in treating this type of polyneuropathy. Their influence on the pathophysiology of this condition has been controversial. Steroid induction has been beneficial in hastening recovery in patients with multiple relapses. In one study of 13 patients, all showed improvement coincident with steroid induction. Although some of these may have spontaneously remitted, the high percentage of responses suggests that steroids play some role in reversing disability. Additionally, eight of the 13 showed relapse as soon as the steroid dose was reduced and, in this sense, were termed "steroid dependent" (31). Significantly, four of these patients had previously shown spontaneous remissions; their dependence on steroids to maintain improvement was a new phenomenon. It is unclear whether this change represents the natural history of these patients' condition, or if the steroids themselves play some role in modifying the pattern of disability. Those patients termed steroid dependent usually remain on steroids for years but show excellent neurologic recovery.

The pathologic alterations seen in this condition have been studied. Some cases demonstrate changes seen with other chronic hypertrophic neuropathies, such as Dejerine-Sottas and Refsum's disease. Segmental demyelination is seen with onion-bulb formation, the latter change relating to repeated episodes of demyelination and remyelination. The question of familial transmission of this condition has been raised, but no epidemiologic data confirm this premise.

The final category of related idiopathic neuropathies is the chronic progressive type. This condition is approximately twice as common in males as females, and childhood onset is more prominent than in the other types of polyneuropathies (40). Some investigators refer to this condition as sporadic Charcot-Marie-Tooth disease; the clinical hallmarks are usually a mixed motor and sensory polyneuropathy, most marked distally with depressed tendon reflexes and occasionally hypertrophic palpable nerves. Spinal fluid protein may be normal or elevated. This chronic idiopathic polyneuropathy may rarely show signs indicative of CNS involvement or almost pure sensory compromise; in these cases, the question of exposure to neurotoxins or a remote effect of underlying carcinoma must be exhaustively studied. Steroids have been advocated in the treatment of chronic polyneuropathy, although in many studies, less than 50% of patients respond.

A single pathophysiology may underlie these different polyneuropathies. Thomas et al. (40) have summarized the evidence in support of delayed immunologic hypersensitivity. Waksman et al. (46) succeeded in producing a peripheral neuropathy in animals by the injection of homologous or heterologous peripheral nerve tissue combined with Freund's adjuvants. This neuropathy, termed experimental allergic neuritis (EAN), appears approximately 3 weeks after inoculation and is associated with a rise in CSF protein content. Histologic examination of the peripheral nerves of affected animals shows perivascular foci of inflammatory cells associated with segmental demyelination of nerve fibers and a variable degree of axonal breakdown. The clinical and pathologic features of EAN are similar to those of Guillain-Barré polyneuritis in man. Although not yet fully established, the disease mechanism probably is the same in both. EAN is similar to experimental allergic encephalomyelitis (EAE), in which demyelination of the brain and spinal cord occurs in relation to perivascular foci of inflammatory cells, following inoculation of homologous or heterologous CNS tissue combined with adjuvants.

EAN can be transmitted by sensitized lymphocytes but not by serum. The initial histologic lesion appears to be the accumulation of lymphocytes in the tissues, the demyelination being a later event. EAN is usually self limiting; the animals recover fully after a few weeks, provided they survive the initial illness. Some, however, follow a chronic relapsing course after either single or repeated inoculations (45). This situation likely provides an experimental model applicable to human cases. Considered together, these data are strong evidence that cell-related immunologic mechanisms are related in the induction and progress of certain polyneuropathies. Steroids may interrupt these mechanisms by their effects of lymphocytes. No direct activity on axonal or neurotransmitter mechanism by steroids has been identified, although preliminary evidence suggests a possible effect by the drug on demyelinated axons of the peripheral nervous system. Arnason and Chelmincka-Szorc (4) have proposed that steroids acutely improve conduction velocity in demyelinated nerve, an effect too rapid to be accounted for by antiinflammatory activity. No further corroborative studies are available.

IDIOPATHIC FACIAL PARALYSIS

Unilateral weakness of the facial muscles occurs when the seventh cranial nerve (facial nerve) is damaged. Disease at the pontine nucleus of the nerve causes the same distribution of facial paresis but is uncommon when compared to the more peripherally placed lesions. Tumors, abscesses, vascular disease, or trauma can cause this distribution of complete unilateral facial paresis, although these etiologies are rare. Bell's palsy is the term used to describe facial paralysis of undetermined origin which occurs acutely and has a usual natural history of good recovery (19). The popularized statement that Bell's palsy occurs in the United States every 13 min (20/100,000 persons per year) emphasizes the frequency of this affliction. Because the facial nerve travels through the internal auditory meatus and later gives off branches for taste sensation on the tongue, patients with Bell's palsy may complain of ipsilateral hyperacusis and decreased taste sensibility in addition to weak facial muscles.

The cause of Bell's palsy remains obscure, but modern microsurgical techniques have permitted *in situ* examination of the nerve during paralysis. Marked edema with the nerve under tension is consistently seen during the acute phase (8). The cause of the edema and its relationship, either causal or reactive, to the paralysis is unknown. It is known, however, that pressure on the seventh cranial nerve can compromise its vascular supply and precipitate or aggravate weakness. An ischemic basis for neurologic dysfunction is presumed to underlie Bell's palsy (24), possibly occurring from direct vascular dysfunction and thrombosis of the vaso nervora, the tiny vessels supplying the nerve itself. Alternatively, a primary inflammatory process, viral or immunologic, may induce edema with secondary vascular compromise. The result of both processes is anoxia to the nerve with resultant vasodilatation, transudation of fluid, and further pressure effects in the confined pathway of the seventh nerve.

Steroids have been advocated on the premise that they reduce swelling within the facial canal and thereby diminish vascular compression, so that proper oxygenation occurs (26). Theoretically, this would interrupt the pathologic cycle and inhibit further vasodilation. Adour and Swanson (2) studied the effect of oral prednisone on 194 patients with Bell's palsy compared with 110 untreated patients. Steroid dose was 40 mg for 4 days, tapering within 8 days. The treated group showed fuller recovery and fewer complications, although side effects related to drug treatment occurred in 4% of patients. Furthermore, the two groups were not entirely comparable, since severely affected patients accounted for 42% of the original control group and only 30% of the steroid group. Furthermore, the investigators were so convinced that prednisone was superior to no treatment that they abandoned a double-blind format midway into the study. Complete facial recovery was seen in 89% of steroid-treated and 64% of nontreated patients (4). Some investigators have suggested that the positive steroid effect is maximal if the treatment is started within the first few days of facial weakness; others find steroids to be of benefit at all stages of illness (3).

Not all investigators agree that steroids are selectively effective in Bell's palsy. May et al. (27) treated a small group of patients with vitamins; 65% recovered fully, compared to 60% in the steroid group. In a large prospective and randomized study by Wolf et al. (48), 88% of steroid-treated and 80% of nontreated control patients recovered full strength. The incidence of residual autonomic synkinesis from probable regenerating neural fibers was less prominent in the steroid-treated group.

The overall excellent prognosis of Bell's palsy with or without steroid treatment is confirmed in all studies. Approximately 15 to 30% show some residual weakness, but severe weakness is usually seen in only 2 to 4%. The pharmacologic basis of steroid activity focuses on general antiinflammatory or vasoactive properties, with no presumed activity on neuronal function per se.

DEMYELINATING DISEASES OF THE CNS: MULTIPLE SCLEROSIS

The demyelinating diseases represent an assortment of acquired conditions in which there is loss of myelin in the CNS, while other elements (axons, neurons, and blood vessels) remain relatively well preserved. MS, the most common of these diseases, has a prevalance of 40 to 60/100,000 in the United States population and is usually first apparent in individuals between 20 and 40 years of age (5). MS usually cripples rather than kills its victims. The pathologic lesions are discrete, irregularly shaped plaques of demyelination that are multiple and do not necessarily appear simultaneously. These features are the basis for the adage: "MS represents CNS multifocal disease separated in time and space." The most common neurologic problems in MS include: (a) loss of central vision, associated with demyelination of the optic nerve, (b) diplopia, often with weakness of the adducting eye and nystagmus of the abducting eye (internuclear ophthalmoplegia), (c) tingling paresthesia, especially with neck flexion (L'Hermitte sign) associated with demyelination in the dorsal column, (d) weakness and spasticity or ataxia associated with pyramidal and cerebellar dysfunctions, (e) lancinating pain in the distribution of the trigeminal nerve called tic douloureux, and (f) bladder incontinence.

Clearly, while many different syndromes are seen in MS, certain patterns are distinctly uncommon. Because this is a disease of CNS myelin, lesions of the peripheral nervous system would not be seen. Furthermore, aphasias, indicative of dominant cortical damage and "crossed syndromes" seen in brainstem stroke patterns, are possible but rare.

Treatment of MS involves integration of pharmacologic therapy, physical rehabilitation medicine, and psychologic counseling in many cases. Numerous drug combinations have been suggested to treat various aspects of neurologic dysfunction, bladder incontinence, neurogenic pain syndromes, flexure spasms, and vertigo (23). Such therapies do not aim to alter the demyelinating process itself but only to abate the resulting clinical problems. In contrast, steroids have been advocated as a specific putative treatment for the demyelination, although their precise mechanism of action relative to the disease is not clear (43).

Many investigators assert that the pathophysiology of MS relates to autoimmune mechanisms (44). The animal model for MS has traditionally been EAE, which relates cell-mediated delayed hypersensitivity. In these animals, steroids abate the condition, an effect that relates primarily to antiinflammatory effects. Steroids presumably reduce secondary, nonspecific inflammation; edema and pressure thus are aborted, and nerve function is thereby improved (42).

Spinal fluid gamma-globulin concentrations are usually elevated in MS patients, a finding that has been used to support the concept that immunologic mechanisms are intimately involved in the pathophysiology of the disorder (41). In human studies of MS patients, ACTH and steroids change oligoclonal IgG synthesis, but concentrations remain detectable even when patients clinically recover (42). The relationship of oligoclonal IgG to the manifestations of MS is not yet known, but these proteins may be disease "markers." That steroids alter their concentration suggests that these drugs may be interrupting primary aspects of the condition. Further details remain to be established.

The national cooperative ACTH study reported that treated patients in relapse with MS showed more rapid and complete improvement with short-term followup, but that in long-term studies, final outcome did not differ between ACTH and placebo groups (34). ACTH is usually given in doses of 40 to 120 U/day i.v. or i.m. for 7 to 30 days during an exacerbation. When therapy is given for only 1 week, no tapering of ACTH is needed; prednisone 60 mg twice daily for 10 days, then tapered at a rate of 20 mg/day, has been recommended (42). Prednisone, 100 mg/day orally, or decadron, 16 mg/day for 10 days with tapering and alternate day therapy afterwards for approximately 21 days, has been used with reports of success in acutely exacerbating MS (42). These latter regimens have not been studied under controlled, double-blind conditions; thus specific doses should not be considered as absolute or firmly established.

There is little to recommend ACTH over oral steroids, except that ACTH is given in the hospital where active physical therapy and often secondary psychiatric supportive care can be administered simultaneously. Oral steroids are usually synthetic glucocorticoids, which are readily absorbed from the gastrointestinal tract and are bound highly to proteins. Their plasma half-life is 1 to 3 hr. Methylprednisolone has a longer half-life than either prednisone or prednisolone; along with dexamethasone, it causes very little water and salt retention. These drugs easily cross the blood-brain barrier; 4 mg methyprednisolone is equivalent to 5 mg prednisone or 0.75 mg dexamethasone.

Noncontrolled studies have been performed using ACTH gel or corticosteroids (methylprednisolone, prednisone, or dexamethasone) for 1 to 2 years to abate chronic progressive disability in MS (42). These patients have been reported to show some abatement of their problems, but investigators caution against too-rapid tapering of steroid drugs in this group. A seeming exacerbation of MS can be seen if the steroid dose is lowered precipitously; often, slow tapering is required after long-term exposure.

The mechanism of steroid or ACTH activity on CNS function remains elusive. It is known that the drugs do have CNS activity, since sleepiness or excessive energy can be side effects of steroid administration. Whether they alter the pathophysiology of MS via direct CNS activity on axonal or synaptic function is unknown. The antiinflammatory activity of these drugs has already been discussed.

POLYMYOSITIS—DERMATOMYOSITIS

Idiopathic inflammatory muscle disease was identified in the 19th century. Four main groups of patients are now considered under the combined polymyositis-dermatomyositis (PM-DM) heading: (a) PM may occur alone and be acute with myoglobinuria, subacute or chronic, (b) dermatomyositis, or myositis with prominent skin changes, (c) PM often with skin rash but associated with an underlying malignancy, and (d) PM associated with evidence of other collagen vascular disorders (6,11). Because these categories often are overlapping and evolve from one into another, the descriptive subdivision should not be too strictly viewed. The unifying clinical and histologic picture of muscle involvement suggests that common pathogenic or pathophysiologic factors, not yet identified, may link these overlapping disorders (9).

The muscle involvement in this group of conditions is remarkably consistent, except in rare instances. Over several weeks, proximal muscle weakness becomes apparent to the patient, and ambient pain or tenderness with palpation may be present (11). Such tasks as rising from a chair, walking up steps, or brushing one's hair are characteristically difficult, since they require use of proximal muscle groups. Dysphagia may be evident, although other facial muscles and cranial nerve function remain normal. Deep tendon reflexes are preserved, and atrophy is seen only late. Cases of acute myositis can occur, especially in the pediatric population, and are associated with massive myoglobinuria and renal failure. In both adults and children, associated systemic alterations, including fever, arthralgias, and elevated erythrocyte sedimentation rate, suggest the diagnosis of inflammatory myopathies as opposed to muscular dystrophies. Muscle enzymes (creatine phosphokinase, aldolase, and, serum glutamic-oxaloacetic transaminase [SGOT]) are elevated, and the electromyographic picture is one of myopathy with small amplitude bursts of activity. Muscle biopsy shows intense inflammation in active lesions; in chronic PM, however, atrophy and only minimal inflammation may be evident (1).

DM may originally present as myositis without rash and only later demonstrate the clear dermatologic abnormalities. Violaceous or erythematous, edematous lesions especially involve the eyelids and periorbital skin, but periungual and upper chest regions may also show prominent skin changes.

The age distribution of DM suggests a bimodal curve, with a pediatric peak at ages 5 to 15 and a second peak of 50 to 60 years. One feature that distinguishes the pediatric group is the severe necrotizing vasculitis that accompanies the clinical DM. Intimal proliferation in small vessels and resultant infarctions in skin, muscle, and viscera may be fatal (25).

Underlying neoplasm has been estimated to occur in 7 to 34% of patients with PM or DM. In men over the age of 40, a tumor search is warranted in a patient with proximal weakness and muscle tenderness with or without skin rash. Nevertheless, as Bohan and Peter (6) stress, the association between the two phenomena has not been unequivocally confirmed, and hypotheses linking the etiologies of cancer to muscle disease are premature.

Patients with DM generally fare significantly worse than those with myositis alone. In the former group, approximately one-third of patients will recover with treatment, one-third will show remaining significant disability, and one-third will die. The disease does not last indefinitely. Usually, the initial episodes last 1 to 2 years, after which the disease is more quiescent. Death is usually due to pulmonary infection but may also relate to cancer (6).

The final syndrome is proximal myopathy occurring in the context of other collagen vascular disease, systemic sclerosis, systemic lupus erythematosis, rheumatoid arthritis, or polyarteritis nodosa. The muscle biopsy may not distinguish this group from the others. Occasionally, however, only focal lymphocytic infiltration, patchy atrophy, and perifascicular atrophy may be found, which establishes this myopathy as separate from PM.

The cause or causes of PM-DM are unknown. Humoral factors, which have been extensively investigated, do not appear to be primarily responsible. While anti-muscle antibodies are found in PM, these proteins are not cytotoxic and are seen in numerous other noninflammatory myopathies and neurogenic disorders (12,35). Hence their presence does not correlate with the necrosis, the inflammation, or the myopathy. Data regarding antigen-antibody complexes in muscles or vessels are conflicting, but IgG, IgM, and C_3 have been detected in some patients with PM-DM. DM has been seen in a patient with agamma-globulinuria suggesting that globulins are not prerequisite to the development of muscle dysfunction (18).

Stronger evidence is available to support the concept that cellular immune mechanisms may be involved in the pathophysiology of PM or DM. Repeated injections of muscle homogenates in Freund's adjuvant cause myositis and lymphocytic infiltrates in guinea pigs (10). Lymphoid cells from these animals are cytoxic to fetal muscle culture (21). Prednisolone inhibits this cytotoxic reaction. Viral infections have been implicated in the pathophysiology of these muscle disorders, since possible viral particles have been identified in biopsy materials. These findings are intriguing, but there is no firm causal relationship between viral infection and eventual myositis.

Corticosteroids are generally considered to be beneficial in the treatment of PM-DM. One problem in evaluating clinical data is that the natural history of the fused conditions is not well enough understood to conclude that any given therapy is efficacious. No large controlled studies testing steroids in these diseases are available. Perhaps in terms of steroid efficacy, the individual syndromes should be separated. With neoplasm-associated myositis, case reports suggest that resolution of myositis occurs after treatment of the cancer (47). Childhood DM has not been studied in a controlled setting, but dramatic reports of improvement after steroid induction strongly suggest that these drugs are beneficial in these cases.

High-dose prednisone (60 to 100 mg daily with changes to alternate day therapy as soon as sedimentation rate returns to a low range) is the usual recommendation. Over 2 to 3 months, 5 to 15 mg alternate day doses are characteristic (50).

The mechanism of action of steroids in treating PM-DM is elusive, but immunosuppression and antiinflammatory effects are suggested (29). When steroids do not improve a patient's status, other immunosuppressive measures are instituted, including methotrexate and chlorambucil (6). Steroids do affect muscle and in fact can be associated with a drug-induced myopathy. In patients with PM-DM treated with long-term, high-dose steroids, the original myopathy could have been treated with a second drug-induced myopathy superimposed. This differential diagnosis can be difficult and is addressed below.

TOXICITY OF STEROID MEDICATIONS

Two categories of toxic signs are seen in steroid-treated patients: those that result from (a) medication withdrawal and (b) continued high-dose exposure. Withrawal states replicate the clinical feature of Addison's disease and include fever, myalgia, arthralgia, malaise, and mental confusion. These problems are prevented by slow withdrawal of medication, which may require months of gradual dose tapering.

Prolonged therapy with steroids can be associated with complications that are nonneurologic or neurologic (5). Hyperglycemia and increased susceptibility to infections, including tuberculosis, peptic ulcers, and osteoporosis, are characteristic systemic side effects of steroid drugs, as well as the Cushing's habitus (moonface, central obesity, and hirsutism).

Neurologic complications include drug-induced myopathy, altered mentation, increased intracranial pressure, and secondary effects, including compressive neuropathic syndromes and vascular accidents. The myopathy has been briefly discussed and may appear clinically similar to PM with profound proximal weakness (9). Selective type II atrophy without inflammation is the classic histologic appearance at biopsy, but this pattern is not universal (16). The management problem in discriminating between PM or steroid myositis can be difficult when the classic biopsy patterns are not seen. Steroid-induced muscle changes relate to electrolyte alterations and decreased potassium in the muscle cells. Steroids also accelerate breakdown or decrease synthesis of essential muscle proteins (30).

Psychiatric alterations are frequent and can be dangerous. Nervousness, insomnia, mania, hallucinosis, and severe depression with suicidal ideation may be seen (39). No specific cellular effect explains the steroid-induced behavioral changes, and no toxic metabolite has been identified. Neither dose nor duration of therapy influences the likelihood of steroid behavioral changes, which can be seen early or late in therapy. The important factor is the patient's prior psychiatric status, since those patients with previous mental or emotional instability are more susceptible to psychiatric complications of steroids. Recovery from steroid-induced psychosis may require several months; slow withdrawal is needed to prevent steroid withdrawal syndromes, which also can be associated with behavioral changes (14).

Increased intracranial pressure and papilledema (pseudotumor cerebri) can be seen in infants and adults treated with chronic steroids. Although the pathophysiology of this syndrome is not known, it may be related to water intoxication (36).

Finally, steroids can induce neurologic dysfunction on a secondary basis, since they alter the osseous and hematologic systems. Vertebral compression with resultant myelopathies or compressive radiculopathies can occur, as can thromboembolic cerebrovascular accidents related to steroid-induced hypercoaguability (15).

SUMMARY

Present knowledge regarding steroid pharmacology in relation to neurologic disease is incomplete. Antiinflammatory effects and changes in immunologic physiology have been suggested, but these remain hypotheses; the primary basis of steroid efficacy has not yet been identified. Whether this primary effect is the same for the four neurologic conditions discussed or differs depending on the pathologic substrate is again undetermined. Research in these areas is actively underway.

REFERENCES

1. Adams, R. D. (1973): The pathologic substratum of polymyositis. In: *The Striated Muscle*, edited by C. M. Pearson and F. K. Mastofi, pp. 292–300. Williams & Wilkins, Baltimore.
2. Adour, K. K., and Swanson, P. (1971): Facial paralysis in 403 consecutive patients. *Trans. Am. Acad. Ophthalmol. Otolaryngol.*, 75:1284–1301.
3. Adour, K., Wingerd, M., Bell, D., et al. (1972): Prednisone treatment for idiopathic facial paralysis. *N. Engl. J. Med.*, 287:1268–1272.
4. Arnason, B. G. W., and Chelmincka-Szorc, E. (1974): Experimental peripheral nerve segmental demyelination induced by intraneural diphtheria toxin. *Arch. Neurol.*, 30:157.
5. Baker, A. B., and Baker, L. H. (eds.) (1975): *Clinical Neurology, Vols. 1–3*. Harper & Row, Hagerstown, Maryland.
6. Bohan, A., and Peter, J. B. (1975): Polymyositis and dermatomyositis. *N. Engl. J. Med.*, 292:344–347; 403–407.
7. Bransome, E. D., Jr. (1968): Adrenal cortex. *Am. Rev. Physiol.*, 30:171–212.
8. Cawthorne, T. (1946): Peripheral facial paralysis, some aspects of pathology. *Laryngoscope*, 56:653–664.
9. Coomes, E. N. (1965): Corticosteroid myopathy. *Ann. Rheum. Dis.*, 24:465.
10. Dawkins, R. L. (1965): Experimental myositis associated with hypersensitivity to muscle. *J. Pathol. Bacteriol.*, 90:619–625.
11. Eaton, L. M. (1954): The perspective of neurology in regard to polymyositis: A study of 41 cases. *Neurology (Minneap.)*, 4:245–263.
12. Fessel, W. J., and Raas, M. C. (1968): Autoimmunity in the pathogenesis of muscle disease. *Neurology (Minneap.)*, 18:1137–1139.
13. Frick, E., and Angstwurm, P. (1968): Zur Kortikosteroid-Behandlung der idiopathischen polyneurites. *Munch. Med. Wochenschr.*, 110:1265–1271.
14. Glatzel, J., and Penn, H. (1967): Klinisch-elektroencephalographische verlaufs suntersuchung einer psychose nach hoch dosierter ACTH. *Arch Psychiatr. Nervenkr.*, 209:365.
15. Goetz, C. G., Klawans, H. L., and Cohen, M. M. (1980): Neurotoxic agents. In: *Clinical Neurology, Vol. 2*, edited by A. B. Baker and L. H. Baker. Harper & Row, Hagerstown, Maryland.
16. Golding, D. N., Murray, S. M., Pearce, G. W., et al. (1966): Corticosteroid myopathy. *Ann. Phys. Med.*, 6:171–177.
17. Goodman, L. S., and Gilman, A. (1980): *Pharmacologic Basis of Therapeutics*, sixth edition. MacMillan, New York.
18. Gotoff, S. P., Smith, R. D., and Sugar, O. (1972): Dermatomyositis with cerebral vasculitis in a patient with agammaglobulinemia. *Am. J. Dis. Child.*, 123:53–56.
19. Hauser, W. A., Karnes, W. E., Annis, J., et al. (1971): Incidence and prognosis of Bell's palsy in the population of Rochester, Minnesota. *Mayo Clin. Proc.*, 46:258–264.
20. Hughes, R. A. C., Newson-Davis, J. M., and Perkin, G. D. (1978): Controlled trial of prednisolone in acute polyneuropathy. *Lancet*, 2:750–753.
21. Kakulas, B. A., Shute, G. H., and Leclere, A. L. F. (1971): In vitro destruction of human foetal muscle cultures by peripheral blood lymphocytes from patients with polymyositis and lupus erythematosus. *Proc. Aust. Assoc. Neurol.*, 8:85–92.
22. Lesser, R. P., and Hauser, W. A. (1973): Epidemiologic features of the Guillain-Barré syndrome. *Neurology*, 23:1269–1274.
23. McAlpine, D. M., Lumsden, C. E., and Acneson, E. B. (1972): *Multiple Sclerosis: A reappraisal*, second edition. Williams & Wilkins, Baltimore.
24. McGovern, F. H. (1968): A review of the experimental aspects of Bell's palsy. *Laryngoscope*, 78:324–333.
25. Mastaglia, F. L., and Walton, J. N. (1971): Histological and histochemical changes in skeletal muscle from cases of chronic juvenile and early adult spinal muscular atrophy (the Kugelberg-Welander syndrome). *J. Neurol. Sci.*, 12:15–44.
26. May, M., Hardin, W., Sullivan, J., et al. (1976): Natural history of Bell's palsy. The salivary flow test and other prognostic indications. *Laryngoscope*, 86:704–712.
27. May, M., Wette, R., Hardin, W. B., et al. (1976): The use of steroids in Bell's palsy: A prospective controlled study. *Laryngoscope*, 86:1111–1112.
28. Oh, S. J. (1978): Subacute demyelination of polyneuropathy responding to corticosteroid treatment. *Arch. Neurol.*, 35:509–516.
29. Pearson, C. M. (1966): Polymyositis. *Annu. Rev. Med.*, 17:63–82.

30. Pleasure, D. E., Walsh, G. O., and Engel, W. K. (1970): Atrophy of skeletal muscles in patients with Cushing's syndrome. *Arch. Neurol.*, 22:118–125.
31. Prineas, J. (1970): Polyneuropathies of undetermined cause. *Acta Neurol. Scand.* [*Suppl. 44*], 46:1–75.
32. Quarton, G. C., Clark, L. D., Cobb, S., and Bauer, W. (1955): Mental disturbances associated with ACTH and cortisone: A review of explanatory hypotheses. *Medicine*, 34:13–50.
33. Raven, H. (1967): Neuropathies and steroids. *Acta. Neurol. Scand.* [*Suppl. 30*], 43:1–28.
34. Rose, A. S., Kuzma, J. W., Kurtzke, J. F., Namerow, N. S., Sibley, W. A., and Tourtellotte, W. W. (1970): Cooperative study in the evaluation of therapy in multiple sclerosis: ACTH vs. placebo. Final report. *Neurology (Minneap.)* 20:1–59.
35. Stern, G. M., Rose, A. L., and Jacobs, K. (1967): Circulating antibodies in polymyositis. *J. Neurol. Sci.*, 5:181–183.
36. Sternberg, A., and Bierman, T. (1965): Corticosteroids, pseudotumor cerebri. *Arch. Dermatol.*, 92:746.
37. Stuart, F. P., and Fitch, F. W. (1979): *Immunological Tolerance and Enhancement*. University Park Press, Baltimore.
38. Swick, H. M., and McQuillen, M. P. (1976): Use of steroids in the treatment of idiopathic polyneuritis. *Neurology (Minneap.)*, 26:205–212.
39. Thiele, R. M. (1966): Kortikosteroids in der Neurologie. *Fortschr. Neurol. Psychiatr.*, 34:201.
40. Thomas, P. K., Lascelles, R. G., Hallpike, J. F., and Heuier, R. L. (1969): Recurrent and chronic relapsing in Guillain-Barré polyneuritis. *Brain*, 92:589–606.
41. Tourtellotte, W. W. (1975): What is multiple sclerosis? Laboratory criteria for diagnosis. In: *Multiple Sclerosis Research*, edited by A. N. Davison, J. H. Humphrey, A. L. Liversedge, W. L. McDonald, and J. E. Porterfield, pp. 9–26. Elsevier, New York.
42. Tourtellotte, W. W. (1977): Therapeutics in multiple sclerosis. In: *Clinical Neuropharmacology, Vol. 2*, edited by H. L. Klawans. Raven Press, New York.
43. Tourtellotte, W. W., Murthy, K., Brandes, D., Sajben, N., Ma, B., Comiso, P., Potvin, A., Costanza, A., and Korelitz, J. (1976): Schemes to eradicate the multiple sclerosis central nervous system immune reaction. *Neurology (Minneap.)*, 26:59–61.
44. United States-Japan Conference on Multiple Sclerosis (1976): *Neurology (Minneap.)*, 26:6.
45. Waksman, B. H. (1963): Experimental immunologic disease of the peripheral nervous system. In: *Mechanisms of Demyelination*, edited by A. S. Rose and C. M. Pearson, pp. 170–198. McGraw Hill, New York.
46. Waksman, B. H., Adams, R. D., et al. (1956): A comparative study of experimental allergic neuritis in the rabbit, guinea pig, and mouse. *J. Neuropathol. Exp. Neurol.*, 15:293–314.
47. Williams, R. C., Jr. (1959): Dermatomyositis and malignancy: A review of the literature. *Ann. Intern. Med.*, 50:1174–1181.
48. Wolf, S. M., Wagner, J. H., Davidson, S., et al. (1978): Treatment of Bell's palsy with prednisone: A prospective randomized study. *Neurology*, 28:158–161.
49. Woodbury, D. M. (1958): Relation between the adrenal corticocortex and the central nervous system. *Pharmacol. Rev.*, 10:275–357.
50. Yount, W. J., Utsinger, P. D., and Puritz, E. M. (1973): Steroids and polymyositis. *Med. Clin. North Am.*, 57:1343–1348.

Chapter 32

Myasthenia Gravis

Myasthenia gravis is an autoimmune disease that affects neuromuscular transmission. It is expressed clinically by fluctuating degrees of weakness of involved muscle groups, which occurs with a characteristic distribution of paresis. Extraocular muscles are the most frequently involved; bulbar, neck, limb girdle, distal limb, and trunk follow in decreasing order. The weakness is further characterized by the influence of fatigue, which invariably worsens the degree of paresis. Neonatal, congenital, juvenile, and adult onsets of myasthenia gravis are known to occur. The similarity between curare intoxication and myasthenia gravis led Jolly in 1895 to suggest that physostigmine, known to be of value in the treatment of curare poisoning, might be of value in the treatment of myasthenia gravis. The initial, often dramatic response of patients with myasthenia gravis to physostigmine focused scientific interest on the neuromuscular junction. Although the neuromuscular junction was recognized to be involved in the pathophysiology of this disease, the exact site of abnormal function was unknown. Initial interest was focused on presumed abnormal presynaptic mechanisms; in recent years, altered function and availability of postsynaptic acetylcholine (ACh) receptor sites has been identified as the basic defect in this disease.

To discuss the pharmacology of this disorder, it is necessary to understand some mechanisms of neuromuscular transmission. ACh, the neurotransmitter at the neuromuscular junction, is synthesized in the presynaptic nerve terminal and then stored for subsequent release within vesicles. When an electrical impulse is propagated down the nerve, ACh vesicles are released. The released ACh diffuses across the synaptic cleft, where it randomly interacts with postsynaptic ACh receptor sites. This interaction alters postsynaptic membrane permeability and results in electrical depolarization of that membrane to varying degrees. When ACh is released randomly without a specific presynaptic electrical impulse, the amount released and the degree of electrical depolarization of the postsynaptic membrane are less (miniature end plate potential). When presynaptic ACh is released in sequence with a presynaptic nerve impulse, the amount released and the degree of postsynaptic electrical depolarization are greater (end plate potential). An end plate potential usually triggers a muscle action potential, which is propagated along the muscle membrane. This muscle action potential subsequently invades the muscle and initiates excitation contraction coupling, and muscle contraction ensues. The effect of ACh at the ACh receptor is terminated in part by the activity of the enzyme cholinesterase and in part by diffusion. Interference with this sequence of neuromuscular transmission can result in weakness (Fig. 1).

The striking clinical finding that administration of anticholinesterase produces marked improvement in muscle strength in patients with myasthenia gravis brought attention to the neuromuscular junction. This observation did not clarify whether myasthenia gravis was a presynaptic problem with ACh release, a problem of overactive cholinesterase activity, or a problem of defective ACh receptors. Early studies reported no abnormalities in the activity of cholinesterase, nor has this been advanced as an etiologic factor in myasthenia gravis. Recent interest in acetylcholinesterase activity is discussed below.

Early electrophysiologic studies demonstrated smaller than normal miniature end plate potentials, which were interpreted as demonstrating smaller than normal amounts of spontaneously released ACh. This, coupled with reports that myasthenic end plate regions displayed normal sensitivity to ACh, led to the concept that myasthenia gravis was a disorder of presynaptic ACh release and storage. The advent of new techniques to evaluate the ACh receptor resulted in the finding that myasthenia gravis is related to defects in the postsynaptic ACh receptor. The introduction of alpha-bungarotoxin binding techniques (the toxin binds irreversibly

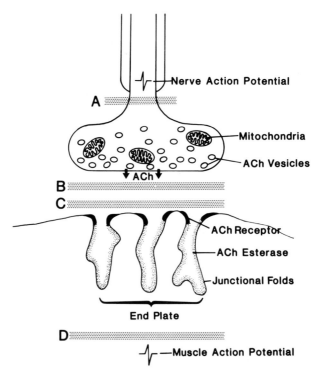

FIG. 1. Sequence of neuromuscular transmission. **A, B, C,** and **D** indicate potential sites for disruption of the normal physiologic process.

to the ACh receptor) has resulted in a quantitative and direct assessment of functional ACh receptors in striatal muscle. Patients with myasthenia gravis have a significant reduction in the number of ACh receptor sites when compared to nonmyasthenic controls (9). In addition, microiontophoretic studies demonstrated decreased sensitivity to ACh at the myasthenic end plates. Also, electron microscopic studies revealed structural changes in the end plate region of myasthenic muscle. These studies have clarified that the abnormalities in neuromuscular function in this disorder reside in the altered function of the postsynaptic ACh receptor site.

Circumstantial clinical evidence implicated involvement of the immunologic system in this disorder. Myasthenia gravis is associated with other autoimmune diseases (systemic lupus erythematosus, pernicious anemia, agamma-globulinemia, thyroiditis, rheumatoid arthritis). A large percentage of patients with myasthenia gravis have thymic abnormalities; and there is a favorable association between thymectomy and remission of myasthenic symptoms. The finding of alterations in the postsynaptic ACh receptor site led to investigations directed at determining whether or not autoimmune mechanisms might be involved. Several studies have reported detectable antireceptor antibody in the serum of myasthenic patients. The antibody titer was found to be weakly correlated with the degree of severity of the disease. When individual cases were examined, a correlation was found between total amount of receptor antibody and symptomatology.

The demonstration of immunoglobulin at the postsynaptic membrane is additional evidence in support of the role of antibodies in the production of the defect in myasthenia gravis. In fact, patients with thymoma had higher levels of antibody than those without. Thymectomy and/or immunosuppressive therapy led to reduced antireceptor antibody levels. Whether these humoral antibodies are a primary or a secondary phenomenon in myasthenia is uncertain. It has been suggested that the immune response is secondary to an initial event that damages the end plate region and triggers an antigenic response. This theory arose from the study of two patients with recent onset of myasthenia who had no IgG antibody to the receptor but had IgM antibody to the receptor. Over the course of a few months, IgG antireceptor antibody appeared, and IgM antireceptor antibody disappeared. This was suggestive of the immunization response and resulted in the postulate that the immune response is secondary (15).

The effect of the antibody ACh receptor interaction appears to be a blockade of the receptor. In addition, this interaction results in destruction of the receptor and produces an overall increase in the degradation of the receptor population. These circulating antibodies are probably responsible for the long-known, clinically postulated humoral transfer factor which is responsible for transient neonatal myasthenia.

Cell-mediated immune mechanisms also may be involved in myasthenia gravis. The frequent role of thymic abnormalities has been one source of circumstantial evidence that some cell-mediated immune mechanisms may be involved. It has been suggested that a break in immunotolerance occurs in the thymus in relationship to primitive myoid cells. Human thymus tissue was examined for the presence of

ACh receptors; none were detected in either normal or myasthenic thymus tissue, despite the finding that cultured thymus can grow out muscle fibers with ACh receptors present (19). Other evidence implicating cell-mediated immune responses includes alteration in lymphocyte-mediated reactions. An example of this phenomenon is the stimulation of lymphocytes from myasthenic patients when cultured with ACh receptors (11). The occasional finding of lymphorrhages (local collections of lymphocytes) in myasthenic muscle also suggests a role for a cell-mediated process.

The pharmacologic treatment of myasthenia is directed at altering aspects of both neuromuscular transmission and the immunologic response. Until recently, the mainstay of therapy consisted of the use of acetylcholinesterase inhibitors (Table 1). Since the postsynaptic ACh receptors are partially blocked by antibody, the usual amount of ACh released produces an ineffective or only partially effective response in the muscle, which is observed clinically as weakness. If cholinesterase, which rapidly inactivates ACh and terminates the ligand receptor interaction, is inhibited, ACh in the synaptic cleft may remain active for a longer period. This increased number of ligand receptor interactions may allow normal muscle activity, despite the reduced number of effectively functioning ACh receptors. This pharmacologic approach to treatment in myasthenia gravis, while often clinically effective, does not alter the underlying process affecting the ACh receptor.

Short- and long-acting cholinesterase inhibitors are useful in clinical practice. The shorter-acting inhibitor endrophonium (Tensilon®) is useful as a pharmacologic diagnostic test for myasthenia. The complete clinical details of the Tensilon test and the ancillary electrical diagnostic tests useful in the diagnosis of myasthenia gravis are beyond the scope of this chapter. Endrophonium is an extremely short-acting cholinesterase inhibitor, which produces enzyme inhibition within 10 to 30 sec; its action is reversed within 5 minutes. The test requires intravenous administration of the drug and the identification of a clinically observable and reliable end point (e.g., ability to open the eyes, amelioration of nasal speech). A test dose of 2 mg followed 60 sec later by a bolus of 8 mg is administered, and the clinical end points are observed. If the test is positive, clinical improvement, often of a dramatic nature, will occur within 30 sec. The Tensilon test also can be used to judge the adequacy of treatment with longer-acting anticholinesterases.

TABLE 1. *Acetylcholinesterase agents*

Generic	Trade name	Onset of distress	Duration of action
Pyridostigmine	Mestinon	10–30 min	4 hr
Neostigmine	Prostigmine	10–20 min	3–4 hr
Ambenonium	Metelase	20–30 min	4–5 hr
Endrophonium	Tensilon	30–60 sec	2–4 min

After the diagnosis of myasthenia gravis is established, the institution of the appropriate dosage of cholinesterase inhibitor therapy is an empiric judgment based on patient response. The most widely used anticholinesterase is pyridostigmine (Mestinon®), which begins to be effective 10 to 30 min after oral administration, peaks at 2 hr, and is over at 4 hr. It is usually possible to arrive at an appropriate dose strictly based on clinical response. Attempts have been made to correlate plasma pyridostigmine levels and therapeutic response. These studies have not demonstrated a positive correlation between pyridostigmine plasma concentration and clinical effect in myasthenia. In patients who were clinically stable, the plasma level of pyridostigmine ranged between 20 and 60 ng/ml despite an 11-fold difference in daily drug intake (60 to 660 mg/day). The investigators (4,5) concluded that the differential effective dosage reflects not only disease severity but also individual variations in drug absorption and disposition. At present, these plasma determinations are of doubtful clinical usefulness.

On occasion, a Tensilon test may be useful to assess whether or not maximally tolerable and effective inhibition of cholinesterase has been achieved. When this extra refinement of therapeutic adjustment is required, the Tensilon test should be performed at 2 hr after administration of pyridostigmine, at the time of its maximum anticholinesterase activity. The most common clinical mistake is to perform a Tensilon test either before or after peak action of the long-acting cholinesterase has been achieved. This invariably leads to a positive Tensilon test and the erroneous assumption that the dose must be increased. An additional danger inherent in this test is that a given patient may be underdosed with respect to one group of muscles but overdosed with respect to a different group of muscles. An overdramatic example of this might be interpreting the Tensilon test to increase anticholinesterase dosage to correct ptosis, while respiratory function declines in response to the increased dose. A sustained release preparation of anticholinesterase is available but should be employed only at bedtime when it is necessary to maintain early morning strength and to permit restful sleep.

Since it is well known that excessive cholinesterase ingestion can produce signs of cholinergic toxicity (Table 2) including voluntary muscle weakness, it occasionally becomes necessary to distinguish between cholinergic and myasthenic crises. Although this often can be done clinically, a Tensilon test can help to distinguish these two states. In myasthenic crises, Tensilon will improve symptomatology. If the patient is in a cholinergic crisis, Tensilon may exacerbate the symptoms. If endrophonium is used in this setting, all ancillary help and expertise to manage a respiratory arrest must be present. It is often simpler, more effective, and safer to manage an acutely ill myasthenic patient with respiratory distress by withdrawing all pharmacologic agents and mechanically assisting respiration rather than performing a Tensilon test in an ambiguous situation.

The chronic use of cholinesterase inhibitors often results in a situation in which the patient requires increased inhibitor therapy in order to improve functional strength. When anticholinesterase dose is increased, muscarinic cholinergic side effects may appear and become dose limiting. In this situation, it is often possible

TABLE 2. *Symptoms and signs of cholinergic toxicity*

Muscarinic symptoms and signs
   Salivations
   Abdominal cramps, nausea, vomiting
   Involuntary defecation
   Involuntary urination
   Sweating
   Lacrimation
   Bradycardia
   Hypertension
Nicotonic symptoms and signs
   Fatigue and generalized weakness
   Involuntary twitching
   Fasciculation
   Paralysis
Cholinergic CNS toxicity
   Confusion
   Ataxia
   Slurred speech
   Seizures

to administer an anticholinergic agent (atropine) in low doses to ameliorate unpleasant muscarinic side effects. There is an obvious danger in going too far with this approach, since the appearance of signs of cholinergic toxicity is an indication that the maximum tolerated dose is being approached. If the dose of an anticholinergic is used to entirely suppress these early symptoms, and anticholinesterase inhibitor therapy is advanced, cholinergic crisis, as discussed previously, could be precipitated.

An additional pharmacologic diagnostic test is the curare test. Since this involves potential risk to the patient, and useful, accurate alternatives are available, it is rarely employed. Nevertheless, it is illustrative of the postsynaptic ACh receptor deficit seen in this disorder. The test is performed by intravenously administering 1/10 the normal curarizing dose. Curare is a postsynaptic blocking agent; in a normal individual, the small dose administered has no effect. In a myasthenic patient who already has reduced numbers of functioning ACh receptor sites, however, the additional blockade of receptors will further decrease the safety factor and can result in weakness. Obviously, the degree of weakness produced can be variable, and the ability to support respiratory function is mandatory if the curare test is employed. The use of the regional curare test is an attempt to make this a safer test.

An entirely different although not necessarily separate approach to the pharmacologic treatment of myasthenia gravis is the use of steroids. As early as 1935, the potential usefulness of corticotropins was recognized. In the 1950s and 1960s, numerous reports of the experience of ACTH administration in patients with myasthenia varied greatly. The use of high-dose (100 U), short-course (10 to 12 days) ACTH was established as an effective but variable treatment in some severely ill myasthenic patients (10,26). The use of ACTH was often associated with severe exacerbation of weakness, often necessitating ventilatory assistance. Improvement in strength following ACTH was variable not only in the percentage of patients responding but also in duration of improvement.

The use of oral prednisone in the treatment of myasthenia gravis was introduced in the early 1970s. Early reports of its effectiveness in producing relief of symptoms were favorable. In fact, in the last decade, the overwhelming experience has been favorable, and more than 70% of patients have been reported to improve (7,12, 13,23). However, despite these reports, the pharmacologic mechanism of action and which myasthenic patients should receive this treatment remain unclear. The mechanism of action of prednisone in this disorder is unknown, although its beneficial effect is often related to immunosuppression. Few clinical data support this, and the use of prednisone has been another example of an empiric advance in pharmacologic treatment of a syndrome. There are two general approaches to pharmacologic treatment of these patients: (a) initial use of anticholinesterase and use of prednisone only in those patients who are treatment failures on anticholinesterases, and (b) use of prednisone as the first line of treatment with anticholinesterases only being added when needed as a supplementary form of therapy.

Initiation of prednisone treatment in these patients is also associated with exacerbation of weakness. Approaches to avoid this include gradually increasing the steroid dose and the alternate day prednisone plan proposed by Seybold and Drachman (23). Either can be employed. When prednisone is added to the treatment of a myasthenic patient already receiving anticholinesterases, signs of cholinergic toxicity (Table 3) may appear during the course of improvement, necessitating careful monitoring of all active pharmacologic agents. Although the rationale for the use of prednisone in myasthenia is not well understood, it is often proposed as a more logical approach to therapy since it is directed more closely at the "primary" cause of the disease (dysfunction of the immune system), as opposed to simply treating a secondary effect—the apparent lack of response to ACh.

Thymectomy, obviously a nonpharmacologic treatment, has been reported to produce favorable clinical response in 50% of patients within 5 years (21). Although the exact therapeutic mechanism involved in remission postthymectomy is also unknown, it has been proposed that its effect is related to the immunologic system. It is clear that the use of prednisone prior to thymectomy has decreased the surgical and postoperative morbidity of this procedure. This has been related to the induction by prednisone of remission or marked improvement in the patient prior to major surgery. The management of postoperative thymectomy patients also has been facilitated by preoperative prednisone therapy.

Other pharmacologic agents that have been used as minor clinical adjuvants include ephedrine, potassium chloride, calcium, and guanidine. These agents have been employed in clinical practice in some patients to further increase muscular strength in those being treated with anticholinesterases. These agents, although of relatively minor importance, are all felt to enhance acetylcholine release. Potassium chloride has also been proposed to act by replacing intracellular potassium lost

TABLE 3. *Drugs reported to precipitate myasthenia gravis or to induce a myasthenic syndrome*

Antibiotics	Psychotropics	Antirheumatics	C.V.	Anticonvulsants	Hormones	Miscellaneous
Colistin	Chlorpromazine	Chloroquine (?)	Procainamide	Phenytoin	ACTH	Acetylcholinesterase inhibitors
Kanamycin	Lithium	D-Penicillamine	Propranolol	Trimethadione	Corticosteroids	Methyoxyflurane
Streptomycin			Quinidine		Thyroid hormones	Tetanus antitoxin
Tetracyclines			Oxprenolol		Oral Contraceptives	
					(?)	
Gentamicin			Practolol			
Neomycin			Trimethaphan			
Polymyxin B						

during motor end plate depolarizations. Additional drugs proposed as adjuvants to therapy include theophylline and 4-aminopyridine. Theophylline has been reported to increase ACh release; a triad of theophylline, ephedrine, and neostigmine might offer clinical advantage, but no clinical evidence supports this (3). A new experimental drug that also results in increased transmitter release at the motor nerve terminals is 4-aminopyridine. This agent, tried in six patients with myasthenia, resulted in improved strength both alone and in conjunction with cholinesterase inhibition (16).

Other immunosuppressive agents, besides prednisone, have been tried on a more limited basis. 6-Mercaptopurine and azothioprine have been reported to be of benefit in a majority of patients (17,18). In fact, Mertens and colleagues (18) reported that 32 of 38 patients, including some thymectomy failures, had a favorable response to these immunosuppressives. In addition, five patients with myasthenia who, despite thymectomy, prednisone, and cholinesterase inhibitor therapy remained severely disabled, were treated with a combination of plasmapheresis, prednisone, and azothioprine. This combined therapy resulted in striking clinical improvement and an associated fall in antireceptor antibody titers (6). A different immunosuppressive therapeutic approach was employed by Pirofsky and colleagues (22), who used antihuman thymocyte antiserum globulin. They reported that eight of 10 myasthenic patients had some variable clinical response to this treatment, including remission of up to 2 years. These agents and techniques generally have not been used, except for unusual treatment failures with the more generally accepted pharmacologic and surgical approaches to myasthenia gravis.

Another novel approach to the treatment of intractable myasthenia was reported by Bingle et al. (2). Their patient was a 27-year-old female with thymic carcinoma and myasthenia. Despite oral neostigmine, pyridostigmine, prednisone, azothioprine, and plasmapheresis, she was still unable to sit up and still suffered respiratory embarrassment. The physicians employed a battery-operated infusion pump to deliver variable and continuous amounts of subcutaneous neostigmine, which led to resumption of normal motor activities.

Although it was mentioned earlier that abnormalities of cholinesterase do not play a major role in the pathophysiology of myasthenia, several circumstances indicate that altered activity of the esterase may be important. It has been recognized that as many as 25 to 50% of women with myasthenia may experience a cyclic monthly remission of their symptoms associated with their menstrual cycle. A recent investigation interviewed 12 female myasthenics and discovered three who had cyclic monthly remission. In these three women, assay of the activity of RBC acetylcholinesterase showed a marked reduction in acetylcholinesterase activity at the time of the menstrual remission of myasthenic symptoms. One conclusion of this study was that there might be altered neuromuscular acetylcholinesterase activity as well, which might explain the altered symptoms (25).

A new myasthenic syndrome, with abnormalities of acetylcholinesterase, has been reported (8). This patient's symptoms began shortly after birth and consisted primarily of generalized weakness, which was exacerbated by exertion and was refractory to anticholinesterase inhibitor therapy and guanidine. In an extensive clinicopathologic study, the major feature of this unusual myasthenic syndrome included electron microscopic demonstration of marked decrease in presynaptic nerve terminals, degenerative changes in the postsynaptic end plate region, normal concentrations of ACh receptors, and absence of acetylcholinesterase from the end plate region. In addition, total muscle acetylcholinesterase activity was markedly reduced.

Evaluation of the cholinergic system in myasthenia has also included examination of plasma precursors of ACh. However, choline concentration in myasthenia has been reported to be normal (24).

Since the mechanism of neuromuscular transmission is highly dependent on the proper metabolic function of nerve and muscle, as well as on the proper ionic conditions in the environment, it is not surprising that the administration of pharmacologic agents can sometimes unexpectedly interfere with this process. On the other hand, other than those pharmacologic agents specifically designed to alter aspects of neuromuscular transmission, it is relatively uncommon for clinically used drugs to cause dysfunction of neuromuscular transmission. Approximately 30 drugs, other than anesthetics, interfere with neuromuscular transmission. In addition, more than 200 cases have been reported in which pharmacologic alterations in neuromuscular transmission have resulted in clinical syndromes (23). A general proposal to explain drug-induced neuromuscular dysfunction proposes that the mechanism of action of the drug might involve four basic steps in the physiologic process of neuromuscular transmission (Fig. 1) (1). Drugs can interfere with presynaptic mechanisms either by altering the propagation of the nerve action potential (Fig. 1A) or interfering with ACh release (Fig. 1B). Drugs might also interfere with postsynaptic mechanisms by either blocking or interfering with the ACh receptor (Fig. 1C) or by interfering with electrical impulse propagation along the muscle membrane (Fig. 1D). When a specific drug produces a myasthenic-like syndrome in a given patient, an alteration exists in that patient of the usual excessive safety factor which allows for normal neuromuscular transmission.

Two separate types of myasthenic syndromes are induced. One is the precipitation or aggravation of myasthenia gravis; the second is the induction of a myasthenic syndrome. In the first instance, the special circumstance that has made the patient more susceptible to the specific drug is obvious: the presence of myasthenia gravis. When the patient has never before had myasthenia, the failure of the symptomatology to resolve when the offending drug is withdrawn is accepted as indicating that the patient presumably had subclinical myasthenia gravis. In the second instance in which a drug induces a myasthenic syndrome, patients have been previously normal, and the symptomatology resolves when the drug is withdrawn. Something must make these patients different from the general population; although this may be explained on the basis of age or unsuspected poor renal clearance of a specific drug, it does not provide an adequate explanation for most of these occurrences. The proposed mechanism of action and the drugs responsible for producing myasthenic-like syndromes are listed in Table 3. Although numerous preclinical reports have explored the action of various drugs on neuromuscular transmission, whether or not these reports are directly translatable to the clinical disorders induced by these same drugs is not clear; a much lower concentration of the drug is often found in tissue when it is used clinically.

In situations in which a pharmacologic agent induces a myasthenic syndrome, it is usually sufficient to withdraw the implicated drug. Symptoms will then abate, unless a precipitation of subclinical myasthenia has occurred. In more severe and dramatic instances (e.g., antibiotic-induced postoperative respiratory depression), respiratory support will be needed. The use of calcium gluconate in this situation has been advocated and has been reported to promptly reverse the respiratory depression. It is presumed that the reversal of paresis by calcium in this situation is related in part to reversal of presynaptic inhibition of neuromuscular transmission produced by the offending antibiotic. In any situation in which a drug-induced myasthenia is reversible by the use of Tensilon and which does not resolve promptly, the use of long-acting anticholinesterase agents may be required.

A final situation that involves dysfunction of neuromuscular transmission and fluctuating weakness is the Eaton-Lambert syndrome (ELS) (myasthenic syndrome). ELS (14) is characterized by easy fatigability and weakness of proximal muscles. It is often distinguished from myasthenia gravis by the lack of involvement of ocular and bulbar musculature, transient increase in strength of the involved muscle on repetitive activity, and poor response to endrophonium. Electrodiagnostic criteria also serve to distinguish the two entities. ELS is most often seen in patients with malignancies, usually small cell carcinoma of the lung. The clinical and electrical characteristics of ELS are thought to result from dysfunction of release mechanisms related to presynaptic ACh. Guanidine, which has been reported to be effective in the treatment of ELS, has been reported to increase the quantity of ACh liberated at nerve terminals (20). It is of interest that a patient's favorable response to guanidine treatment may take 3 to 4 days and that after discontinuing the drug, its effects may persist for 3 to 4 days. Although initially thought to be relatively innocuous, guanidine toxicity has been increasingly recognized and includes minor problems (parathesias, mild gastrointestinal symptoms) and more serious problems (weakness and liver, bone marrow, and nervous system toxicity).

REFERENCES

1. Argov, Z., and Mastaglia, F. L. (1979): Disorders of neuromuscular transmission caused by drugs. *N. Engl. J. Med.*, 301:409–413.
2. Bingle, J. P., Rutherford, J. D., and Woodrow, P. (1979): Continuous subcutaneous neostigmine in the management of severe myasthenia gravis. *Br. Med. J.*, 1:1050.
3. Burn, J. H. (1978): Early observations and their importance today. *J. Pharm. Pharmacol.*, 30:779–780.
4. Calvey, T. N., and Chan, K. (1977): Plasma concentration and pharmacological effects of pyridostigmine in patients with myasthenia gravis. *Br. J. Clin. Pharmacol.*, 4:404.
5. Chan, K., and Calvey, T. N. (1977): Plasma concentrations of pyridostigmine and effects in myasthenia gravis. *Clin. Pharmacol. Ther.*, 22:596–601.
6. Dau, P. C., Lindstrom, J. M., Cassel, C. K., Denys, E. H., Sher, E. E., and Spitler, L. E. (1977): Plasmopheresis and immunosuppressive drug therapy in myasthenia gravis. *N. Engl. J. Med.*, 297:1134–1140.

7. Drachman, D. B. (1978): Myasthenia gravis. *N. Engl. J. Med.*, 298:185–193.
8. Engel, A. G., Lambert, E. H., and Gomez, M. R. (1977): A new myasthenic syndrome with end plate acetylcholinesterase deficiency, small nerve terminals and acetylcholine release. *Ann. Neurol.*, 1:315–330.
9. Fambrough, D. M., Drachman, D. B., and Satyamurti, S. (1973): Neuromuscular junctions in myasthenia gravis: decreased acetylcholine receptors. *Science*, 182:293–295.
10. Freydberg, L. D. (1960): The place of corticotrophin in the treatment of myasthenia gravis. *Ann. Intern. Med.*, 52:108–118.
11. Havard, C. W. (1977): Progress in myasthenia gravis. *Br. Med. J.*, 2:1008–1011.
12. Howard, F. M., Jr., Duane, D. D., Lambert, E. H., and Daube, J. R. (1976): Alternate-day prednisone: Preliminary report of a double-blind controlled study. *Ann. N.Y. Acad. Sci.*, 274:596–607.
13. Kjaer, M. (1971): Myasthenia gravis and myasthenic syndromes treated with prednisone. *Acta Neurol. Scand.*, 47:464–474.
14. Lambert, E. H. (1966): Defects of neuromuscular transmission in syndromes other than myasthenia gravis. *Ann. N.Y. Acad. Sci.*, 135:367–384.
15. Lefvert, A. K., Bergstrom, K., Motell, G., Osterman, P. O., and Pushanern, C. (1978): Determinations of acetylcholine receptor antibody in myasthenia gravis: Clinical usefulness and pathogenetic implication. *J. Neurol. Neurosurg. Psychiatry*, 41:394–403.
16. Lundh, H., Nilsson, O., and Rosen, I. (1979): Effects of 4-aminopyridine in myasthenia gravis. *J. Neurol. Neurosurg. Psychiatry*, 42:171–175.
17. Matell, G., Bergstrom, K., Franksson, C., Hammarstrom, L., Lefvert, A., Moller, E., Reis, G., and Smith, E. (1976): Effects of some immunosuppressive procedures on myasthenia gravis. *Ann. N.Y. Acad. Sci.*, 274:659–676.
18. Mertens, H. G., Balzereit, F., and Leipert, M. (1969): The treatment of severe myasthenia gravis with immunosuppressive agents. *Eur. Neurol.*, 2:321–339.
19. Nicholson, G. A., and Appel, S. H. (1977): Is there acetylcholine receptor in human thymus? *J. Neurol. Sci.*, 34:101–108.
20. Oh, S. J., and Kim, K. W. (1973): Guanidine hydrochloride in the Eaton-Lambert syndrome. *Neurology*, 23:1084–1090.
21. Papatestas, A. E., Alpert, E. I., Osserman, K. E., Osserman, R. S., and Karak, A. E. (1971): Studies in myasthenia gravis: Effects of thymectomy. *Am. J. Med.*, 50:465–474.
22. Pirofsky, B., Reid, C. H., Bardana, E. J., and Boker, R. L. (1979): Myasthenia gravis treated with purified antithymocyte antiserum. *Neurology*, 29:112–116.
23. Seybold, M. E., and Drachman, D. B. (1974): Gradually increasing doses of prednisone in myasthenia gravis: Reducing the hazards of treatment. *N. Engl. J. Med.*, 290:81–84.
24. Stein, C., Moor, W., Weinreich, D., and Mayer, R. (1978): Choline levels in plasma of myasthenia gravis patients and normal individuals. *Ann. Neurol.*, 4:290–291.
25. Vijayan, N., Vijayan, K., and Dreyfus, P. M. (1977): Acetylcholinesterase activity and menstrual remission in myasthenia gravis. *J. Neurol. Neurosurg. Psychiatry*, 40:1060–1065.
26. Von Reis, G., Liljestrand, A., and Matell, G. (1965): Results with ACTH and spironolactone in severe cases of myasthenia gravis. *Acta Neurol. Scand. [Suppl. 13]*, 41:463–471.

Chapter 33

The Periodic Paralyses

A number of different disease states are associated with clinical episodes of periodic paralyses (Table 1). It is generally accepted that the individual episodes of paralysis in most if not all these disorders are related in some way to potassium; however, the hypokalemic syndromes are the only ones in which there is a clearcut relationship between demonstrable levels of serum potassium and each attack.

HYPOKALEMIC PERIODIC PARALYSIS

As in all periodic paralyses, the pathophysiology is not known, although potassium is involved. Urinary excretion of potassium falls prior to the onset of an attack of paralysis, and potassium moves into the skeletal musculature at the onset of weakness (17). It is not clear whether this movement is the cause of the weakness or is secondary to some other process (13). The clinical characteristics that aid in the differential diagnosis of the periodic paralyses are beyond the scope of this review (see ref. 13). A number of provocative procedures will often elicit paralysis and clarify the diagnosis and relationship to potassium. In hypokalemic periodic paralysis, the following procedures are helpful: (a) oral glucose, 1.5 g/kg up to 100 g, (b) intravenous glucose, 1.5 to 3.0 g/kg over 60 min, and (c) intravenous glucose, as above, with insulin (0.1 U/kg at 30 and 60 min; this often results in postinfusion hypoglycemia. These are usually recommended in the order listed. In all, maximum lowering of potassium is seen in 90 to 150 min.

TABLE 1. *Classification*[a]

Hypokalemic
Familial
Thyrotoxic
Hyperkalemic (potassium sensitive)
Normokalemic
Paramyotonia associated with periodic
paralysis
Paramyotonia congenita
Paralysis periodica paramyotonia

[a]Adapted from Riggs and Griggs (13).

Treatment

Potassium salts will invariably stop an acute attack of hypokalemic periodic paralysis, but their chronic use is of no prophylactic value (5). It is safest, if possible, to give potassium orally. Intravenous potassium itself can be dangerous, and the other components of the solution (glucose or saline) may actually increase weakness for a time (8). The recommended dose of potassium is 60 mg i.v. to be given slowly in 500 ml normal saline.

For chronic prophylaxis, the carbonic anhydrase inhibitor acetazolamide appears to be the drug of choice (5,12). Efficacy is observed in most patients with a dose range of 125 to 1,500 mg daily and is often apparent in the first 24 hr of therapy. Tolerance is not a problem. Withdrawal can be associated with precipitation of an attack within 2 to 4 days, especially in patients who normally have frequent episodes. The mechanism of action of acetazolamide is unknown. It is classically thought that there is no carbonic anhydrase in muscle, and efficacy can occur at doses that probably do not completely inhibit carbonic anhydrase. Acetazolamide does cause acidosis, which may protect against the shift of potassium from serum to muscles (7,12).

Chronic acetazolamide therapy is often associated with paresthesias, dysgeusia, nausea, anorexia, and mild weight loss. For unknown reasons, the paresthesias are more common and severe when acetazolamide is used in patients with hyperkalemic periodic paralysis. Since renal calculi have been reported, the dosage should be kept as low as possible, and fluid intake must be maintained. Concomitant sulfonamide therapy should be avoided.

Spironolactone has been shown to be of value in the the prophylaxis of recurrent episodes of hypokalemic periodic paralysis. This is usually felt to be related to antagonism of aldactone and potassium retention, but this agent does cause a mild metabolic acidosis. Spironolactone can cause gynecomastia, hirsutism, and occasionally impotence. More significantly, if an episode of periodic paralysis occurs in a patient on spironolactone, potassium administration can be more dangerous.

THYROTOXIC PERIODIC PARALYSIS

The pathophysiology of episodic weakness in thyrotoxicosis is unknown. As in hypokalemic periodic paralysis, however, the episodes are associated with a shift of potassium from the serum into the skeletal muscles (14). Potassium salts usually abort acute attacks (3). The attacks invariably cease when the patient becomes euthyroid; thus long-term specific therapy is not required. It is important to note that acetazolamide usually has a deleterious effect here (16). Spironolactone does have some prophylactic efficacy, but potassium salts do not. Propanolol can also be used as a prophylactic agent (3,16).

HYPERKALEMIC PERIODIC PARALYSIS

The exact relationship between potassium and attacks of weakness in hyperkalemic periodic paralysis is less clear. The term hyperkalemic may not be completely applicable, since the potassium level is not necessarily elevated during an attack (4). Careful study, however, usually shows an increase of potassium during an episode, even though the entire change may be within the usual normal range for serum potassium. All patients with hyperkalemic periodic paralysis are sensitive to oral potassium ingestion and develop weakness from serum levels of potassium that would not cause weakness in normal individuals (11). Overall, the pathophysiology is not understood. The finding that the resting membrane potential of skeletal musculature is decreased before and during episodes suggests that this disorder could be associated with increased passive loss of potassium from muscle cells (7).

Oral potassium loading, using between 0.5 and 1.5 g/kg potassium chloride, may precipitate weakness. In using this provocative procedure, the lower dose must be used first. The maximum elevation of potassium occurs at 90 to 180 min. Oral glucose and insulin also may elicit an attack.

Most acute attacks are so brief that no treatment is necessary. As most patients have learned, consumption of glucose at the first sign of weakness will usually stop an episode. In severe attacks, intravenous glucose can be used (6). The efficacy of glucose is due to a rapid lowering of circulating potassium levels, with a shift of potassium from serum to musculature. Other agents with similar effects, including epinephrine, insulin, glucagon, and calcium gluconate, also have been used (13).

Acetazolamide is an effective prophylactic agent in most but not all patients (9,11). Paresthesias may be troublesome and thereby preclude its use. These patients and those who do not respond to acetazolamide often improve on thiazide diuretics (10). Whether the efficacy of the thiazides is due to their kaliuretic action or to metabolic alkalosis is unclear. Occasional patients do best on 9-α-fluorohydrocortisone.

NORMOKALEMIC PERIODIC PARALYSIS

Many patients with normokalemic periodic paralysis are sensitive to the administration of oral potassium salts and may actually have a form of hyperkalemic periodic paralysis. Occasional patients have episodes that have no relationship to potassium levels. Most patients do resemble those with the hyperkalemic form, and the treatment is identical.

PARAMYOTONIA WITH PERIODIC PARALYSIS

Episodes of weakness in patients with paramyotonia have been reported with either hypokalemia or hyperkalemia (15), reflecting the fact that there are two separate forms of paramyotonia (1): (a) paramyotonia congenita, associated with hypokalemic episodes of weakness, and (b) paralysis periodica paramyotonia, associated with episodes of hyperkalemic periodic paralysis. Since many reports of the treatment of paramyotonic periodic paralysis have not made this differentiation, the pharmacology is not clearly defined. In general, potassium-sparing agents, such as spironolactone, are of value in the long-term treatment of paramyotonia congenita; kaluretic agents, such as thiazides, are useful in paralysis periodica paramyotonia. In general, acetazolamide has not been helpful in either form.

BIBLIOGRAPHY AND *SELECTED REVIEWS

1. Becker, P. E. (1971): Genetic approaches to the nosology of muscle disease: Myotonias and similar diseases. *Birth Defects*, 7:52–62.
*2. Bradley, W. G. (1969): Adynamia episodica hereditaria. Clinical, pathological and electrophysiological studies in an affected family. *Brain*, 92:345–378.
3. Conway, M. J., Seibel, J. A., and Eaton, R. P. (1974): Thyrotoxicosis and periodic paralysis: Improvement with beta blockade. *Ann. Intern. Med.*, 81:332–336.
4. Gamstorp. I. (1956): Adynamia episodica hereditaria. *Acta Paediatr. [Suppl. 108]*, 45:1–126.
5. Griggs, R. C., Engel, W. K., and Resnick, J. S. (1970): Acetazolamide treatment of hypokalemic periodic paralysis. *Ann. Intern. Med.*, 73:39–48.
6. Herman, R. H., and McDowell, M. K. (1963): Hyperkalemic paralysis (adynamia episodica hereditaria). Report of four cases and clinical studies. *Am. J. Med.*, 35:749–767.
7. Jarrell, M. S., Greer, M., and Maren, T. H. (1976): The effect of acidosis in hypokalemic periodic paralysis. *Arch. Neurol.*, 33:791–793.
8. Kunin, A. S., Surawicz, B., and Sims, E. A. H. (1962): Decrease in serum potassium concentrations and appearance of cardiac arrhythmias during infusion of potassium with glucose in potassium-depleted patients. *N. Engl. J. Med.*, 266:228–233.
9. Layzer, R. B., Lovelace, R. E., and Rowland, L. P. (1967): Hyperkalemic periodic paralysis. *Arch. Neurol.*, 16:455–472.
10. Lewis, E. D., Griggs, R. C., and Moxley, R. T. (1981): Regulation of plasma potassium in hyperkalemic periodic paralysis. *Neurology (in press)*.
11. McArdle, B. (1962): Adynamia episodica hereditaria and its treatment. *Brain*, 85:121–148.
12. Resnick, J. S., Engel, W. K., Griggs, R. C., and Stam, A. C. (1968): Acetazolamide prophylaxis in hypokalemic periodic paralysis. *N. Engl. J. Med.*, 278:582–586.
*13. Riggs, J. E., and Griggs, R. C., (1979): The diagnosis and treatment of the periodic paralyses. In: *Clinical Neuropharmacology, Vol. 4*, edited by H. L. Klawans. Raven Press, New York.
14. Shizume, K., Shishiba, Y., Sakuma, M., Yamuchi, H., Nakao, K., and Okinaka, S. (1966): Studies and electrolyte metabolism in idiopathic and thyrotoxic periodic paralysis. *Metabolism*, 15:138–162.
15. Thursh, D. C., Morris, C. J., and Salmon, M. V. (1972): Paramyotonia congenita: A clinical, histochemical and pathological study. *Brain*, 95:537–552.
16. Young, R. T. T., and Tse, T. F. (1974): Thyrotoxic periodic paralysis. Effect of propranolol. *Am. J. Med.*, 57:584–590.
17. Zierler, K. L, and Andres, R. (1957): Movement of potassium into skeletal muscle during spontaneous attack in family periodic paralysis. *J. Clin. Invest.*, 36:730–737.

Chapter 34

Dementia and Other Problems in Geriatric Neuropharmacology

Dementia is a progressive decline in higher cortical function. The relative degree to which each aspect of cortical function (cognitive abilities, judgment, etc.) is affected varies in any individual patient, but the most prominent early dysfunction involves memory. The incidence of dementia rises dramatically in the aging population. Alzheimer's disease is characterized by a specific neuropathologic constellation of neuronal dropout, neurofibrillary tangles, senile plaques, and granulovacuolar degeneration. The cause of this common form of dementia remains obscure, although possible toxic or viral etiologies as well as a hereditary component have been suggested. There are multiple causes of dementia, including infections, deficiency states, endocrinologic and metabolic abnormalities, benign and malignant CNS tumors, normal pressure hydrocephalus, and vascular disease (multi-infarct dementia). Those patients with progressive idiopathic (Alzheimer's) dementia are usually those who are included in clinical pharmacologic studies of dementia.

Unfortunately, it is clear that no truly successful form of therapy exists for the all-too-common dementias of the aging population. It is equally true no rational pharmacology is available for this problem. Despite these handicaps, sufficient data have accrued, warranting presentation. The various pharmacologic agents used (or promoted) for the treatment of dementia in the aging population are listed in Table 1.

TABLE 1. *Drugs employed in the treatment of dementias in the aged*

Drug	Proposed mechanism
Hydergine	Stimulant of cerebral metabolism
Papaverine	Vasodilator
Cyclandelate	Vasodilator
Pentylenetetrazol	Stimulant
Gerovital H-3	Unknown, possible MAO inhibitor
Choline	Acetylcholine precursor
Lecithin	Acetylcholine precursor

Hydergine is a combination of three hydrogenated ergot alkaloids and is probably the most carefully studied and at the same time most widely used. While its efficacy was originally attributed to a direct increase in cerebral blood flow, it is now presumed that any increase in blood flow and cerebral oxygen consumption is due to a direct effect of neuronal cell metabolism (4). The beneficial effects are limited, but most controlled studies comparing hydergine to placebo have found hydergine to be superior, especially with respect to subjective improvement (1,3,19). Rao and Norris (16) found hydergine to be superior to papaverine. As noted by Raskind and Eisdorfer (17), most of these studies have found improvement in attitude, ward behavior, activities of daily living, and somatic complaints, but long-term quantitative improvement in cognitive functions has never been definitely established. Some investigators (19) have found that hydergine-related improvement was most evident in symptoms commonly associated with depression, such as emotional withdrawal, depressive mood, and motor retardation. This raises the possibility that at least some of the efficacy of hydergine could be a result of antidepressant activity. In this regard, it is important to note that hydergine can inhibit reuptake of norepinephrine *in vitro*, an action similar to that of most tricyclic antidepressants.

Papaverine and cyclandelate are the most widely used cerebral vasodilators and are the only agents of this type which will be discussed. These agents relax the smooth muscle of blood vessel walls in the peripheral circulation and perhaps also in the cerebral vasculature. Theoretically, this could increase cerebral blood flow and oxygenation of brain tissue. This effect has not been demonstrated; even if it were to occur, it would not necessarily result in improved mentation, since any alteration in cerebral oxygen uptake and therefore cerebral blood flow is probably due to the dementing process and not a result of it. It is also clear that reduced cerebral blood flow in the aged may occur without clinical evidence of dementia (22). As reviewed by Yesavage et al. (24), the well-controlled clinical studies of vasodilators in comparison with so-called stimulants of cerebral metabolism significantly favor the latter.

Papaverine is an alkaloid derivative of opium with vasodilator properties. General improvement in behavior, including performance of activities of daily living, has been reported; significant intellectual improvement, however, has not been consistently demonstrated (12,21). Side effects include drowsiness, dizziness, flushing, headache, and hypotension. In rare cases papaverine has also been reported to increase parkinsonian signs and to block the efficacy of levodopa. This must be kept in mind since parkinsonism and dementia overlap.

The action of cyclandelate is similar to that of papaverine. Clinical efficacy has been reported in both uncontrolled and controlled studies, including one in which patients with mild impairment demonstrated some improvement in long-term memory, reasoning, and orientation (20).

In general, any beneficial effect of these agents is limited at best. Consistent, long-term clinical significance has not been proven; thus the chronic use of these agents, probably serves no true therapeutic purpose.

A wide variety of central stimulants, including the amphetamines, methylphenidate, pipradrol, pentylenetetrazol, and magnesium pemoline, have been studied as possible pharmacologic agents to improve cognitive function. While many of these have been reported to increase activity level, alertness, and attention to stimuli, improve recall and recognition, and decrease lethargy, there is little if any evidence that these improvements can be maintained over time (23).

The drug of this type that is probably most widely used in the geriatric population is pentylenetetrazol, but any efficacy of this agent is limited. Lehman and Ban (10) reviewed 16 controlled studies of pentylenetetrazol and found that only five of these (less than one-third) showed definite efficacy. Other agents in this group have not been studied and have little if any reason to be used (14,24).

For over two decades, a Romanian buffered form of procainamide (Gerovital H-3) has been enthusiastically promoted for aging and dementia. It is usually given intramuscularly 3 times per week for 12 weeks. Following such administration, it is probably completely hydrolyzed in minutes. Many uncontrolled studies, mostly performed in Europe, claim efficacy in a wide range of physical and mental disorders. Controlled studies of procainamide have not confirmed these claims.

Jarvik and Milne (8), in an extensive review, found six well-controlled studies of procainamide in the elderly which showed no benefit (9). Two recent controlled studies of the Romanian procainamide in depression did show some improvement, possibly related to the reported effect of this drug as an MAO inhibitor. More conclusive evidence is needed to demonstrate that Gerovital H-3 is more than an expensive placebo.

Interest in the study of cholinergic mechanisms in Alzheimer's disease began when Perry et al. reported reduction of choline acetyltransferase (CAT) and acetylcholinesterase in demented patients at autopsy (12a). Cholinergic mechanisms have been associated with memory function, and improvement in memory has been reported in normal patients after administration of physostigmine or arecoline, two cholinergic agents. Numerous studies have since been conducted to assess the effects of presumed dietary precursors to acetylcholine in demented patients. Phosphatidylcholine (lecithin) and choline chloride increase brain acetylcholine in experimental animals, and it has been suggested that they serve as precursor substrates in man for central synthesis of acetylcholine (4a). This latter hypothesis has not been proven. Results in clinical trials of these two agents have not shown consistent improvement in the memory or global function of Alzheimer patients (2a). Since it remains unknown if in fact these agents lead to enhanced cholinergic activity in the brain, these equivocal results do not weaken a cholinergic hypothesis for Alzheimer's disease.

Two other problems commonly associated or confused with dementia often require pharmacologic intervention: (a) disturbed or psychotic behavior, and (b) depression. Unfortunately relatively few data have been published on psychopharmacology in this population. Neuroleptics in adequate dosages are probably effective for symptom relief in both elderly chronic schizophrenics and behaviorally disturbed elderly patients with dementia, especially if the patients are acutely disturbed. The beneficial effects, however, are less consistently achieved than they are in younger patients (17). There is also no evidence at this time that one antipsychotic agent is more effective than another in this age group. This is similar to the lack of any drug specificity among neuroleptics for particular subgroups of younger psychotic patients.

Depression can accompany or even mimic dementia in older patients. The MAO inhibitors are probably least suitable for use in the elderly (13). Psychostimulants cannot be advocated as antidepressant agents. Although some clinicians have used them successfully over brief periods for the treatment of mild depression, few clinical studies have specifically examined their efficacy in depressed geriatric patients. The tricyclic antidepressants are widely used in the elderly, with apparently reasonable efficacy (15). In general, tricyclics are the pharmacologic treatment of choice for depression in elderly patients with or without dementia (see Chapter 21).

One other major pharmacologic problem of the elderly is their increased susceptibility to adverse effects, especially toxic confusional states. Demented patients are, of course, even more susceptible than normal aged individuals. This is especially true of any agents with central anticholinergic activity, including the tricyclic antidepressants.

PHARMACOKINETIC PROBLEMS OF AGING

In general, clinical studies have pointed out a number of age-related pharmacokinetic problems, including alterations in (a) absorption, (b) drug metabolism, (c) protein binding, and (d) renal clearance. Changes in absorption with increasing age are probably not very significant but may be an occasional cause of ineffective therapy. The effects of increasing age on drug absorption have not been thoroughly studied. Bender (2) has noted the general paucity of such information but maintains that there was an overall suggestion of reduced absorption in the elderly. Age-related decreases in the absorption of glucose and calcium (specifically transported substances, unlike most drugs, which are passively absorbed) are of uncertain significance, but the decreased absorption of xylose and iron with increasing age may indicate some decrease in the efficiency of drug absorption. Decreased intestinal blood perfusion may be responsible for decreased drug absorption. While circulation to the coronary and cerebral regions is only slightly changed in the elderly, intestinal blood flow is decreased by 40 to 50%.

The duration of action of many drugs is determined by the rate at which they are metabolized by the hepatic enzymes. In elderly patients, both decreased hepatic enzymatic activity and reduced hepatic circulation can occur, with significant effects on drug metabolism. Plasma binding of drugs is often decreased because of decreased plasma protein levels. This can affect both blood levels and the percentage of the plasma content that is bound. The elimination of many drugs or metabolites from the body is via the kidneys, usually as a result of simple glomerular filtration but at times involving active tubular excretion. Urinary excretion obviously limits the pharmacologic effect of all nonmetabolized drugs and also controls the elimination of metabolites of other drugs. Renal function is probably the factor most responsible for altered drug levels and effects in the aging population. The age-related decrease in renal perfusion is estimated to be 1.5% per year during adult life, resulting in an overall decrease of roughly 40 to 50% from age 25 to age 65. This decrease results in a similar drop in both glomerular filtration rate and urea clearance, with a corresponding 50% increase in blood urea nitrogen. Even in the absence of any active intrinsic renal disease, creatinine clearance is reduced in normal elderly individuals to about one-half the rate of normal young adults. Creatinine clearance can serve as an index of drug clearance capacity. This age-related decrease in kidney function can lead to prolonged drug half-life and increased blood levels (18).

Adequate studies of these problems have been carried out only for a few neuropharmacologic agents. Some of these agents are listed in Table 2. As can be seen with phenytoin, these changes can be multiple and the total effect complex. Hayes et al. (5) found that the plasma binding of phenytoin was decreased by about 20% in people over age 65 as compared to those under 45. This difference was due to reduced concentrations of albumin. Increased phenytoin clearance in the older group is probably related to decreased binding; thus more unbound drug can be metabolized. Other clinical studies with phenytoin indicate that serum levels are increased in older patients. It is possible that the more rapid metabolism of phenytoin in younger subjects would lead to both lower serum levels and a lower drug clearance rate. Because of decreased binding in elderly patients, any serum level would represent a greater amount of unbound active drug. Older individuals, therefore, may be more likely to have greater efficacy and toxicity at any particular level than younger patients. The situation is less complex for phenobarbital, where the half-life increases with age. The same phenomenon occurs with diazepam. Amantadine hydrochloride is excreted unchanged in the urine. Elderly patients with decreased creatinine clearance may quickly accumulate toxic levels of this agent. It is of interest that most reports of amantadine hydrochloride-induced seizures have involved elderly patients. Decreased lithium clearance is uniform in the elderly, so

TABLE 2.

Drug	Observation
Phenytoin	On same daily maintenance dosage, drug levels increased twofold due to decreased metabolism (7); increased plasma clearance with aging and decreased plasma binding due to decreased plasma albumin concentration (5)
Phenobarbital	Half-life increases from 71 hr (ages 20 to 40) to 107 hr (ages greater than 70) (7)
Lithium	Clearance decreases with age from 41.5 ml/min (age 25) to 7 ml/min (age 63) (11); thus the dose required to achieve therapeutic plasma levels decreases by about 30% from age 20 to 80 (6)
Diazepam	Half-life increases with age from 20 hr at age 20 to 80 hr at age 70 due to altered liver metabolism (9)

that the daily dosage needed to maintain therapeutic levels decreases with increased age.

BIBLIOGRAPHY AND *SELECTED REVIEWS

1. Banen, D. M. (1972): An ergot preparation (Hydergine) for relief of symptoms of cerebrovascular insufficiency. *J. Am. Geriatr. Soc.*, 20:22–24.

2. Bender, A. D. (1968): Effect of age on intestinal absorption: Implications for drug absorption in the elderly. *J. Am. Geriatr. Soc.*, 16:1131–1139.

2a. Christie, J. E., Blackburn, I. M., and Glen, A. I. M. (1979): Effects of choline and lecithin in presenile dementia. In: *Nutrition and the Brain*, edited by A. Barbeau, J. H. Growdon, and R. J. Wurtman, pp. 377–387. Raven Press, New York.

3. Ditch, M., Kelley, R. J., and Resnick, O. (1971): An ergot preparation (Hydergine) in the treatment of cerebrovascular disorders in the geriatric patient: Double-blind study. *J. Am. Geriatr. Soc.*, 19:208–217.

4. Emmenegger, H., and Meier-Ruge, W. (1968): The actions of Hydergine on the brain. *Pharmacology*, 1:65–78.

4a. Haubrich, D. R., Gerber, N. H., and Pflueger, A. B. (1979): Choline availability and synthesis of acetylcholine. In: *Nutrition and the Brain*, edited by A. Barbeau, J. H. Growdon, and R. J. Wurtman, pp. 57–72. Raven Press, New York.

5. Hayes, M. J., Langman, M. J. S., and Short, A. H. (1975): Changes in drug metabolism with increasing age. 2. Phenytoin clearance and protein binding. *Br. J. Clin. Pharmacol.*, 2:73–79.

6. Hewick, D. S., and Newbury, P. A. (1976): Age: Its influence on lithium dosage and plasma levels. *Br. J. Clin. Pharmacol.*, 3:354P.

7. Houghton, G. W., Richens, A., and Leighton, M. (1975): Effect of age, height, weight, and sex on serum phenytoin concentration in epileptic patients. *Br. J. Clin. Pharmacol.*, 2:251–256.

8. Jarvik, L. F., and Milne, J. F. (1975): Gerovital H-3: A review of the literature. In: *Aging, Vol. 2*, edited by S. Gershon and A. Raskin, pp. 203–228. Raven Press, New York.

9. Klotz, U., Avant, G. R., Hoyumpa, A., Schenker, S., and Wilkinson, G. R. (1975): The effects of age and liver disease on the disposition and elimination of diazepam in adult man. *J. Clin. Invest.*, 55:347–359.

10. Lehman, H. E., and Ban, T. A. (1975): Central nervous system stimulants and anabolic substances in geropsychiatric therapy. In: *Aging, Vol. 2*, edited by S. Gershon and A. Raskin, pp. 179–202. Raven Press, New York.

11. Lehman, K., and Merten, K. (1974): Die elimination von lithium in abhangigkeit vom lebensalter bei gesunden und niereninsuffizienten. *Int. J. Clin. Pharmacol.*, 10:292–298.

12. Lu, L. M., Stotsky, B. A., and Cole, J. O. (1971): A controlled study of drugs in long-term geriatric psychiatric patients. *Arch. Gen. Psychiatry*, 25:284–288.

12a. Perry, E. K., Perry, L. H., Blessed, G., and Tomlinson, B. E. (1977): Necropsy evidence of cholinergic deficits in senile dementia. *Lancet*, 1:889.

13. Prange, A. J. (1973): The use of antidepressant drugs in the elderly patients. In: *Psychopharmacology and Aging*, edited by C. Eisdorfer and W. E. Fann, pp. 114–127. Plenum Press, New York.

*14. Prien, R. F. (1973): Chemotherapy in chronic organic brain syndrome—A review of the literature. *Psychopharmacol. Bull.*, 9:5–20.

15. Prien, R. F., Haber, P. A., and Caffrey, E. M. (1975): The use of psychoactive drugs in elderly patients with psychiatric disorders: Survey conducted in 12 Veterans Administration hospitals. *J. Am. Geriatr. Soc.*, 23:104–112.

16. Rao, D. B., and Norris, J. R. (1972): A double-blind investigation of Hydergine in the treatment of cerebrovascular insufficiency in the elderly. *Johns Hopkins Med. J.*, 130:317–324.

*17. Raskind, M., and Eisdorfer, C. (1976): Pharmacology of the aged. In: *Drug Treatment of Mental Disorders*, edited by L. L. Simpson, pp. 237–267. Raven Press, New York.

*18. Richey, D. P., and Bender, A. D. (1977): Pharmacokinetic consequences of aging. *Ann. Rev. Pharmacol. Toxicol.*, 17:49–65.

19. Roubicek, J., Geiger, C. H., and Abt, K. (1972): An ergot alkaloid preparation (Hydergine) in geriatric therapy. *J. Am. Geriatr. Soc.*, 20:222–229.

20. Smith, W. L., Lowrey, J. B., and Davis, J. A. (1968): The effects of cyclandelate on psychological test performance in patients with cerebral vascular insufficiency. *Curr. Ther. Res.*, 10:613–618.

21. Stern, F. H. (1970): Management of chronic brain syndrome secondary to cerebral arteriosclerosis, with special reference to papaverine hydrochloride. *J. Am. Geriatr. Soc.*, 18:507–510.
22. Wang, H. S. (1973): Evaluation of brain impairment. In: *Mental Illness in Later Life*, edited by E. W. Busse and E. Pfeiffer, p. 83. American Psychiatric Association, Washington, D. C.
23. Weiss, B., and Laties, V. (1972): Enhancement of human performance by caffeine and the amphetamines. *Pharmacol. Rev.*, 14:1–36.
*24. Yesavage, J. A., Hollister, L., and Buriane, E. (1979): Vasodilators in senile dementia. A review of the literature. *Arch. Gen. Psychiatry*, 36:220–223.

Chapter 35

Neurologic Side Effects of Nonneuropsychiatric Agents

Neurologic complications have been reported from a wide variety of therapeutic agents. Such problems are more common with drugs used in the treatment of neurologic or psychiatric disorders. These and certain other specific problems, such as drug-induced movement disorders and myotonia, are discussed in previous chapters and are not included here. Certain side effects, which occur with diverse drugs, are listed in Tables 1 through 6.

ANTIBIOTICS

Penicillins

Penicillin G and related agents have been reported to cause central nervous system (CNS) toxicity (14,27). Myoclonus, seizures, asterixis, hallucinations, and coma

TABLE 1. *Iatrogenic neuromuscular blockade or other causes of flaccid weakness*

Colchicine	Polymyxin B
Colistimethate sodium	Procainamide
Corticosteroids	Streptomycin
Diphenylhydantoin	Sulfonamides
Kanamycin sulfate	Tetracycline
Meprobamate	Lincomycin
Neomycin	Clindamycin
Oxytetracycline	Quinine

TABLE 2. *Iatrogenic involvement of the eighth cranial nerve*

Chloroquine	Erythromycin
Gentamicin	Amakacin
Kanamycin sulfate	Ethacrynic acid
Nitrogen mustard	Furosemide
Quinidine sulfate	Chloropropramide
Quinine	*cis*-Platinum
Large doses of salicylates	Tobramycin
Streptomycin	Sulindac

TABLE 3. *Iatrogenic optic neuropathy*

Penicillamine	Ethambutal
Chloramphenicol	Vincristine
Chloroquine	Digitalis
Isoniazid	Quinine

TABLE 4. *Iatrogenic peripheral neuropathy*

Vincristine	Streptomycin
Isoniazid	Polymyxin B
Nitrofurantoin	Sulfonamides
Gold	Penicillin
Allopurinol	Chloroquine
Chloramphenicol	Nitroglycerine
Ethambutal	5-Fluororacil
Hydralazine	cis-Platinum
Nitrogen mustard	Procarbazine
Disulfuram	Metronidazole
Kanamycin	

TABLE 5. *Iatrogenic disorders of taste*

Penicillamine	Ethambutal
Phenylbutazone	Metronidazole
Amphotericin B	Lincomycin
Griseofulvin	Allopurinol
Azulfadine	Carbamazine
Gold	Baclofen

TABLE 6. *Iatrogenic pseudotumor cerebri*

Vitamin A	Penicillin
Tetracycline	Sulfamethoxazole
Naladixic acid	Oral contraceptives

have been associated with methicillin, ampicillin, carbenicillin, and penicillin G. Meningeal inflammation may enhance neurotoxity of penicillins by promoting penetration of these drugs into the nervous system and decreasing transport from the cerebrospinal fluid (CSF) (14). Neurotoxic reactions to penicillin rarely occur with usual doses (20 million U daily) in patients without underlying cerebral and renal diseases. Doses of penicillin G in excess of 20,000 U intrathecally cause convulsions. Since that route of administration is of no greater therapeutic benefit than peripheral injection, it should never be used. The mechanism of neurotoxicity of penicillin is as yet unexplained, although alteration in electrolytic flux at the cellular level of cortical tissue has been demonstrated *in vitro* after penicillin administration.

Sulfonamides and Folate Inhibitors

Sulfonamides, pyramethamine, and trimethoprim inhibit the synthesis of tetrahydrofolinic acid, the one-carbon donor needed for the synthesis of methionine, serine, and purines. These drugs are associated with a low incidence of neurotoxicity, including headache, fatigue, tinnitus, and acute psychosis (25). The pathogenesis of these is unclear.

Erythromycin

Erythromycin is probably the least toxic of the commonly used antibiotics but can occasionally cause temporary hearing loss (23). This has been reported during treatment with 4 g or more per day of the lactionate derivative of oral erythromycin and is reversible with dosage reduction or discontinuation.

Lincomycin and Clindamycin

Lincomycin and clindamycin are remarkably free from adverse reactions, other than pseudomembranous colitis and diarrhea. Potentiation of neuromuscular blockade is rare but can occur and may be life threatening (37). These agents can cause prolonged postoperative respiratory depression in patients receiving curare-like neuromuscular-blocking agents. Lincomycin has been reported to cause gustatory dysfunction.

Chloramphenicol

Other than aplastic anemia, chloramphenicol causes few undesirable reactions. Toxic encephalopathy with symptoms of confusion and delirium has been reported after use of more than 8 g/day chloramphenicol. Underlying neoplastic disease and liver and renal dysfunction may predispose to excessive blood levels and subsequent encephalopathy (30). Prolonged therapy and excessive daily dosage have been associated with the production of reversible optic neuritis, especially in patients with cystic fibrosis.

Tetracyclines

The toxicity of the tetracyclines is relatively low, and the neurotoxicity is rare. The syndrome of benign intracranial hypertension, characterized by headache, papilledema, and elevated CSF pressure, has been reported. Infants are most susceptible, although in rare instances this may be seen in adults (4). Signs and symptoms disappear within a few days of drug withdrawal.

Aminoglycosides

All aminoglycoside antibiotics (neomycin, kanamycin, streptomycin, gentamicin, tobramycin, and amikacin) have similar toxic profiles. The adverse neurologic effects are potentiation of neuromuscular weakness and eighth nerve involvement, producing decreased hearing, tinnitus, dizziness, and vertigo. Both cochlear and vestibular damage are the result of direct toxicity of these drugs. The incidence and severity of damage to the eighth cranial nerve increase with patient age, total dose, cumulative dose, and concomitant use of other ototoxic drugs. Auditory toxicity is more common with amikacin and kanamycin, whereas vestibular toxicity predominates following gentamicin therapy. Tobramycin is associated with equal degrees of vestibular and auditory damage. The incidence of clinical ototoxicity due to aminoglycosides ranges from 5 to 25%, depending on whether audiometry is used to detect hearing deficits (29). Aminoglycoside hearing loss is usually irreversible and may even progress following discontinuation of drug therapy.

A potentially fatal neurotoxic effect of all aminoglycosides is neuromuscular blockade. Rapid absorption from a large epithelial surface (as in the case of neomycin administration) or rapid intravenous infusion may result in respiratory paralysis. Neuromuscular block results from a curare-like effect of the aminoglycosides. Ether and drugs used to induce muscular relaxation during anesthesia are potentiated by aminoglycosides. Therefore, prolonged respiratory depression in the postoperative period should suggest additive effects of nonanesthetic drugs. Sudden or prolonged respiratory paralysis due to aminoglycosides may be reversed by calcium or neostigmine administration. These drugs are contraindicated in patients with myasthenia gravis.

Aminoglycosides do not penetrate the subarachnoid space upon systemic administration. In treating gram-negative meningitis due to susceptible bacteria, intrathecal administration of aminoglycosides may be required. Arachnoiditis with polyradiculitis has resulted from prolonged intrathecal administration of a parenteral gentamicin preparation. A preservative-free preparation is preferable when using intrathecal gentamicin.

Polymyxins

Polymyxins are closely related to the aminoglycosides in structure and neurotoxicity. The incidence of neurotoxic reactions to the polymyxins has been estimated at 7% (26). Most of the reactions are transient and completely reversible with discontinuation of therapy. These include paresthesias, peripheral neuropathy, diplopia, dysphagia, muscle weakness, dizziness, seizures, confusion, and psychosis. Respiratory paralysis is the most serious neurotoxic reaction. Underlying renal dysfunction predisposes to this neuromuscular blockade. Prodromal symptoms of dyspnea, restlessness, diplopia, and weakness may precede respiratory paralysis. The mechanism of this drug-induced respiratory depression is unknown. Treatment consists of ventilatory support and drug withdrawal. Like the aminoglycosides, polymyxins may increase the effect of neuromuscular blocking agents used during anesthesia.

Isoniazid

Direct toxic effects of isoniazid are related to its binding of pyridoxine, resulting in excessive urinary excretion and subsequent depletion of this vitamin. A multitude of neurologic symptoms is associated with isoniazid-induced pyridoxine deficiency. Peripheral neuropathy, manifested by paresthesias, sensory loss, and eventually weakness, is the most common problem. Seizures, emotional irritability, euphoria, depression, headache, and acute psychosis may occur. All neurotoxic reactions due to isoniazid are dose related, are more common in slow inactivators, and are prevented by concomitant administration of pyridoxine at a dose of 50 mg daily (16).

Ataxia, generalized seizures, and coma have been observed within hours of acute isoniazid intoxication secondary to overdosage. Pyridoxine inactivation and metabolic effects of isoniazid itself are responsible for such acute neurologic symptoms. Pyridoxine (1 g/g ingested isoniazid or 5 g if the isoniazid dose is unknown), standard anticonvulsants, and supportive measures are recommended.

Rifampin

Neurologic side effects, although uncommon, include headache, dizziness, drowsiness, inability to concentrate, confusion and fatigue. Rarely, paresthesias and complaints of pain suggestive of peripheral neuropathy have been reported.

Ethambutol

Reversible optic neuritis occurs uncommonly at a dose of 25 mg/kg day. In patients with normal renal function receiving the usual recommended dose (15 mg/kg day), visual disturbances should not occur. Periodic visual acuity determinations are suggested in patients on prolonged ethambutol therapy. Ethambutol also may cause a more general peripheral neuropathy, which is reversible upon discontinuation of the drug. A metallic taste in the mouth is not uncommon (40).

Nitrofurantoin

Prolonged therapy has been associated with the production of a peripheral neuropathy (47). Sensorimotor polyneuropathy characterized by paresthesias and dysethesias in the stocking-glove distribution may occur as early as the first week of treatment and appears to be unrelated to dosage. Upon discontinuation of the drug, one-third to one-half of the patients recover completely, although 10% of affected patients may remain symptomatic.

Metronidazole

A wide variety of neurotoxic reactions to metronidazole has been reported, including confusion, irritability, depression, and headache. A peripheral neuropathy, predominantly distal sensorimotor and clinically relatively mild, is not uncommon. Although full recovery occurs upon withdrawal of metronidazole, it is important to recognize early symptoms, since pathologic investigation has shown a major degree of nerve degeneration in affected patients (5). Metronidazole is also associated with an unpleasant sharp or metallic phantoguesia, which is readily reversible upon cessation of therapy (40).

Chloroquine

Neurotoxic reactions associated with chloroquine in the treatment of malaria are relatively rare and usually mild. These include headache, visual disturbances, and nausea. Tinnitus with progressive hearing loss may occur with high-dose therapy and is usually reversible. Optic nerve dysfunction may appear as scotomatous field defects, decreased acuity, or, rarely, optic atrophy (44). Abnormal involuntary movements have occurred during chloroquine therapy (12). Most of the patients developing these movements have been under 30 years of age. The movements have been mainly dystonic in nature, characterized by torticollis, blepharospasm, and tongue protrusion. As with other drug-induced dystonias, intravenous anticholinergic agents reversed the abnormality.

Two related antiparasitic drugs, diiodohydroxyquin and iodochlorhydroxyquin, frequently cause significant neurotoxic effects. Iodochlorhydroxyquin has been withdrawn from use because of a high incidence of subacute myelooptic neuropathy (SMON), which is characterized by progressive blindness and symptoms of spinal cord dysfunction. Diiodohydroxyquin has similar potential, but SMON does not occur during therapy with the recommended adult dose of 650 mg three times daily for 3 weeks (13).

Antibiotic-Related Myasthenia Gravis

Neuromuscular blockade has been mentioned as a side effect of many of the antibiotics, thus leading to prolonged respiratory depression and occasional weakness of various muscle groups (Table 1). It is of equal or greater interest that these drugs may unmask a subclinical myasthenia gravis and, at times, exacerbate a mild to moderate myasthenic weakness to the point of serious, life-threatening, muscular weakness. Lowering the dosage of the implicated drugs, discontinuation of the antibiotic, and anticholinesterase therapy reverse the symptoms.

ANTINEOPLASTIC AGENTS

Certain of the antineoplastic drugs, such as methotrexate (MTX) and the vinca alkaloids, possess specific neurotoxicity, whereas others produce neurologic effects via indirect means (e.g., thrombocytopenia resulting in cerebral hemorrhage). If discovered early enough, neurotoxicity may be reversible but if undetected may produce irreversible damage to the nervous sytem.

Alkylating Agents

The alkylating agents are cell cycle nonspecific drugs that act primarily by alkylating the purine and pyrimidine moieties of DNA, thereby altering synthesis of the DNA proteins. The major toxicity of these agents is bone marrow suppression; in general, neurotoxicity is not a major problem.

Nitrogen Mustard

When given intravenously in a dose of 0.4 mg/kg, nitrogen mustard (NM) is ordinarily not neurotoxic. Hemiplegia and coma have been reported in one patient 7 days after the second of two intravenous doses of NM at the recommended dose schedule. Increased intracranial pressure and CSF pleocytosis with a white blood cell count of greater than 500 were also found. Postmortem examination revealed areas of focal gliosis and neuronal loss within the brain with no evidence of intracranial tumor (3). Massive intravenous injections have caused hearing loss, vestibular dysfunctions, and tinnitus, presumably from damage to the eighth cranial nerve. Intracarotid NM has been associated with hemiplegia, seizures, coma, and death. Clinical evidence of lower motor neuron damage has been observed following high-dose intraarterial perfusion to treat pelvic or limb tumors.

Cyclophosphamide

Cyclophosphamide is associated with little neurologic toxicity. Rapid intravenous infusion has occasionally caused dizziness, a posterior pharyngeal tingling sensation, and a feeling of euphoria (2). These symptoms are all brief, lasting only seconds to minutes, and are completely reversible.

Chlorambucil

Although generally regarded as nonneurotoxic, acute, severe episodes of lethargy, ataxia, seizures, and coma developed in two children inadvertently injected with massive overdoses of chlorambucil (17). Recovery within 1 week occurred without any neurologic sequelae.

Thiotepa

Due to its low neurotoxicity, thiotepa is one of the few drugs that can be given intrathecally. In one series of 10 patients with meningeal leukemia and carcinomatosis treated with multiple courses of intrathecal thiotepa, clinical neurotoxicity developed in only two and consisted of progressive lower extremity weakness, back and leg pain, areflexia, and a progressive myelopathy (20). Gliosis and demyelination in the posterior columns of the spinal cord and the nerve roots of the cauda equina were found.

Methotrexate (MTX)

In the oral or intravenous dosage schedules normally employed, MTX is essentially nonneurotoxic. MTX neurotoxicity has been reported to occur after carotid infusion, when injected directly into the brain tumor bed, following intrathecal injection, and when given in high doses intravenously with citrovorum factor.

Hemorrhagic infarction in both cerebral hemispheres, with fibrinoid degeneratio and hyaline vascular thrombosis, has occurred following intracarotid infusion (18). Cerebral edema with necrosis and reactive astrocytosis with no apparent clinical manifestation has been reported with brain tumor bed infusion of MTX. High-dose intravenous MTX followed by citrovorum rescue occasionally causes a severe, chronic encephalopathy (1). The syndrome is usually permanent and may progress despite discontinuation of therapy. Rarely, improvement occurs over a period of months after the last injection. The incidence of this encephalopathy appears to be less than 2% (1). Although severe encephalopathy is uncommon with high-dose MTX administration, milder forms of encephalopathy undoubtedly occur. Computerized tomographic (CT) scan often demonstrates leukomalacia in the absence of clinical signs (1). These changes, both clinical and by CT scan, increase with the number of treatments.

Most MTX neurotoxicity is now seen during intrathecal administration. The acute effects include a mild to moderate but transient meningoencephalitis, usually beginning within hours of intrathecal administration and characterized by headache, nausea, vomiting, nuchal rigidity, lethargy, and fever (46). The illness usually lasts 1 to 3 days but may persist for 2 weeks. CSF examination frequently reveals a moderately severe pleocytosis. This reaction is relatively uncommon and rarely recurs upon subsequent administration. Intrathecal MTX may cause an acute transverse myelopathy with paraplegia, which may be permanent (15). Transient radiculopathies, possibly related to epidural or subdural injection, have also been described. Intrathecal injection can cause spinal subdural hematomas resulting in either myelopathy or radiculopathy (10). These acute problems are all uncommon.

Delayed neurotoxic reactions to intrathecal MTX are more frequent. Of these, encephalopathy is the most important and usually follows repeated doses of MTX into the lateral ventricle or lumbar subarachnoid space. The clinical syndrome is characterized by slowly progressive confusion, dementia, somnolence, tremor, ataxia, and seizures; less commonly, sudden onset of hemiplegia and coma eventuate in death (43). Pathologically, the lesion is usually a leukoencephalopathy with areas of coagulative necrosis and demyelination similar to the changes seen in radiation damage to the CNS. These alterations may occur throughout the white matter after intrathecal administration but have a predilection for the periventricular areas when given intraventricularly.

Stupor, coma, persistent vegetative state, and death have been observed in patients given long-term intrathecal treatment, usually in association with radiation therapy. In some cases, the onset is subacute with progressive deterioration. CT scans often show extensive patchy white matter attenuation, again mostly in the periventricular area. In milder forms of encephalopathy, CT scans show abnormalities similar to those seen in patients without neurologic findings. Autopsy material has shown variable changes in the cerebral white matter, including gliosis, spongy changes, and altered neuronal structure. Optic atrophy with blindness and cerebellar dysfunction have been described in patients treated with multiple therapeutic regimens, including intrathecal MTX (40).

Antipurines and Antipyrimidines

The antipurines have limited usage in the treatment of neoplasia. In addition, neurologic side effects of these agents, such as 6-mercaptopurine, are rare.

The antipyrimidine 5-fluoracil (5-FU) is commonly associated with neurotoxicity, which is characterized by gait ataxia, ataxia of the extremities, dysmetria, hypotonia, and coarse nystagmus, all of which are attributable to cerebellar dysfunction. The onset of these symptoms is subacute and potentially reversible (39). These cerebellar signs have been reported in as many as 7% of patients receiving 5-FU, but more recent studies suggest an incidence of 1 to 2%. Symptoms occur within hours to days of administration, often last only a few days, and in most cases are completely reversible. Further treatment with the drug may again cause the syndrome. The use of a lower dosage prevents recurrence, as does increasing the interval between treatments.

Other neurotoxic reactions reportedly associated with 5-FU include memory loss and mild to moderate encephalopathy. Blurring of vision and diplopia have also been reported, both of which clear upon cessation of therapy.

Plant Alkaloids

Vincristine (VCR) and vinblastine (VBL) are alkaloid derivatives of the periwinkle plant. The mechanism of action of these drugs is not known, although they may interfere with DNA and RNA synthesis. Vinca alkaloids are toxic to both the central and peripheral nervous systems.

The major limiting factor in the use of VCR is its neurotoxicity. The average required dose invariably results in a sensorimotor peripheral neuropathy. In addition, VCR affects the cranial nerves and central and autonomic nervous systems. VCR neuropathy may occur after only one or two weekly treatments, often beginning with decreased ankle jerks. Paresthesias in the fingers and toes followed by distal sensory loss and distal weakness complete the clinical picture. Deep tendon reflex abnormalities reach a peak approximately 2 weeks after a single dose and may return to normal in 1 to 3 months after a single dose (41). Weekly doses appear to have a cumulative effect; as additional doses are given, depression of all reflexes occurs with complete areflexia being quite common (7). Weakness is usually minimal in the routine dose schedules. The feet are almost invariably affected, especially the dorsiflexors and evertors. If more severe, the extensors of the fingers and wrists may become involved.

Nerve conduction studies show some reduction in motor nerve conduction as well as sensory nerve velocities. A progressive decrease in conduction velocities occurs during VCR therapy but may remain in the normal range despite obvious clinical neuropathy. Needle electromyography demonstrates denervation in distal musculature. Reduction in amplitude of sensory evoked potentials and prolonged distal motor latencies are often found in these patients, suggesting that the pathology is one of axonal degeneration with a component of "dying back" phenomenon (42).

VCR is also associated with an autonomic neuropathy. Constipation is the most common problem, occurring in almost one-third of patients in one large series (21). Mild abdominal pain is also common. The autonomic side effects appear to be dose related and dose limiting. Patients. usually children, may present with the clinical picture of acute abdominal pain due to a paralytic ileus. Bladder dysfunction, impotence, and orthostatic hypotension have been reported with VCR administation but are quite rare.

Cranial nerve dysfunction is rare. Bilateral seventh nerve paresis occurs occasionally (41). The facial weakness is usually symmetric, helping to differentiate this VCR reaction from meningeal seeding of tumor. Oculomotor paresis, usually presenting as ptosis, has been reported in as many as 10% of patients receiving VCR (41). Abnormalities of the brain and spinal cord are rare when VCR is given intravenously because of its poor permeability across the blood-brain barrier. Seizures have been reported with VCR, at times in association with the syndrome of inappropriate ADH secretion (8). Seizures occur in up to 4% of patients without underlying metabolic or structural abnormalities, usually about 5 days after administration of this drug.

VBL has similar neurotoxic reactions to those of VCR. These occur only at high doses, which usually cannot be used because of hematologic toxicity.

Antibiotic Antineoplastic Agents

Bleomycin

Since bleomycin is ordinarily used in conjunction with other chemotherapeutic agents, pure bleomycin-related neurotoxicity is uncertain. Abnormalities in mental status have been reported when the drug is given in combination with other agents but are reversible with discontinuation of only bleomycin. Peripheral neuropathy has been associated with bleomycin therapy. No pathologic changes have been reported in brain or peripheral nerves.

Adriamycin and Actinomycin D

In the doses usually employed in clinical practice, adriamycin and actinomycin D produce no neurologic side effects because of their inability to cross the blood-brain barrier.

Miscellaneous Antineoplastic Agents

Nitrosoureas: BCNU and CCNU

The nitrosoureas have not been reported to produce neurologic toxicity in the recommended dosage regimens.

cis-*Platinum*

cis-Platinum is often grouped under alkylating agents, but its mechanism of action is unknown. It causes profound nausea and vomiting. The most disturbing neurotoxic effect is ototoxicity; although this side effect may be dose limiting, the development of transient partial deafness is usually not an indication for cessation of therapy. Deafness often begins within 3 to 4 days of the initial treatment, slowly improving over succeeding weeks after treatment is stopped. In most cases, deafness is reversible; but when profound, it may be permanent. Direct toxicity of *cis*-platinum on the organ of Corti appears to be the cause of the deafness, since nystagmus and vertigo have not been reported (36). A final side effect of *cis*-platinum is peripheral neuropathy, mainly sensory in nature and characterized by paresthesias in a stocking-glove distribution and diminished proprioceptive abilities (24).

CARDIOVASCULAR AND ANTIHYPERTENSIVE AGENTS

Cardiac Glycosides

Neurologic complications of digitalis therapy have been recognized for almost 200 years and are characterized by nausea, vomiting, visual disturbances, seizures, and syncope. Adverse effects on the CNS reportedly occur in 40 to 50% of patients with clinical digitalis toxicity. Symptoms referrable to CNS dysfunction may occur prior to, simultaneously, or following signs of cardiac toxicity (28,32). Explanations for the dramatic incidence of neurotoxicity of digitalis have been inadequate. The few pathologic studies have shed little light on the pathogenesis of the neurotoxic reactions.

The most frequent neurotoxic reaction and often the first sign of clinical digitalis toxicity is nausea, which is probably centrally mediated. Digitalis apparently stimulates the chemoreceptor trigger zone, which lies in the floor of the fourth ventricle. Nausea associated with digitalis toxicity is often accompanied by vomiting; when chronic, it may lead to malnourishment, cachexia, and a Wernicke's encephalopathy (38).

Visual disturbances are common in digitalis toxicity, occurring in up to 40% of such patients. The manifestations include blurred vision, reversible scotomas, diplopia, and defects of color vision. The pathogenesis of these visual disturbances is unknown.

Seizures are known to occur as a result of digitalis toxicity and are most commonly seen in the pediatric population. The incidence of digitalis-related seizures is difficult to estimate because of the frequency of other possible mechanism (e.g., arrhythmia).

Transient mental aberrations resembling transient global amnesia with complete remission have been reported (19). Syncope, probably due to conduction delay or hyperactivity of baroreceptors, has also occurred in digitalis toxicity. Other neurotoxic reactions include paresthesias, headache, weakness, and fatigue. Cerebral symptoms, consisting of confusion, delirium, mania, and hallucinosis, have been reported in as many as 15% of patients with digitalis toxicity. Although the mechanism for the symptoms is unknown, they probably are not the result of altered cardiac function.

Methyldopa

The adverse effects of methyldopa on the CNS may be related to the synthesis of false catecholamine neurotransmitters, methylnorepinephrine, and methyldopamine. The most frequent such side effect is sedation, which is usually transient in nature but may persist in as many as 5% of patients. Mood alterations usually characterized by depression are not uncommon. Most patients in whom behavior changes develop usually have a prior history of affective illness. The depressive state is completely reversible upon withdrawal of the drug. Parkinsonism, resulting from dopamine depletion, has been reported but, considering the widespread use of this agent, is rare (45). Usually beginning within 1 to 4 months of therapy, parkinsonian symptoms resolve relatively soon after methyldopa is discontinued. Other minor neurologic complaints associated with methyldopa include confusion, dizziness, headaches, and syncope.

Clonidine

Clonidine acts as an alpha-adrenergic agonist. It has been suggested that this stimulation may result in an overall decrease in norepinephrine release, possibly via presynaptic inhibition. The most common adverse neurologic effect is sedation. Other less common neurotoxic reactions include depression, nightmares, and a reversible dementia syndrome which occurs as a result of reduction in cerebral blood flow.

Hydralazine

Hydralazine is the only direct-acting vasodilator generally available for the treatment of chronic hypertension. The neurologic side effects are quite uncommon, peripheral neuropathy characterized by diffuse numbness and tingling being the only consistent neurotoxic reaction. The neuropathy may be due to a toxic effect of hydrazine, the same moiety present in isoniazid.

Reserpine

Reserpine prevents the reuptake of norepinephrine, dopamine, and serotonin into their respective storage granules, thus causing depletion of these neurotransmitters. CNS side effects are common and include depression, excessive drowsiness, parkinsonism, and headache (35). A change in affect may occur in up to 10% of patients and manifests itself as early morning awakening, melancholy, loss of appetite, and loss of self-confidence. This effect is more common with higher doses and usually is seen in patients with a history of prior affective disturbance. Drug withdrawal does not always result in immediate reversal; early symptoms of depression should alert the physician to discontinue therapy. Characteristic parkinsonism occurs much less often on therapeutic reserpine dosages and is always reversible upon drug withdrawal (see Chapter 1).

Propranolol

CNS toxicity is uncommon, despite the widespread use of propranolol and its high degree of penetration across the blood-brain barrier. Neurotoxic reactions are often quite mild and nonspecific in nature. These consist of sleeplessness, excessive drowsiness, dizziness, lightheadedness, and symptoms of global dysfunction characterized by depression, confusion, delirium, and hallucinations (48).

Miscellaneous Agents

The other antihypertensive agents (nitroprusside, guanethedine, and diazoxide) have almost no direct, adverse effect on the CNS. All are associated with headache and syncope, the latter on the basis of orthostatic hypotension.

ANTIARTHRITIC AGENTS

Salicylates

Salicylate toxicity can result from acute ingestion of large quantities or from the cumulative effect of chronic, high-dose therapy. Many of the toxic effects of these agents are on the neurologic system of man, but considerable variation in the development and manifestations of salicylate toxicity exists.

The most common early and prominent neurotoxic effect is ototoxicity, represented by tinnitus, hearing loss, and vertigo. The typical pattern of salicylate-induced hearing loss shows greater losses at the higher frequencies and is of the sensorineural type. This sensorineural hearing loss may be reversible within days after cessation of therapy and may be related to salicylate-depression of afferent auditory nerve impulses, increased labyrinthine pressure, or direct toxicity to cochlear hair cells (34).

Nausea and vomiting are frequently associated with salicylate toxicity. Both central neurogenic and peripheral gastrointestinal effects play a role. Other central neurotoxic effects of salicylates include encephalopathy characterized by drowsiness, lethargy, confusion, delirium, tremor, and, rarely, visual hallucinations. Seizures also have been reported. Severe salicylate intoxication leads to coma, pyramidal tract signs, fixed pupils, and, at times, death. Almost all these encephalopathic effects of salicylates are the result of acid-base alterations and metabolic derangements at the neuronal level.

Chloroquine

Chloroquine, originally an antimalarial agent, is now employed in the therapy of rheumatoid arthritis. The most common adverse effects are gastrointestinal, but numerous neurologic side effects also occur during therapy. The more common neurotoxic effects are headache, lassitude, irritability, emotional lability, and visual disturbances. Peripheral neuropathy has been reported in rheumatoid patients receiving chloroquine (31). These patients complained of paresthesias and weakness in the lower extremities with objective decrease in muscle power and absent knee and ankle reflexes. Withdrawal of therapy leads to full restoration of neurologic function. Bilateral abducens nerve paralysis, which is completely reversible upon discontinuation of therapy, is rare.

Optic neuritis with pallor of the optic discs, retinitis, and visual field defects have been associated with chloroquine therapy (44). In many patients, the visual loss has remained permanent.

Administration of chloroquine for prolonged periods in high doses may lead to myopathy. This is initially characterized by proximal weakness, although generalized (distal and bulbar) weakness has been reported. Rapid development over a few weeks is characteristic. Histologic examination reveals a vacuolar muscle degenerative process (22).

Penicillamine

Although not officially approved in the United States until quite recently for the treatment of rheumatoid arthritis, penicillamine has shown efficacy in clinical trials dating back to 1970. The toxic effects have been especially prominent in patients with connective tissue disorders.

The most frequently encountered neurotoxic effect is loss or abnormality of taste, which has been correlated with high doses and long duration of therapy (9). Hypoguesia occurs in 25 to 30% of patients at doses of 1 g/day within 6 weeks. It may be reversible with decreasing the dosage or discontinuation of the drug and may not occur in dosages of 500 mg or less. Zinc infiltration of taste receptors has been postulated to cause the hypoguesia induced by penicillamine (40).

Dermatomyositis and polymyositis characterized by typical tender proximal muscle weakness with elevation of serum aldolase and CPK may occur during penicillamine therapy. This rare side effect is usually associated with serologic abnormalities resembling lupus erythematosis. Drug-induced myasthenic reactions often presenting with ptosis, diplopia, and dysphagia have been reported (6). Generalized weakness usually follows, especially if early signs are undetected. Reversibility with endrophonium confirms the diagnosis. Whether penicillamine uncovers preexisting subclinical myasthenia gravis by causing neuromuscular blockade similar to certain antibiotics is as yet unknown. Withdrawal of the drug reverses the weakness.

Penicillamine therapy can cause optic neuritis and seizures, both thought to be a result of an antipyridoxine effect of penicillamine (49). Both are rare and can be prevented by concurrent pyridoxine administration.

Gold

Neurologic complications of gold therapy are uncommon. Cerebral irritation characterized by delirium, agitation, and seizures has been rarely reported (11).

Isolated cases of ascending polyneuropathy simulating Gullain-Barré, cranial nerve palsies, and transverse myelopathy have been reported with gold therapy in rheumatoid arthritis. Occasional signs and symptoms of diffuse symmetric sensorimotor peripheral neuropathy have been seen in association with this drug regimen.

Indomethacin

CNS toxicity is the factor that precludes the use of indomethacin in 30 to 50% of patients. The neurotoxic effects are usually mild to moderate and consist of headaches, depression, agitation, and, rarely, hallucinations. Slow increases in dosage may prevent these effects. Other neurotoxic effects of indomethacin include ataxia, clumsiness, and impaired postural reflexes.

Phenylbutazone

Neurotoxicity is not commonly associated with phenylbutazone. Alteration in taste sensation, although rare, is the most common neurologic side effect.

Naproxen

Adverse neurologic reactions have been reported in approximately 8% of patients receiving naproxen and consist of headache, drowsiness, vertigo, inability to concentrate, and depression. Because of its protein binding affinity, it may displace phenytoin; thus patients on chronic phenytoin will have a higher percentage of unbound phenytoin, possibly resulting in toxicity with what are usually therapeutic levels.

Sulindac

The neurotoxicity of sulindac has been estimated at between 1 and 10%, with headache and dizziness being most common. Vertigo, tinnitus, and decreased hearing occur in less than 1% of reported patients. Paresthesias, peripheral neuropathy, and transient blurring of vision are quite rare, but more clinical experience is needed to confirm the true incidence of these reactions.

Allopurinol

The neurologic side effects of allopurinol are rare, even during prolonged therapy, and consist of hypoguesia and sensorimotor peripheral neuropathy. Both are reversible with a decrease in the daily dosage.

ORAL CONTRACEPTIVES

The oral contraceptive agents have been shown to predispose to four separate types of neurologic complications: (a) strokes, especially in women who smoke; (b) increase in the frequency or severity of migraine headaches or the initial precipitation of migraine; this often precedes the onset of a stroke. Any worsening of migraine is a contraindication to the continuation of oral contraceptives; (c) chorea (see Chapter 3); and (d) pseudotumor cerebri, which always reverses upon discontinuation of the medication.

BIBLIOGRAPHY AND *SELECTED REVIEWS

*1. Allen, J. C. (1978): The effects of cancer therapy on the nervous system. *J. Pediatr.*, 93:903–909.
2. Arena, P. J. (1972): Oropharyngeal sensation associated with rapid intravenous administration of cyclophosphamid. *Cancer Chemother. Rep.*, 56:779–780.
3. Bethlenfalvay, N. C., and Bergin, J. J. (1972): Severe cerebral toxicity after intravenous nitrogen mustard therapy. *Cancer*, 29:366–369.
4. Bhowmick, B. K. (1972): Benign intracranial hypertension after antibiotic therapy. *Br. Med. J.*, 4:30.
5. Bradley, W. G., Karlson, I. J., and Rassol, C. G. (1977): Metronidazole neuropathy. *Br. J. Med.*, 2:610–611.
6. Brucknall, R. C., Dixon, A., Glick, E. N., Harris, A. M. (1976): Myasthenia gravis associated with penicillamine treatment for rheumatoid arthritis. *Br. Med. J.*, 2:600–602.
7. Casey, E. G., Jellife, A. M., LeQuesne, M., LeGarde, T. S. (1973): Vincristine neuropathy: Clinical and electrophysiological observations. *Brain*, 96:69–86.
8. Cutting, H. O. (1971): Inappropriate secretion of antidiuretic hormone secondary to vincristine therapy. *Am. J. Med.*, 51:269–271.
9. Day, A. T., and Golding, J. R. (1973): Reaction of D-penicillamine in rheumatoid arthritis. *Br. Med. J.*, 3:593.
10. Edelson, R. W., Chernik, N. L., and Posner, J. B. (1974): Spinal subdural hematomas complicating lumbar puncture. *Arch. Neurol.*, 31:134–137.
11. Endtz, L. J. (1958): Complications to the nervous system of gold therapy. *Rev. Neurol. (Paris)*, 99:395–310.
12. Eronini, E. A., and Umez-Eronini, E. M. (1977): Chloroquine-induced involuntary movements. *Br. Med. J.*, 1:945–946.
13. Fleischer, E. I., Helper, R. S., and Landau, J. W. (1974): Blindness during diiodohydroxyquin (Diodoquin) therapy: A case report. *Pediatrics*, 54:106.
14. Fussieck, B., and Parker, R. H. (1974): Neurotoxicity during intravenous infusion of penicillin: A review. *J. Clin. Pharmacol.*, 14:504–510.
15. Gagliano, R. G., and Costanzi, J. J. (1976): Paraplegia following intratheca imethotrexate. *Cancer*, 37:1663–1668.
16. Goldman, A. L., and Braman, S. S. (1972): Isoniazid: A review with emphasis on adverse effects. *Chest*, 62:71–79.
17. Grees, A. A., and Naiman, J. L. (1968): Chlorambucil poisoning. *Am. J. Dis. Child.*, 116:190–191.
18. Greenhouse, A., Newberger, K. J., and Bowerman, D. L. (1964): Brain damage after intracarotid infusion of methotrexate. *Arch. Neurol.*, 11:618–625.
19. Greenlee, J. E., Crampton, R. S., and Miller, J. Q. (1975): Transient global amnesia associated with cardiac arrhythmia and digitalis intoxication. *Stroke*, 6:513–516.
20. Gustin, P. H., Levi, J. A., Wiernik, P. H., and Walker, M. D. (1977): Treatment of malignant meningeal disease with intrathecal tiotepa: A phase II study. *Cancer Treat. Rep.*, 1:885–887.
21. Holland, J. F., Scharlan, C., Gaolani, S., and Falkson, G. (1973): Vincristine treatment of advanced cancer: A cooperative study of 392 cases. *Cancer Res.*, 33:1258–1264.
22. Hughes, J. T., Esiri, M., Oxbury, J. M., and Whitty, C. W. N. (1971): Chloroquine myopathy. *Q. J. Med.*, 40:85–93.
23. Karmody, C. S., and Weinstein, L. (1977): Reversible sensorineural hearing loss associated with intravenous erythromycin lactobionate. *Ann. Otolaryngol.*, 86:9–10.
24. Kedar, A., Cohen, M. E., and Freedman, A. F. (1978): Peripheral neuropathy as a complication of cis-dichlarodiamine platinum treatment: A case report. *Cancer Treat. Rep.*, 62:819–821.
25. Koch-Weser, J., Sidel, V. W., Dexter, M., and Federman, E. B. (1971): Adverse reaction to sulfisoxazole, sulfamethoxazole and nitrofurantoin. *Arch. Intern. Med.*, 128:399–403.
26. Koch-Weser, J., Sidel, V. W., Federman, E. B., and Dexter, M. (1970): Adverse effects of sodium colistemethate: Manifestations and specific reaction rates during 317 courses of therapy. *Ann. Intern. Med.*, 72:857–861.

27. Kurtzman, N. A., Rogers, P. W., and Harter, H. R. (1970): Neurotoxic reaction to penicillin and carbenicillin. *JAMA*, 214:1320–1322.
28. Lely, A., and VanEnter, C. (1970): Large scale digitalis intoxication. *Br. Med. J.*, 3:737–740.
29. Lerner, S. A., Seligsohn, R., and Matz, G. J. (1977): Comparative clinical studies of ototoxicity and nephrotoxicity of amikacin and gantamicin. *Am. J. Med.*, 62:919–924.
30. Levine, P. H., Regelson, W., and Holland, J. F. (1970): Chloramphenicol associated encephalopathy. *Clin. Pharmacol. Ther.*, 11:194–198.
31. Loftus, C. R. (1963): Peripheral neuropathy following chloroquine therapy. *Can. Med. Assoc. J.*, 89:917–920.
32. Lyon, A. F., and DeGraff, A. C. (1963): The neurotoxic effects of digitalis. *Am. Heart J.*, 65:839–840.
*33. Meadows, A. T., and Evans, A. E. (1976): Effects of chemotherapy on the CNS. *Cancer*, 37:1079–1085.
34. Myers, E. N., Berstein, J. M., and Fostiropolous, G. (1965): Salicylate ototoxicity, a clinical study. *N. Engl. J. Med.*, 273:587–590.
35. Pfeifer, H. J., Greenblott, D. J., and Koch-Weser, J. (1976): Clinical toxicity of reserpine in hospitalized patients. *Progr. Am. J. Med. Sci.*, 271:269–276.
36. Piel, I. J., Meyer, D., Perlia, C. P., and Economou, P. G. (1974): Effects of cis-platinum on hearing function in man. *Cancer Chemother. Rep.*, 58:871–875.
*37. Pittinger, C., and Adamson, R. (1972): Antibiotic blockade of neuromuscular function. *Ann. Rev. Pharmacol.*, 12:169–178.
38. Richmond, J. (1959): Wernicke's encephalopathy associated with digitalis poisoning. *Lancet*, 1:344–345.
39. Riehz, J. L., and Brown, W. J. (1964): Acute cerebellar syndrome secondary to 5FU therapy. *Neurology*, 14:961–967.
40. Rollin, H. (1978): Drug-related gustatory disorders. *Am. Otolaryngol.*, 87:37–43.
41. Sandler, S. G., Tobin, T., and Henderson, E. S. (1969): Vincristine-induced neuropathy: A clinical study of fifty leukemic patients. *Neurology (Minneap.)*, 19:367–374.
42. Schochet, S. S., Lampert, P. W., and Earle, K. M. (1968): Neuronal changes induced by intrathecal vincristine sulfate. *J. Neuropathol. Exp. Neurol.*, 27:645–658.
43. Shapiro, W. R., Chernik, N. Z., and Posner, J. B. (1973): Necrotizing encephalopathy following instillation of methotrexate. *Arch. Neurol.*, 28:96–102.
44. Smith, J. L. (1962): Chloroquine macular degeneration. *Arch. Ophthalmol.*, 68:186–190.
45. Strang, R. R. (1966): Parkinsonism occurring during methyldopa therapy. *Can. Med. Assoc. J.*, 110:928–929.
46. Sullivan, M. P., Vietti, T. J., Fernbach, D. J., Griffith, K. M., Hardy, T. B., and Watkins, W. L. (1969): Clinical investigations in the treatment of meningeal leukemia: Radiation therapy vs. conventional intrathecal methotrexate. *Blood*, 34:301–309.
47. Toole, J. F., and Parrish, M. L. (1973): Nitrofurantoin polyneuropathy. *Neurology*, 23:554–557.
48. Waal, H. J. (1967): Propranolol-induced depression. *Br. Med. J.*, 2:50.
49. Walshe, J. M. (1968): Toxic reactions to penicillamine in patients with Wilson's disease. *Postgrad. Med. J.*, 44(S):6–8.

Subject Index